Nurse Practitione

This book is dedicated to the memory of Mike McNulty whose teaching is remembered with fond affection by many and also to the life of Jack Reveley, who will be sadly missed

Nurse Practitioners

Clinical Skills and Professional Issues

Edited by

Mike Walsh PhD, BA (Hons), RGN, PGCE, DipN (London)
Reader in Nursing, St Martin's College, Carlisle

Alison Crumbie MSN, BSc, RGN, DipNP, Dip App ScN
Senior Lecturer Nurse Practitioner, St Martin's College, Lancaster

Shirley Reveley PhD, MA, BA, RGN, RM, RHV, DipN (London), CertEd
Principal Lecturer, Primary Health Care, St Martin's College, Carlisle

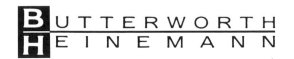

OXFORD   AUCKLAND   BOSTON   JOHANNESBURG   MELBOURNE   NEW DELHI

Butterworth-Heinemann
Linacre House, Jordan Hill, Oxford OX2 8DP
225 Wildwood Avenue, Woburn, MA 01801-2041
A division of Reed Educational and Professional Publishing Ltd

A member of the Reed Elsevier plc group

First published 1999

British Library Cataloguing in Publication Data
Nurse practitioners: clinical skills and professional issues
    Nurse practitioners
    I. Walsh, Mike *1949–*   II. Crumbie, Alison
    III. Reveley, Shirley
    610.7'30692

Library of Congress Cataloguing in Publication Data
Nurse practitioners: clinical skills and professional issues/edited
    Mike Walsh, Alison Crumbie, Shirley Reveley
    p.   cm.
    Includes bibliographical references and index
    1. Nurse practitioners.   2. Clinical competence.   I. Walsh, Mike,
    SRN.   II. Crumbie, Alison.   III. Reveley, Shirley
    [DNLM: 1. Nurse Practitioners. 2. Clinical Competence.
    3. Patient Care.   WY 128 N9733 1999]
    RT82.8.N864   1999
    610..73'06'92–dc21

ISBN 0 7506 3990 3

Typeset at Replika Press Pvt Ltd, Delhi 110 040, India
Printed and bound in Great Britain

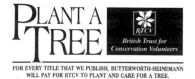

Contents

Part Two   Professional and legal issues

Contributors

Scott Bowman

Scott Bowman is currently an Associate Professor and also the Head of the School of Clinical Sciences at Charles Sturt University in Australia. He trained as a diagnostic radiographer at Northampton and Kettering General Hospitals in the UK and he has worked as a radiographer in a number of London Hospitals. After training as a teacher he became a Principal Lecturer at Guy's Hospital and South Bank University before taking up the post of Head of the Department of Radiography and Imaging Sciences at the University College of St Martin in Lancaster. He moved to Australia in 1998. Scott's research interests are in professional decision making, skill mix and patient–radiographer interactions.

Christina Clark

Christina Clark trained in the UK but moved to the USA in 1978 as a staff nurse to work in Texas. In 1986 she qualified as a nurse practitioner in San Francisco with an MSc in Nursing. Her subsequent experience as a nurse practitioner in California was mostly in the field of family care and also working on an AIDS home care team. She came to the UK in 1996 to help develop the St Martin's BSc Nurse Practitioner course (franchized from the RCNI) before returning to the USA in 1998. She is currently employed as a nurse practitioner in San Francisco.

Alison Crumbie

Alison Crumbie is a nurse practitioner and senior lecturer at St Martin's College, Lancaster. She has worked and studied in Australia, the United States and Britain and has a breadth of experience in both the hospital and community setting. Alison is the course leader for the nurse practitioner course at St Martin's College and plays an important role in courses for nurses who work with people who live with chronic conditions. As a founding member of the Northern Nurse Practitioner Association she has been instrumental in developing a network for nurse practitioners across the north of Britain.

Joy Duxbury

Joy Duxbury is currently a Senior Lecturer at Bolton Institute. She has worked in higher education for six years since attending Hull University as a postgraduate where she gained a First Class Honours Degree. Joy lectures on a variety of topics such as health psychology and communication and she continues to pursue her research interests, particularly in violence and aggression, via her PhD studies and ongoing publications.

Lesley Kyle

During the last ten years, Lesley Kyle has worked as a community nurse/midwife, a practice nurse and a research nurse for the British Family Heart Study. She is currently working as a nurse practitioner in Canonbie, a small village in the Scottish Borders, caring for a farming community with two dynamic and innovative General Practitioners. She also lectures at St Martin's College in Carlisle, which gives her the opportunity to teach clinical skills to student nurse practitioners.

Shirley Reveley

Shirley Reveley trained as a nurse in the 1960s and became involved in community nursing soon afterwards as a school/clinic nurse. A spell as a home nursing sister was followed by midwifery training and later health visitor training. After several years of health visiting practice she undertook a Diploma in Nursing at London University and, in the mid-1980s, an Open University Degree in Education Research. She is currently Principal Lecturer in Primary Health Care at St Martin's College, Carlisle, where she manages community nursing courses. She was responsible for setting up a nurse practitioner programme in Carlisle and Lancaster in association with the RCN Institute, a popular programme that has primary care and hospital routes. Shirley's research interests include evaluating the nurse practitioner role and she is completing her doctoral thesis on this subject.

Charles Sloane

Charles Sloane qualified as a radiographer in 1989 and obtained his first post working in the Radiology Department at Stoke Mandeville Hospital, Buckinghamshire. Since then he has gained a wide variety of experience in radiography working with a number of imaging specialities as well as maintaining an interest in plain radiography and trauma imaging. He is currently on secondment from his post as Clinical Tutor at the Royal Lancaster Infirmary, working as a Lecturer in Radiography at St Martin's College, Lancaster. Charles is keen to see radiographers and nurses improve their knowledge of the radiographic appearances of trauma and other pathologies as he feels this will inevitably lead to an improvement in the service offered to patients.

Fiona Smart

Fiona Smart is a Senior Lecturer in Child Health and Children's Nursing at St Martin's College. She is based in Carlisle, Cumbria. Fiona qualified as a Registered General and Children's Nurse in 1983 and practised in a variety of settings before entering the world of education in 1988. Most recently, her concern for the health and well-being of children and young people has led to a number of curriculum developments at St Martin's College; of these it has been the construction of a School Nursing pathway through the Specialist Practitioner programme in particular that has enabled thinking to develop in respect of a public health role for nursing. Currently Fiona is engaged in MPhil/PhD studies on a part-time basis.

Mike Walsh

As Reader in Nursing, Dr Mike Walsh's main work is in the field of research and practice development. He has been heavily involved in nurse practitioner education since 1995 and has several research projects underway evaluating the impact of innovative nurse practitioner roles. His background is in A&E nursing, his PhD investigating the use made by the general public of the A&E service in Bristol and he still maintains his A&E clinical practice on a sessional basis at the Cumberland Infirmary A&E Department in Carlisle. He is the author of a range of books and journal articles on both clinical and professional issues.

Introduction

No man has a right to fix the boundary of the march of a nation; no man has a right to say to his country – thus far shalt thou go and no further (Charles Stewart Parnell 1885).

Nurse practitioners today are pushing hard at the traditional boundaries of practice: the words of Parnell, whilst originally uttered as part of his peaceful campaign for Irish independence, have a definite resonance today. Nurse practitioners are operating at the boundaries between medicine and nursing – this is a very exposed and, at times, difficult place to be. It is also a complicated place to be as boundaries between systems do not consist of the simple clear cut demarcation lines that people used to imagine. Jack Cohen and Ian Stewart have written eloquently of the new and emerging disciplines of complexity and chaos theory. They show how boundaries between dynamic systems are chaotic places where even simple rules and assumptions can create unimaginable complexity (Cohen and Stewart 1994). There is another problem with boundaries and that is that they demand recognition; it is then an easy step to insist that they be protected and defended. If we retreat behind them they become potential zones for conflict: the nurse practitioner could be forgiven for being afraid of being caught in the crossfire.

It is a truism to say that health care is changing rapidly today, as never before. The provision of health care depends on staff placing the patient's best interests first and living with the inevitable changes this perspective will produce. This means *all* health staff must move away from striving to preserve professional status, the traditional monopoly of practice and the status quo. The patient's best interests must come ahead of professional self-indulgence. Care should be delivered by whoever is most appropriate, acceptable to the patient and best trained for the job, rather than by a member of the professional group who traditionally delivered that care.

In many cases that can only be the doctor, so there is no need for medical colleagues to fear redundancy. We can understand doctors looking anxiously at other professional groups seeking to expand the boundaries and borders of their practice. They would be entitled to feel concern if the field of health care were a fixed static area, as they would see their territory being eroded by the expansion of others. But health care is an expanding universe growing bigger by the day as new discoveries, techniques and challenges present themselves. Other professional groups can widen their practice without threatening the viability of medicine because the whole field of health care is also expanding at a dramatic rate.

Doctors should only be doing things when they are the most appropriate person to do so, not because they have always done them. The same comment is equally true in nursing. In trying to decide which clinician does what, the acid test should be what is in the best interests of the patient, rather than the professional group involved.

Medicine today faces an enormous challenge. It can no longer continue to deliver all the services to patients as it has traditionally done in the past. The dramatic growth in the demand for and complexity of health care, set against a static and in some areas declining number of doctors ensures this is so. Medicine has a dilemma, neatly expressed to us by a hard-pressed SHO who said doctors want nurses to take over more medical tasks, but not take over medicine!

The issue has not been helped by the inability of the United Kingdom Central Council to follow up their liberating *Scope of Professional Practice* document published in 1992. It is as if they let the genie out of the bottle and don't know what to do with it – hence their sluggish and unhelpful response to the burgeoning nurse practitioner movement.

This book is an attempt to deal with the clinical and professional issues raised by the thousands of nurses who want to push on and challenge the traditional boundaries of care. Public safety demands that nurses have the knowledge necessary to work in new and different ways from traditional nursing. The nurse practitioner sees patients with undifferentiated health problems, often as a first point of contact, and works with far greater autonomy, often discharging the patient from care without referral to another health professional. As a result s/he requires new assessment skills and problem-solving techniques for effective and safe practice. The nurse practitioner must remember that s/he is always a nurse and remain true to the holistic concept of care, seeing the patient as a partner in care. This will allow the nurse practitioner to avoid simply carrying out tasks that junior doctors are too busy to do. The new nurse practitioner roles must also be located within the framework of professional and legal accountability.

This book attempts to chart a path through these challenges. It is based on the authors' experience as teachers, researchers and practitioners in this new field of health care. In the physical and social sciences it has long been known that it is at the boundaries of systems that creative interaction takes place, often with startling and unpredictable results, which may have very positive outcomes. This is what is happening in health care today and why the words of Parnell are so appropriate. Traditional professional boundaries are artifacts; as long as nurse practitioners develop practice so that the patient's best interests always come first, nobody has the right to say: 'thus far and no further'.

Mike Walsh

References

Cohen J., Stewart I. (1994) *The Collapse of Chaos*. New York: Penguin.

United Kingdom Central Council (1992) *The Scope of Professional Practice*. London: UKCC.

Part one

CLINICAL PRACTICE

CHAPTER 1
Problem-solving

Alison Crumbie

Nurse practitioners consult with patients who have undifferentiated, undiagnosed conditions. Patients are assessed, receive a diagnosis and are offered education, treatment, referral or discharge. This type of activity exemplifies the autonomous practice which characterizes the work of a nurse practitioner. In order to remain within the United Kingdom Central Council's scope of professional practice (United Kingdom Central Council 1992), the nurse practitioner should accept responsibility for autonomous decision-making. It is therefore essential that the nurse develops an effective and secure clinical reasoning strategy to guide the problem-solving process.

Problem-solving is not unique to nursing. Indeed, most professionals face problems in their area of practice. A detective is an obvious example of a person presented with a problem who works through a certain process in order to arrive at a solution to a crime. Engineers are faced with problems of constructing bridges across increasingly large stretches of water; a builder faced with the problem of a leaking roof has to employ a problem-solving strategy to discover the leak and repair it. There is an enormous amount of literature relating to theories of problem-solving and clearly different approaches are valuable in different settings. The problem-solving process which is most appropriate for nurse practitioners may not be the same as for nurses working in other areas of practice.

Hurst *et al.* (1991) carried out a series of interviews with nurses to gain insight into their understanding of the problem-solving process. They found that nurses gave a high degree of attention to the implementation stage of problem-solving but attached little importance to evaluation. Hurst *et al.* suggest that this may be because nurses concentrate on the 'doing' aspects of nursing, at the expense of the analytical processes of problem-solving. Nurse practitioners, however, are making autonomous decisions and therefore have to address the analytical processes of problem-solving rather than adopting the traditional approach of 'doing things' for the patient. The nurse practitioner will take a history

from the patient, carry out appropriate physical examination techniques and make decisions about further tests, referral or treatment regimes. This process may involve doing things with and for the patient but the expertise lies in the analysis of problems and the ability to arrive at accurate diagnoses in an efficient and effective manner. A problem-solving strategy which underpins the nurse's clinical decision-making will ensure that diagnoses are more accurate and treatment regimes are more effective. The nurse will learn from the process, building up a level of expertise for future encounters with clients. A secure clinical reasoning strategy enables the nurse to progress as far as his or her level of knowledge will allow.

There are two major theories of problem-solving – the *information-processing* system theory (Newell and Simon 1972) and the *stages model* theory. The information-processing system is based on the theory that problem-solving is a product of two processes – understanding and solving. Understanding is based on your immediate thought processes when you meet a problem and your knowledge and experience of similar situations. The solving process is a search for the solution using your experience of similar situations, identifying, analysing and synthesizing knowledge gathered during the understanding process (Hurst *et al.* 1991). Hurst *et al.* state that there is little research to support the application of the information-processing system to real-life problems such as those found in dealing with patients. The information-processing system theory is most often associated with well-defined problems; frequently, the problems faced by nurse practitioners are complex and ill-defined.

Hurst (1993) points out that a review of the literature relating to stages model theory over the last 50 years elicited 55 different representations of stages models. The stages theory of problem-solving is a stepwise process involving different stages and different numbers of steps depending on the model used. According to Hurst (1993), the stages model encourages systematic thinking which can be applied to each new problem. It is flexible: when problem-solving is unsuccessful, it is possible to isolate the weak link in the process and therefore its use can facilitate learning.

There are, however, several criticisms of the stages model. It is suggested that the stages represent a rigid process of discrete steps and that this does not adequately reflect what really happens in practice (Hurst 1993). In clinical practice the stages become blurred and there is a dynamic process which does not necessarily follow a logical stepwise approach. Barrows and Pickell (1991) developed a model of clinical problem-solving which is presented as a stages approach to the clinical decision-making process. The model is built up in a series of steps; however, the authors suggest that it is a dynamic process including ongoing feedback and development of the initial impressions of the patient. The clinician may work through the steps in a matter of seconds, and then work through the steps again as more information becomes available through the patient inquiry.

The Barrows and Pickell model was primarily written for medical students. It incorporates issues of patient education, compliance, physical examination, diagnosis and viewing the problem from the patient's perspective and therefore has relevance to the work of nurse practitioners. Barrows and Pickell point out that there are two components of clinical problem-solving which are inexorably linked. One component is *content*, which is the knowledge base of the practitioner. The second component is *process*, which is the method of manipulation used by the practitioner to apply knowledge to the patient's problem. A well-developed problem-solving process enables the practitioner to utilize knowledge and experience to provide the most effective care for patients. Barrows and Pickell suggest that effective, efficient and fast clinical reasoning skills are the skills behind intuition. Intuition is not a magical phenomenon representing the art of clinical practice – it can be developed and taught. According to Barrows and Pickell, the more a practitioner focuses on the skills of problem-solving, the more intuitive his or her practice will become. The skills of the problem-solving process within Barrows and Pickell's model of clinical reasoning will now be applied to the problems faced by nurse practitioners in the clinical setting.

Forming the initial concept

It is essential that each part of the encounter with a patient is an active process on the part of the nurse practitioner. The first impressions of the patient provide the nurse with an enormous amount of information which should be noted and which will form part of the initial concept. All significant factors should be considered, including quality of the patient's voice, smell, appearance, movements and the people accompanying the patient. This information is gathered in seconds and provides the basis for the practitioner's initial perceptions. The practitioner analyses these perceptions and develops the initial concept (Barrows and Pickell 1991, p. 34):

Patient information available at the outset
↓
Perceptions
↓
Analysis
↓
Initial concept

The patient's appearance, age, sex and opening comments add to the initial concept developing in the mind of the practitioner. A patient who walks into the consulting room and sits down before complaining of hip pain will provide a different picture to the patient who limps in with the help of a relative and gingerly lowers himself down on to the chair with an outstretched leg and then complains of hip pain. A patient who comments of feeling tired and low and is judged to be approximately 55 years of age, female and slightly overweight will create a different initial concept to a patient who complains of feeling tired and low, is judged to be approximately 25 years of age, female and very thin.

The initial concept is gradually developed from deliberately sought observations. For example, in the case of the female patient who is 55 years of age, slightly obese, tired and low, the nurse may particularly concentrate on observing her hair for quality and quantity, looking at her skin for hydration and listening to the quality of her voice. All of this information can be added to the initial concept. In the case of the 25-year-old female who is tired and low and very thin, the nurse may in particular observe her facial expressions, general appearance and manner of approach to the consulting room and add this information to the initial concept of the patient. In each of these cases the practitioner is gathering information which is relevant to the presenting complaint and, whilst avoiding the dangers of jumping to conclusions too quickly, a focused exploration for the signs of hypothyroidism in the first case and for depression in the second expedites the problem-solving process.

It is also important to note the demeanour of those who have accompanied the patient. Observations of body language and listening carefully to the speech of the carer or relative will provide further information about the patient's problem. Patients quite frequently attend the surgery because they have been asked to do so by friends or relatives. It is important to ascertain this fact as it provides information about the patient's perception of the problem.

A threat to this process is prejudice and bias. The practitioner's own beliefs and assumptions will weaken the effectiveness of the assessment. It is clearly important to become self-aware and to recognize any prejudice which may cloud judgement in the clinical setting. This differs from the need to be aware of culturally specific disease processes. For example, if a 50-year-old Asian person complained of feeling tired and low it would be quite reasonable to entertain an initial hypothesis of diabetes mellitus. The analysis of the patient's problem must remain objective in order to preserve accuracy and therefore other assumptions about culture, gender, sexual orientation and class should be deliberately checked for elements of personal bias which could contaminate the problem-solving process.

A further threat to the process of developing an initial concept is the possibility of making a translation error. This occurs when a patient uses a term which the practitioner immediately translates into something which does not accurately represent the patient's experience. For example, a patient may complain of being sick and the practitioner notes nausea and vomiting. The patient could mean feeling ill, feeling nauseous, feeling guilty or depressed or feeling feverish and therefore it is essential for the practitioner to check the meaning of the patient's words with him or her before making assumptions.

It is important at this stage to keep tentative hypotheses separate from the initial concept. The initial concept includes information gathered from the patient's appearance, observations of people accompanying the patient, awareness of a hidden agenda, the patient's perception of the problem and any evidence which may support initial hypotheses.

For example, in the case of the woman who complains of feeling tired and low, the nurse practitioner can collect information and develop a summarized version of observed facts:

A 55-year-old Caucasian woman who states she is feeling tired and low, appears to be slightly overweight, has coarse thin hair, has dry skin and a hoarse voice, is not accompanied by a relative, walked into the consulting room with no restrictions and states she doesn't know what is wrong.

It would be a mistake at this stage to note 'a 55-year-old woman with hypothyroidism'. Hypothyroidism is simply one of several potential hypotheses. Similarly, with the 25-year-old woman who is complaining of feeling tired and low, it would be a mistake to note 'a 25-year-old depressed woman'. It is more accurate to note: 'a 25-year-old woman who states she is tired and low, appears to have a low body mass index, has slow speech and movement, with a depressed appearance'. Depression is a potential diagnosis for this woman and is

one of several hypotheses until further evidence can be added to the initial concept.

Generating hypotheses

A hypothesis is a provisional explanation for the occurrence of the patient's problem. It provides a label for the information which has been collected and allows the practitioner to focus a line of enquiry in a certain direction. Once the initial concept has been formulated, several different hypotheses may spring to mind. This can happen in a matter of seconds and the number and type of hypotheses will vary according to the clarity of the patient's complaint. The generation of hypotheses will also depend upon the experience and clinical knowledge of the practitioner. A nurse who has little experience of women's health and the menopause, for example, may come up with differential diagnoses of anxiety disorder or depression for a woman who complains of sleeplessness and feelings of distress during meetings at work. A nurse with experience in caring for women experiencing the symptoms of the menopause may generate hypotheses of menopause, anxiety disorder or depression and the subsequent enquiry will have a broader perspective covering different issues.

Nurse practitioners are frequently presented with vague complaints from patients such as 'I feel tired all the time', 'I have been experiencing headaches' or 'I have been feeling dizzy'. For each of these vague complaints there are many potential hypotheses and once the initial concept has been developed, the hypotheses have to be narrowed down to provide a focus for the consultation. For the complaint of 'dizzy', for example, the nurse has to ask initial questions to help focus the enquiry. 'When does it occur?' 'What makes it better and what makes it worse?' 'Are there any other symptoms associated with the dizziness?' 'Can you describe the feeling?' The questions at this stage are broad and should not bias the responses of the patient. For example, asking the question 'Are there any other symptoms associated with the dizziness?' is different to asking 'Do you feel nauseous when you are dizzy?' Questions which are too focused at this stage can contaminate the patient's story and lead the patient into providing information which does not necessarily represent the reality of his or her experience but rather tells the practitioner what he or she wants to hear.

It is possible to generate broad hypotheses which can be focused after gathering further information from the patient. For example, if a patient complains of pain in the hand and the forearm, the practitioner may generate a hypothesis of 'painful forearm'. Further information may lead the practitioner to generate several more focused hypotheses. If the patient states that he doesn't remember sustaining an injury but the pain has been present for many months and is now stopping him in his work, the hypotheses of 'nervous injury to the median nerve, radial nerve or ulnar nerve' could all be generated. These hypotheses then provide the basis for further enquiry and the practitioner needs to generate a strategy to provide evidence which may support or refute the hypotheses generated so far.

Formulating an enquiry strategy

The initial concept and the hypotheses must remain flexible and open to change in the light of new information. As the nurse becomes aware of new information, this must constantly be checked against the initial concept and the hypotheses. Hypotheses may be ruled out or substantiated by further enquiry and it is here that the nurse practitioner must utilize physical examination skills and focused history-taking to elicit the information required to generate a working hypothesis which will underpin the subsequent management plan. The aspects of physical examination to be carried out, the tests which may need to be performed and the sequence of questions to be asked form the enquiry strategy.

The enquiry strategy is a process of analysis and synthesis of information. For example, in a patient who complains of headache, the initial concept may be: 'Woman who appears to be 30 years old states she has been experiencing headaches with increasing frequency over the last 12 months but does not have one today'. On asking broad questions the woman states that she feels nauseous with the headache, paracetamol has helped slightly, the headache is made worse by noise and she tends to go to bed if she has one, the headaches seem to come on in the evenings and she has never experienced anything like this before. At this stage the hypotheses could be focused to 'migraine', 'tension headache', 'cluster headache', 'eye strain', 'sinusitis', 'side-effects of medications' or, less likely, 'brain tumour' or 'severe hypertension'. The differential diagnosis of 'meningeal irritation' has already been ruled out as meningitis presents with a sudden severe, generalized headache which would have been present during the consultation.

The nurse practitioner's knowledge of anatomy and physiology, pathophysiology and previous experience will then guide the history-taking process to ask some more focused questions, such as: 'Please show me where you feel the pain.' 'Do you notice any other symptoms with the headache?' 'When did you last have an eye examination?' 'What type of work do you do?' 'Are you on any other medications?' 'Do you have any neck pain?' 'How long do the headaches last for?' 'What do you think your headaches are related to?' 'Do any of your family members have problems with headaches?' 'Is there any link between the headaches and your menstrual cycle?' Several of these questions will allow the practitioner to rule out some of the potential generated hypotheses. For example, if there is a negative reply to 'Are you on any other medications?', side-effects of medications can be ruled out. A positive response to the question relating to neck pain enhances the possibility of tension headache. The associated symptom of nausea may heighten the possibility of migraine, while the location of the headache bilaterally around the occipital region may support tension headache. If the woman reports that the headaches last for 4–6 hours and there is no history of family migraine or similar headaches, tension headache may again be considered. In response to the menstrual cycle question, the patient answers that she would not know as she hasn't had a period for a few months. This information clearly changes the initial concept and generates further hypotheses relating to potential pregnancy for analysis and synthesis with the original concept.

The enquiry strategy is a deductive process. The information obtained will allow the practitioner to reject some hypotheses, support others or generate new ones in the light of fresh information. Some questions will effectively rule out certain hypotheses. Patients who attend the clinic with headaches are often concerned that they may have hypertension. Practitioners are aware that hypertension is an unlikely cause of headache, however, it takes only a few moments to check a patient's blood pressure and this will quickly reassure the patient on being told that the reading is normal. Similarly, some patients fear a brain tumour with unexplained headaches, so it is worthwhile addressing this and enquiring about the type of headache (deep, steady and dull); what makes it worse (coughing or straining); when it is worse (worse on waking and often improves with upright position), and then letting the patient know that a headache which has been intermittent over 12 months and worse in the evenings is unlikely to be associated with a brain tumour.

The methods described in the enquiry strategy are described by Barrows and Pickell (1991) as a searching process. Searching is focused on the particular presenting problem. Scanning is another process used by practitioners to scan the horizon for further clues. This includes the review of systems, review of past medical history, family history, demographics and social situation. This may produce useful information which may generate new hypotheses or support the present hypotheses. The scanning process also provides the nurse with information which is incredibly valuable when considering treatment options. If in the scanning process the nurse finds that the patient left home when she was 16 and now lives in shared accommodation with four other women, is employed at present but only on the minimum wage and has no savings, this will have serious implications for suggestions regarding treatment options.

After searching and scanning, the practitioner may need to redesign the enquiry strategy. Clearly, in the case of the woman with the headache, the new hypotheses may include 'pregnant' and experiencing 'tension headaches'. This would have to be checked with further history-taking, now focused on sexual activity, the nature of the nausea, weight loss or weight gain and the possibility of being pregnant. The process remains dynamic and flexible and the practitioner must be open to change and regeneration of new hypotheses throughout the process.

Applying appropriate clinical skills

Clinical skills include the ability to carry out an appropriate physical examination and to focus the history to dissect and elaborate on the patient's complaint. Most of a diagnosis is made on the history alone and much of the physical examination is conducted to support or refute hypotheses generated during the enquiry and history-taking process. History-taking skill involves the ability to adapt to the particular patient's communication style. The use of broad questions followed by more focused questions helps to elicit as much information as possible in the patient's own words. Barrows and Pickell (1991) suggest that direct questions help to dissect the specifics of the patient's problem. Direct questions should cover reasons for the encounter, onset of the problem, quality and intensity of the symptoms, associated symptoms, sequence and localization of symptoms, physical or emotional stress preceding the problem and relieving or palliation factors. The history-taking process is covered in greater detail in Chapter 2.

In taking the patient's history questions should generally be open, as closed questions tend to bias the patient's responses. Open questions allow patients to elaborate on their symptoms and to tell their story. There are some occasions, however, when closed questioning is appropriate. In an emergency situation such as an acute asthmatic episode a closed question, 'Have you already taken your blue inhaler?', will help the practitioner to understand the severity of the attack. In a consultation with a patient who does not easily elaborate on the story of the problem, closed questions may be necessary to elicit responses to specific questions.

The history-taking process in a person with headaches might start with an open question such as 'How do your headaches affect you?' This may be followed by a series of more focused questions, including: 'When do they occur? Where do you feel the pain? How long have you been experiencing them for? Do you experience any other symptoms?' Depending on the responses to the more focused questions, the practitioner might want to go on to ask a series of closed questions to confirm or rule out certain hypotheses, for example 'Do you find the light makes it worse?' or 'Does your neck feel painful?' It is important not to channel the patient down a specific line to support the hypotheses that were generated in the first few seconds. Open questioning avoids this problem and allows the practitioner to build a broad picture of the patient's problem. This will reduce the likelihood of missing a vital clue.

The physical examination is guided by the generated hypotheses. Physical examination is a further searching process and is most often carried out simply to confirm the hypotheses. Physical examination can be carried out after the history-taking process or the two processes can be carried out at the same time. If a patient complains of abdominal pain but is unable to describe the exact location of the pain, is in his mid 40s, tells you that the pain sometimes keeps him awake at night and sometimes makes him vomit, the hypotheses of pancreatitis, peptic ulcer, intestinal obstruction, gastroenteritis, reflux oesophagitis, irritable colon and ureterolithiasis are all possible. For efficient use of time it is worthwhile examining the patient's abdomen whilst carrying out further questioning. The physical examination helps to provide more precise information about the location of the pain. When the patient places his hand over the epigastric area of his abdomen and does not complain of any tenderness in the costovertebral angles or in the lower abdomen, several of the hypotheses can be rejected and the practitioner can focus the history-taking and further physical examination on the remaining hypotheses. This very brief initial examination can assist the history-taking process and, whilst it is important to carry out a thorough abdominal examination and urinalysis and it is important to take a thorough history including systems review, allowing the patient to point to the area of discomfort on his exposed abdomen will help focus the searching techniques during the consultation. When the patient points to the epigastric area, the initial concept of the patient is developed further, the practitioner employs the enquiry strategy to collect more information, analyses the information, utilizes further searching techniques of physical examination and history-taking and adds all the information to the initial concept. Eventually enough data will have been gathered to analyse and resolve the patient's problem. At this point the practitioner can develop a problem synthesis.

Developing the problem synthesis

Once the initial concept has been developed and refined and the information has been checked for accuracy with the patient, the enhanced initial concept develops into the problem synthesis. This is a representation of the patient's problem. Once a problem synthesis has been developed the practitioner should be able to represent the patient's problem with accuracy and clarity. This does not necessarily mean that the practitioner has confirmed a diagnosis. In some cases it is not possible to do so because further tests are needed or because the patient has a rare condition with which the practitioner is unfamiliar. The patient may require referral for a specialist opinion and therefore it is important that the practitioner is able to represent the problem synthesis without necessarily offering a diagnosis.

The problem synthesis is developed from the data-gathering process – the enquiry strategy. The following is an example of the developing problem synthesis. A male patient in his 60s walks into the consulting room complaining of a cough which will not go away. The practitioner develops an immediate initial concept of 'a male patient with a recurrent cough who is in his 60s'. It is possible to develop several hypotheses from this initial information. The patient may have developed chronic bronchitis, chronic obstructive airways disease, congestive heart failure, gastroesophageal reflux, asthma, postnasal drip, a viral upper respiratory tract infection, pneumonia or bronchitis. The patient clearly has a respiratory problem and an experienced practitioner will immediately focus observation on the patient's fingers to look for evidence of nicotine staining, looking at his face, hair and mouth for evidence of the yellow hue of many years of smoking, noting any smell of smoke, observing the lips for signs of pursed-lip breathing and noting the mucous membranes for signs of cyanosis and respiratory distress. The practitioner may also glance at the patient's ankles to see if there is any evidence of peripheral oedema which may provide a clue that the patient has a cardiac condition. This all happens in seconds and immediately the practitioner has developed the initial concept and has gathered vital clues to support or refute the generated hypotheses.

This patient has no signs of smoking and it is not possible to see his ankles underneath his trousers. The practitioner commences with an open questioning style to try and understand more about the nature of the cough. 'Tell me a bit more about your cough'. The patient explains that he has had it for months

and it is bothering him at night. He has fits of coughing and it is keeping his wife awake. The practitioner has gathered vital information here. If the patient has had the cough for months, it is more likely to be a chronic condition and not an acute one. It is therefore possible to focus on the conditions which are more likely to be chronic such as chronic bronchitis, chronic obstructive airways disease, congestive heart failure, gastroesophageal reflux, asthma or postnasal drip and the hypotheses of the acute respiratory conditions, including a viral upper respiratory tract infection, pneumonia or bronchitis are less likely. The initial concept has already changed to 'a man in his 60s who has no signs of smoking, with a cough which he has had for months; the cough is troublesome at night'.

The practitioner must then develop an enquiry strategy which includes history-taking and physical examination. The history will include more focused questions about the cough. Questions about the timing, whether it is productive, whether there are any other associated symptoms, what makes it worse and what makes it better will help to build upon the initial concept. When the patient states that the cough is productive, the practitioner asks an open question to discover exactly what sort of sputum is being produced. When the patient answers that it is 'gooey', that doesn't help the practitioner much. 'What colour is the sputum?', which is different from asking: 'Is the sputum green?' will result in the patient describing the sputum as white, green, yellow, black or red – all of these responses would be significant. If the question had been: 'Is the sputum green?' the patient could answer 'yes' or 'no'. As the patient was not provided with any options the reply may not be an accurate reflection of the nature of his sputum. If he answers 'no' then further questioning is required; if he answers yes, it is possible that the practitioner is leading the patient down a particular path towards a diagnosis and may inadvertently miss a vital clue.

When the patient states that the sputum is white, it is worse at night, nothing seems to help once he has started a coughing fit, sometimes he feels sick and dizzy with the effort of coughing and he often feels short of breath during an attack, he doesn't smoke and his wife is very worried about him, the initial concept has changed again, and the hypotheses can be reviewed. A cough which is aggravated on recumbency can be due to postnasal drip, congestive heart failure or gastroesophageal reflux. There is a possibility that the diagnosis could be asthma, where the cough is triggered by the presence of dust mites in a poorly ventilated bedroom. The presence of white sputum could support the hypothesis of asthma; however, further examination and enquiry are required before eliminating other possible causes of the cough. The initial concept has now developed to 'a man in his 60s who does not smoke has had a cough for months which produces white sputum; the cough is worse at night, nothing relieves it, he feels sick and dizzy during an attack, his wife is worried about his health'.

The enquiry strategy must now go a stage further to ask more searching questions and to carry out the appropriate physical examinations. A practitioner might choose to continue to take the history, including present social situation, past medical history, current medications and relevant family history and follow this with a physical examination. In the history-taking process the nurse finds that the patient has recently retired and moved house, is currently decorating, had a history of 'bronchitis' as a child, has been very fit and well and rarely consults with health care professionals and is not taking any medications. To reject or support hypotheses which now seem to be less likely than at the beginning of the encounter, the practitioner might now specifically ask closed or focused questions about heart or gastric symptoms. 'Do you notice any heartburn?' 'Do you notice a strange taste in your mouth when you lie down?' 'Have you noticed any swelling in your ankles?' 'Do you get breathless when you exercise?' These questions would help rule out with greater certainty gastric reflux and congestive heart disease.

The physical examination component of the enquiry strategy would be focused on the respiratory system and include examination of the cardiovascular system and the sinuses for postnasal drip. It is clear from the history that the practitioner might be working on a preferred hypothesis of asthma and the data-gathering physical examination would be focused on auscultation for bilateral wheezing. Examination of the posterior pharynx for secretions and the mucosa of the nose for cobblestone appearance, followed by palpation of the sinuses for tenderness would help support or rule out the hypothesis of postnasal drip. Examination of the extremities for pitting oedema, assessment of the heart rate for tachycardia and auscultation of the lungs for crackles or wheezes and the heart for extra heart sounds would address the cardiovascular possibilities and add to the initial concept.

Eventually the data-gathering system comes together. Several hypotheses have been rejected and the practitioner can then form a problem synthesis. The problem synthesis represents the patient's problem and therefore in the example of the man in his 60s with a recurrent cough, the practitioner would develop a problem synthesis as follows:

A man in his 60s who does not smoke has had a cough for months which produces white sputum, the cough is worse at night, nothing relieves it, he feels sick and dizzy during an attack, his wife is worried about his health. He has no breathlessness on exercise and does not complain of heartburn. He has a history of bronchitis as a child and no other past medical history. He does not take any medications and is usually well. He has recently retired and moved house. He is currently decorating his present house. There is no evidence of cyanosis in the mucous membranes and no evidence of pursed-lip breathing. Mucous membranes of the oropharynx and nose are pink and moist and there is no evidence of mucoid secretions in the posterior pharynx. He has a pulse rate of 82 and normal heart sounds. He has wheezes throughout both lungs.

Once a problem synthesis has been developed the practitioner can compare the problem synthesis with the generated hypotheses. A judgement is made as to which (if any) of the hypotheses fits the problem synthesis. Drawing on clinical knowledge and experience the practitioner is able to apply the pathophysiological processes to the patient's problem and make a judgement about the possible diagnosis. It may be necessary to utilize a variety of tests or to initiate a trial of treatment to be sure that the diagnosis is correct.

It is essential that throughout the problem-solving process the practitioner is checking the accuracy of the findings with the patient's perception of the problem. Communicating with the patient throughout the process helps him or her to understand the diagnostic process and therefore to understand the treatment plan. It is essential to get to know the patient to help direct subsequent decisions about treatment and tests. If these decisions are made without the patient's contribution, the chances of compliance with the treatment plan are reduced and therefore the success of the intervention will be threatened.

Laboratory and diagnostic findings

It is clearly important in some patient encounters to support or reject the generated hypotheses with tests. For example, in the previous case of the female patient who was 55 years of age, slightly obese, tired and low, the practitioner might want to follow the history-taking process and physical examination with thyroid function tests to support a hypothesis of hypothyroidism. In the example of the man in his 60s with recurrent cough, the nurse may wish to do a reversibility test with pre- and post-salbutamol peak flow readings followed by a week's diary recording of peak flow readings and a follow-up appointment. When deciding which tests to utilize it is important to consider the inconvenience to the patient, the harm caused to him or her, the cost of the test and what information the test is going to provide. Sometimes tests are used as part of the scanning procedure in an attempt to search for other clues, for example, the battery of tests that many clinicians carry out for the complaint of tired all the time (full blood count, urea and electrolytes, thyroid function tests, monospot (or Paul Burnell for glandular fever), erythrocyte sedimentation rate and urinalysis) may help provide a clue where the history-taking and physical examination process have not produced a significant result. It is essential to consider the role of the tests in the enquiry strategy and the relevance of positive or negative results to solving the patient's problem.

The sensitivity, specificity and relevance of the test for the hypothesis must be considered to determine if it is worthwhile proceeding with that test. Sensitivity is measured by the number of false-negatives it might produce. If a test detects most cases of a disease in a tested group of people with few false negative results, then it is sensitive for that disease. If the test is specific for the disease then it will only show a positive result in people who have the disease. If a test shows a positive result in people who do not have the disease then it is not specific. The relevance of a test is the effect it will have on the diagnosis and management of the patient. The reasons for carrying out laboratory testing according to Barrows and Pickell (1991) are to reassure the patient, to provide the practitioner with further evidence to support a hypothesis and to assess the severity of the disease. The results of testing when considered with the rest of the enquiry strategy may support your diagnosis.

Diagnostic decision-making

Eventually the practitioner is faced with the need to make a diagnostic decision. It may not be possible to make an immediate decision about a patient's problem and in some cases it is necessary to live with uncertainty until test results are available or until further evidence comes to light. If the diagnosis is uncertain the clinician has to decide how to progress. It may be that after the enquiry strategy is complete a patient's problem may still have two hypotheses. For example, chronic obstructive airways disease and asthma may be difficult to differentiate in some patients. It may therefore be necessary to implement a course of treatment, monitor the result and then make a diagnostic decision based upon the results of the therapy. If a decision can be made the practitioner then has a further decision-making process to address – how to treat the patient.

Therapeutic decision-making

Evidence which has been collected throughout the patient encounter will have helped the practitioner understand the patient's perception of the problem and learn about the patient's values and beliefs. This is essential when making a decision about treatment with the patient. If a patient has concerns about the overuse of steroids in the treatment of asthma, for example, this issue may have to be addressed and alternatives may have to be explored. Similarly, if the patient expects to receive antibiotics for a cough but the practitioner makes a therapeutic decision to offer no treatment because it is a viral cough of short duration, this decision will have to be considered in the light of the patient's expectations and time will have to be devoted to explaining this decision to the patient.

It is also important to consider the cost of the treatment – both to the patient and to the health service. More expensive treatments are sometimes worthwhile when there is proof that they are more effective. It is essential to consider the patient's perspective and needs here, as a rapid response to an initial treatment may enhance compliance with treatments later in a chronic disease process. The patient must be fully informed of what to expect so that he or she feels there is some partnership in the decision-making process. The practitioner must also consider the risks of the treatment and whether the risks outweigh the benefits. This is not always easy, and, like diagnostic decision-making, it is a dynamic cyclical process which alters according to information gathered from the patient and the knowledge and experience of the practitioner (Figure 1.1).

Reflection in and on practice

The Barrows and Pickell stages model of clinical problem-solving allows the practitioner to reflect upon an encounter with a patient and to consider the stages which went well and stages which did not go well. The model provides a framework for learning from each client encounter and allows the practitioner to identify skills which need to be developed. It is possible to use this framework to carry out reflection in action, as described by Schon (1987). The practitioner can carry out scanning techniques whilst reflecting upon past experiences and synthesizing that knowledge with the information gathered in the present encounter.

The problem-solving process is a dynamic cyclical process which allows the initial concept of the patient to evolve and develop. The whole process may happen in minutes or it may take months, depending upon the need for test results or diagnostic interventions. A structured approach to problem-solving enables the nurse practitioner to utilize the skills of history-taking and physical examination to generate hypotheses and to minimize the possibility of missing a vital clue. A thorough approach will finally enable the nurse practitioner to make diagnostic and

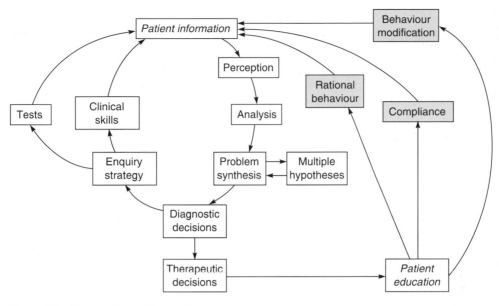

Figure 1.1   Diagnostic decision-making process
Source: Adapted from Barrows and Pickell (1991)

therapeutic decisions with a confidence that enhances the success of the consultation process.

References

Barrows H.S., Pickell G.C. (1991) *Developing Clinical Problem Solving Skills: A Guide to More Effective Diagnosis and Treatment.* New York, Norton Medical Books.

Hurst K. (1993) *Problem Solving in Nursing Practice*, London, Scutari Press.

Hurst, K., Dean, A., Trickey, S. (1991) The recognition and non-recognition of problem solving stages in nursing practice, *Journal of Advanced Nursing*, **16**, pp. 1444–1455.

Newell A., Simon H.A. (1972) *Human Problem Solving*, New Jersey, Prentice-Hall.

Schon D. (1987) *Educating the Reflective Practitioner*, California, Jossey Bass.

United Kingdom Central Council (1992) *The Scope of Professional Practice*, London, UKCC.

CHAPTER 2
Taking a history

Christina Clark

How few there are who, by five or six pointed questions, can elicit the whole case and get accurately to know and to be able to report where the patient is (*Florence Nightingale 1859*).

Introduction

Nurse practitioners must be skilled in taking an accurate history and diagnosing health problems in their clinical setting. All nurses are used to assessing patients and asking questions but the nurse practitioner expands this skill to include an assessment of the medical history. The history-taking interview must be of a high quality so that the patient's symptoms are accurately recorded in a precise, chronological order.

Listening to the patient's story is not just an opportunity for data collection but also for establishing a therapeutic relationship. The encounter may also be an opportunity for a healing or teaching moment. Health care does not have solutions for all the problems that people present with and often all that can be done is to listen and validate the patient's experience. This approach is well summed up by Benner and Wrubel (1989):

> Even when no treatment is available and no cure is possible, understanding the meaning of the illness for the person and for the person's life is a form of healing, in that such understanding can overcome the sense of alienation, loss of self-understanding and loss of social integration that accompany illness.

This chapter will focus on the history-taking aspects of nurse practitioner consultations. The skills of physical examination, health education and the management of many common conditions will be presented in later chapters.

Taking a history is like playing detective – searching for clues, collecting information without bias yet staying on track to solve the puzzle. As the data comes from a human being and is received by another human being, it is subject to error. Patients forget symptoms or get the sequence of events out of order or withhold embarrassing details. Often people may

tell their story in a way they think you want to hear or try to please you, or describe their actions in a way that they think a normal sensible person would behave rather than how events occurred. Clinicians may misunderstand, overlook relevant information, fail to ask key questions or jump to premature diagnostic conclusions. For nursing perhaps more than medicine, the assessment is a continuing process and finding out the patient's story is ongoing rather than being limited to one encounter. Effective communication is clearly the key to success as the history is usually the single most important part of the whole assessment process (Figure 2.1).

Neighbour (1987) reminds us that Milton Erikson stated: 'In therapy, success is a journey, not a destination' pointing out that this applies to the general practice consultation. He states that the consultation is like a journey as it is ongoing with an unfolding of symptoms, problems and feelings which may never come to a firm conclusion as there is always another consultation or further occasion to review a problem. This sense of movement is pertinent to nurse practitioner consultations. In the case of chronic disease management, for example, the nurse practitioner will be meeting the patient at regular intervals over a lengthy period. For practical purposes the clinician will focus on certain aspects to work on in any given consultation, but there will always be more to follow.

The nurse practitioner and patient therefore have to work as a partnership, which involves both acknowledging their differing backgrounds, knowledge and perspectives. For an effective consultation to take place, a rapport has to be established and information has to pass both ways (Figure 2.2). This opens up the possibility of negotiation, understanding and influence leading to change in future behaviour (Neighbour 1987). Both parties are in some way different after the encounter.

The nursing focus of the interview is on the person and his or her experience. It is important to 'stay in the moment' and appreciate the significance of that moment to the patient. Although honesty is essential

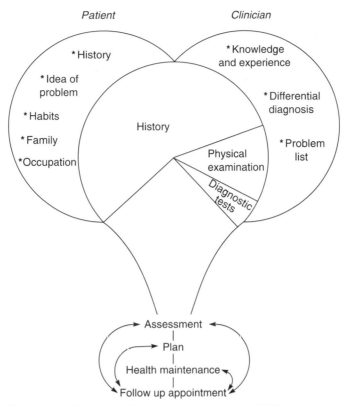

Figure 2.1 Communication between patient and clinician
Source: Adapted from Neighbour (1987)

to understand and validate the person's experience, it may be necessary to suspend judgement and let go of an immediate confronting or judging response. Being there and witnessing the person may be therapeutic in itself when there is no treatment to offer. Simply acknowledging suffering, pain or the wide range of human emotions and social conditions can have a therapeutic effect.

The history should be seen as only one component of assessment and diagnosis; it is the initial stage in data collection. In some instances, such as a chronic disease, the history would be an extensive and important guide to diagnostic tests, whereas a minor skin condition may be diagnosed mainly by visual inspection and only a few questions are needed to reach a conclusion.

The nurse practitioner should start with a fresh mind, collecting information and try to refrain from jumping to conclusions too quickly. Although history-taking may appear to be a daunting task at first, experience and practice will allow the practitioner to focus on the likely cause of the patient's problems with increasing confidence and rapidity. 'In the beginner's mind there are many possibilities, but in the expert's mind there are few' (Suzuki 1986).

History-taking is generally followed by physical examination, which allows the clinician to confirm or reject possibilities raised by the history. There may be a need for further investigations and questions before a diagnosis can be made.

Factors affecting the interview

Self-awareness

Before starting an interview it is important to have taken some time to consider your own feelings, beliefs, values, strengths and weaknesses. Ask yourself what you bring to the relationship both culturally and emotionally, and cultivate interpersonal factors such as liking and respect for others, empathy and the ability to listen. Burnard (1992) presents a model of the outer and inner aspects of self. Outer aspects include facial expressions, gestures, touch, movement and dress; inner aspects include thinking, feeling, sensing, intuition and experience of the body. Through learning about the outer and inner aspects of oneself a sense of self-awareness can be developed.

Taking a complete history can be an intimate experience as you are asking the patient to share personal experiences. It is a privilege to listen and often demands maturity to deal with the information and listen in a non-judgemental way. In a busy clinical

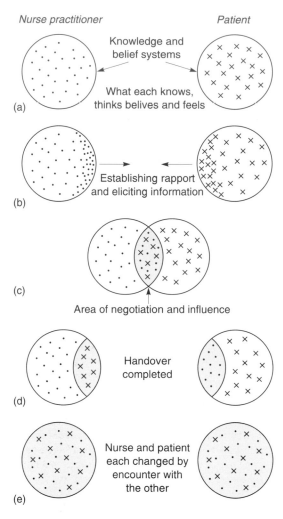

Figure 2.2   Communication – the patient as partner
Source: Adapted from Neighbour (1987)

Personal space

It is worth considering your proximity to the patient. The physical distance between yourself and the patient can send a powerful message and can generate feelings of anxiety or discomfort in some clients. The physical examination takes place in an intimate zone and it is important to remember when moving to this part of the consultation process that you should warn the patient that you are going to move in closer. If a patient feels uncomfortable with the distance from the clinician it may interfere with the development of trust in the relationship.

Personal appearance

Nurse practitioners should think carefully about clothing. Most patients seem to prefer clothing appropriate to the setting, which tends towards conservative, conventional and professional. It is important not to impede or distract patients from being comfortable in telling their story, which may be the case if you are inappropriately dressed.

Other non-verbal communications

Body language can encourage or discourage the flow of conversation. Eye movements, facial expressions, body gestures and posture are all important (Table 2.1). Video-taping consultations can give you useful feedback, especially concerning mannerisms that may discourage patients from talking.

Table 2.1   The interviewer's non-verbal behaviour

Positive	Negative
Professional appearance	Inappropriate dress
Equal-status seating	Standing over or behind desk
Comfortable close proximity	Too close or too far away
Relaxed open posture	Tense
Leaning slightly forward	Slouched away
Occasional facilitating gestures	Critical or distracting
Facial animation or interest	Yawning, pointing, finger-tapping
	Looking at watch
Appropriate smiling	Frowning
Maintaining eye contact	Avoiding eye contact
	Focusing on notes/computer
Moderate tone of voice	Strident or high-pitched
Moderate rate of speech	Too slow or too fast
Appropriate touch	Too frequent or inappropriate touch

situation it is easy to bring charged emotions from a previous encounter with you. Taking a break or a quick refocusing meditation can help bring you back to centre for the next encounter.

Environmental factors

Provide privacy and try to ensure that there are no interruptions from the busy culture of our health care system, such as telephone calls, beepers, mobile phones or colleagues entering the room. Try and discourage interruptions except in cases of emergency. An interruption can disturb concentration and destroy the feeling of a safe environment that takes time to build up and, once lost, may not be fully restored. The room should be a comfortable temperature, with minimal noise. Remove distracting equipment or clutter from view. Arrange the furniture to enable the person to sit comfortably at the same eye level and at an angle which allows eye contact but also allows you to look away easily if desired.

The interview

Medical history-taking has developed into a fairly set format and the nurse practitioner must be sure to include questions pertinent to a medical diagnosis, as this will assist communication with medical practitioners. When appropriate, you should also expand into psychosocial areas of questioning which include more about the person and his or her experiences. Medical diagnosis seeks to find the cause or explanation of the patient's symptoms, whereas nursing assessment is more focused on providing an accurate picture of the person's current condition and experience of the situation. Sometimes the focused questions may seem the same, but the intent and philosophy are slightly different. The skilled nurse practitioner therefore includes sufficient data for a baseline medical assessment but also obtains information that will provide a picture of the patient's experience of the condition.

At the beginning of the interview it is important to consider why the patient is there and what his or her expectations are. The patient also needs to know who you are, why you are there and what your intentions and expectations are. He or she may never have been interviewed in such depth before by a nurse or even heard of a nurse practitioner. The purpose of the interview is to establish a rapport with the patient to gather background information about any problems, current health, past medical history and social history. Patients want someone who is competent to address their concerns. Some may expect to be seen by a doctor and therefore withhold information, thinking a nursing interview is just a preliminary screen. Others may misunderstand time limitations or the expertise of the nurse. It may be helpful to introduce yourself with a simple brief explanation of your role so that patients understand the aim of the interview and its relevance to their care.

Patients must feel comfortable in telling their story and therefore need to know that the interview is confidential. Neighbour (1987) points out that patients have most control over the first part of the interview. Often they modify their first words depending on the environment and their initial unguarded remarks give valuable clues to their inner self. It is helpful to leave as much space as possible for the patient to talk at the beginning of the interview. Simpson *et al.* (1991), in their review of communication, mention one study where patients were interrupted by the clinician on average within 18 seconds of starting to describe their problem and, not surprisingly, failed to go on to disclose significant concerns.

Pendleton *et al.* (1987) identified seven tasks of the consultation:

1 To define the reasons for the patient's attendance
2 To consider other problems
3 To choose with the patient an appropriate action for each problem
4 To achieve a shared understanding with the patient of the problems
5 To involve the patient in the management and encourage him or her to accept responsibility
6 To use time and resources appropriately
7 To establish or maintain a relationship with the patient which helps to achieve the other tasks.

Pendleton's seven tasks can be encapsulated by dividing the interview into three phases – introduction, working phase and termination phase. In the *introduction* phase it is important to take steps to ensure comfort and privacy. The patient should be welcomed and this may involve you introducing yourself and shaking hands with the patient. Social chat is acceptable and is useful when walking from the waiting area to the consulting room. It is particularly important to know and use the patient's name.

During the *working* phase it is necessary to elicit the patient's story by gathering information. The patient's past medical history, family history, psychosocial history, current problem and current health status should be explored and a review of systems carried out. Start with open questions, then become more focused. It is common for patients to have a multitude of problems and it is often impossible to pursue all the problems in one consultation. Therefore it is necessary to prioritize and pursue the most urgent problem. Sometimes a summary of the problems stated so far is helpful to prioritize with the patient. Other problems should be identified and, if they cannot be addressed in this interview, it is important to let the patient know that they will be addressed at a later date.

The termination phase involves a further summary of the important points. The consultation then moves on to physical examination if necessary, a discussion of treatment options and the plan for follow-up if required.

Interview techniques

It is possible to develop interviewing techniques which can assist with the flow of the history-taking process. Helpful techniques are summarized in Table 2.2 and unhelpful techniques in Table 2.3. The nurse practitioner should use reflective practice to analyse the techniques used in each interview and should be able to build on the experience to develop an effective history-taking strategy.

Framework of questions

When interviewing patients it is easy to be sidetracked or omit important questions. Developing a framework of questions can help to gather information in an orderly way. There are many different approaches to history-taking. The traditional medical history is structured so that the clinician can focus easily on the presenting problem and the interviewer

Table 2.2   Helpful interview techniques

- Offer general leads
- Restate in order to clarify
- Reflect
- Verbalize the implied meaning
- Focus the discussion
- Place symptoms or problems in sequence
- Encourage participation and evaluation
- Make observations that may encourage the patient to discuss symptoms
- Use silence
- Summarize

Table 2.3   Interview techniques to avoid

- Asking why or how questions
- Using probing, persistent questions
- Using inappropriate or technical language
- Giving advice
- Giving false assurance
- Changing the subject or interrupting
- Using stereotyped responses
- Giving excessive approval or agreement
- Jumping to conclusions
- Using defensive responses
- Asking leading questions suggesting 'right answers'
- Social chat: the person is expecting professional expertise

Source: Adapted from Morton (1993).

can easily record all data in well-organized sections. Patients tell their stories in different ways and usually not in a structured way. It is up to the clinician to gather the data in a logical sequence. The history obtained should be made up of the components summarized in Table 2.4.

Identifying data
Date, time, age, sex and occupation are usually included, with a brief description of the patient's appearance to help in identification.

Chief complaint
Patients should be encouraged to state the problem in their own words. This statement should be recorded.

Table 2.4   Key elements of a medical history

- Identifying data
- Chief complaint
- Present illness
- Current health and medications
- Past medical history
- Family history
- Psychosocial history
- Review of systems

Present illness
This expands upon the chief complaint, describing it more fully and explaining the chronological development of symptoms. It should include what the patient thinks and feels about the illness and what concerns led to the decision to seek help. The patient's perception of the problem is crucial. Ask patients what they think caused the symptoms and why they have come today for treatment. How the symptoms have affected the person's life should also be checked. Symptoms may become meaningful in a broader sense and may be linked to relationships or significant events in a person's life. It is therefore important to understand the meaning of the symptoms or illness to that person especially, as this may be very different from your perspective as a professional. Remember to allow the patient to speak uninterrupted.

Symptom analysis

In order to encourage patients to describe their symptoms in the most expansive manner, several frameworks have been developed, one of which is PQRST (Morton 1993). This mnemonic is most useful in describing pain but can be used for other symptoms.

P: provocative/palliative
Q: quality
R: region/radiation
S: severity
T: temporal/timing

Provocative/palliative
The nurse practitioner should explore what provokes the symptom or the pain and what relieves it. The patient should be asked if movement, lying down, breathing, over-the-counter medications, heat, cold or any other factors exacerbate or alleviate the symptom.

Quality
The quality of the symptom is a description of how it appears to the patient. Patients use a variety of words to describe their symptoms and this is particularly useful in arriving at a diagnosis. The complaint of crushing chest pain, for example, is almost diagnostic of myocardial infarction.

DeGowin (1987) describes three types of pain:

1. Bright, pricking – often described as sharp or cutting
2. Burning – often described as hot or stinging
3. Deep and aching – often described as gnawing or throbbing

Such is the subjective nature of pain that the patient may use a wide range of words to describe it. McCaffery *et al.* (1994) suggest that if patients are having difficulty in describing the pain, a questionnaire can be used to provide a few words which may help them explain the sensations they are experiencing. For example, throbbing, shooting, stabbing, sharp, cramping, gnawing, hot, burning, aching, heavy, tender, splitting, tiring, exhausting, sickening, fearful, punishing and cruel are all words which can be used to describe discomfort.

Region/radiation

It is important to discover where the pain or symptom is being experienced. Ask the patient if it travels anywhere. This is particularly useful in exploring the pain of shingles or gathering information about skin disorders. A patient may only complain of the acne which appears on his or her face when in fact it has spread to the patient's back. Without asking the relevant questions to explore radiation, the nurse practitioner may never discover the true extent of the problem.

Severity

A rating scale can be used in the assessment of pain. It is important to ensure that all members of the health care team are using the same scale. Most commonly, a scale of 0–10 is used (see p. 234 for a more detailed discussion of the assessment of chronic pain). It is also useful to ask the patient to compare it with other common experiences, such as toothache, menstrual cramp, earache or headache. A rating scale is also a useful tool for the assessment of skin disorders such as psoriasis or eczema and can be applied to any condition which tends to fluctuate over time.

Temporal timing

The timing of the symptom is an important factor in several disease processes. Exploring with the patient when the symptom started, how long it lasted or lasts for, the timing in the day, the pattern of the symptom, its consistency or if it is intermittent, is useful in generating a clear picture of the problem. This can be particularly helpful when exploring symptoms such as a runny nose in allergic rhinitis or cough in asthma, as it can help with the diagnosis and subsequent treatment.

The information comes from the patient but the nurse practitioner must organize the data, clarifying symptoms and quantifying how severe and how frequent they are before finally placing them in order.

Current health

This may be reviewed briefly or expanded to detailed questions depending on the time available. Important topics to review are current medications, allergies,

habits, including tobacco, alcohol and drugs, exercise, diet, sleep and preventive health measures such as screening and immunizations. It is useful to explore the patient's smoking history in some detail. This can be a sensitive issue as people who smoke feel that they are being judged by health care professionals. However, smoking status and history are an important part of the history. You need to ask what is smoked (cigarettes, cigars, etc.), how many and for how long. If the person does not smoke, you need to find out if he or she ever did, for how long and when he or she gave up. It is also worth checking current interest in wanting to stop, enquiring what it would take to make the person stop, possible support and difficulties. Passive smoking should also be explored.

Past medical history

This is needed to put the present illness into context. Here the clinician asks about childhood illnesses, hospitalizations, surgery, blood transfusions and any specialist consultations. Any relevant previous medical history should be explored with the patient.

Family history

You should ask if the patient's parents are alive and if they have any illness. Establish ethnicity and health of blood-related family members. If there is a hereditary disease, enquire about all family members affected for at least two generations. Particularly important diseases to consider include cardiovascular and respiratory disease (including asthma and any cases of sudden death), cancer, diabetes, renal disease, allergies and any mental health disorder.

For diseases which have a genetic component a genogram may be useful: this is a quick visual guide which gives a snapshot of the person's place in the family (Figure 2.3). Genograms are used in family systems theory where the family is viewed as influencing current illness. The family tree can reveal patterns of illness, genetic traits and social and cultural factors. They can be relatively simple with names, dates of birth, death and marriage, or more complex, to include repetitive family themes, genetic traits, alcoholism and marital dysfunction. At least three generations should be studied and presented in the diagram.

Psychosocial history

This section is focused on collecting information to build a picture of how this person functions in society and who is around for social support. There is overwhelming evidence to show that lower social class and poverty are associated with poorer health. Those who are socially connected to others and feel part of a community have better health outcomes.

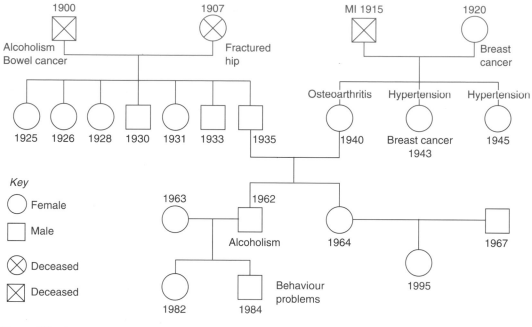

Figure 2.3   A genogram

Clinicians are often unaware of the issues people face in their everyday lives and make assumptions that deter them from revealing intimate problems. This may lead to selective awareness in clinicians. For the nurse practitioner it is important to establish a level of trust that allows patients to reveal problems that may influence their health. From a nursing perspective it is important to build a picture of patients in their social setting so that their experience of health and life is properly understood. Examples of questions that could be used to elicit useful social information can be found in Table 2.5.

To follow on from the information gathered by enquiring about the patient's social history, it may be useful to ask about work environment, recent job changes, work conditions, hours, shifts, chemical hazards, protective clothing required and availability of an occupational health service. Throughout the history-taking process it is important to keep an open mind and not to rush into a diagnosis before all the information is gathered.

Table 2.5   Questions which will elicit a social history

- Tell me about your living situation
- Who lives with you at home?
- What is your occupation?
- Tell me about your hobbies and leisure interests
- How far did you go with education?
- Do you have any financial worries?
- Who would you call if you needed support or in an emergency?
- How stressful has life been recently?
- How do you feel about the future?

Review of systems

A history is not complete without a review of systems. To the beginner it often seems an onerous task to continue with yet more questions, but the idea is to search for hidden clues and double-check that significant information has not been left out in the symptom analysis of presenting illness. It may prompt patients to recall further details about their health, help construct a picture of health and spot areas that might be important to target for health promotion. The review is customarily taken in a logical 'head-to-toe' order. It is limited to subjective data from the person – the response to your questions rather than any observations or objective findings you note on the way. Objective findings should be noted or discussed with the physical examination or investigative tests. As you focus the history and move your line of questioning, it is important to lead into each new section so that the patient has some understanding of the framework and topic to be discussed. This technique may help minimize uneasiness or feeling that the question is not relevant to the original concern.

General

Questions here are focused on general state of health apart from the new symptoms of the presenting illness. Useful questions include:

- Generally, how have you been feeling?
- How is your appetite?
- Is your weight stable ?
- Do you have any fatigue?
- Any fever, chills or night sweats?

Head

Ask the patient if he or she has experienced any headaches, dizziness, faintness or head injury.

Eyes

Any change in vision, redness or irritation, watering or discharge should be explored. The nurse practitioner should check if the patient wears glasses and when the last vision test or glaucoma test was carried out.

Respiratory (including ENT)

Breathing problems such as wheezing, feeling short of breath, cough, production of sputum or coughing up blood should be explored. Ask the patient if there has been any earache, sore throat or hearing problems. Check the date of the last chest X-ray, TB skin test, pneumococcal or flu vaccination.

Cardiac

Enquire about any heart problems or palpitations. Check for high blood pressure, anaemia, recent ECGs or heart stress test.

Gastrointestinal

Check for any difficulties in eating certain types of food, heartburn or indigestion, use of antacids, nausea or vomiting, flatulence, wind or excessive burping and level of appetite. Enquire about any change in bowel movements, constipation or diarrhoea, use of laxatives, rectal problems, haemorrhoids or fissures.

Genitourinary

Recent changes in pattern of micturition should be discussed. Check for symptoms such as frequency, urgency, change in colour or smell of urine or pain. For men it is worthwhile asking if there are any problems in the genital area, any rashes or lumps on the penis, scrotum or testes. Check if the patient carries out regular testicular examination. For women the last menstrual period and the pattern and duration of her cycle should be recorded. Problems with periods, amenorrhoea, mennorhagia, intermenstrual spotting, vaginal discharge, itching, foul smell, pelvic pain, menopause symptoms, use of contraception and date of last cervical smear should all be explored.

Sexual health

It is worth pointing out that you are concerned about *all* aspects of health and that many people have questions about sexual health. This paves the way for asking whether the patient has any concerns in this area.

Musculoskeletal

Ask the patient about pain, stiffness or swelling of the joints and any muscular pain, cramp or loss of strength.

Neurological

Has the patient noticed any numbness, tingling, tremors, weakness, difficulty coordinating movement or other unusual sensations?

Psychological

Start by asking the patient to describe his or her mood. Check how patients generally feels about themselves, what bothers them most about their present condition, how they cope with it and where they look for hope or strength.

The review of the systems concludes the history-taking process. The nurse practitioner should now be in a position to focus more clearly on the physical examination or may feel the need to return to earlier questions to confirm the results with the patient.

Sensitive areas

History-taking may well take you into some sensitive areas but if you are to obtain a holistic picture of the patient's health status, you need to obtain truthful information in such a way that a therapeutic relationship can be established and maintained. The following discussion explores some of these areas, including cultural competence, alcohol and drug use, sexual problems and domestic violence.

Cultural competence

Most nurses would like to think of themselves as sensitive to different cultures. Many nurse scholars have suggested that sensitivity is not enough but that *culturally competent care* is essential to meet the needs of patients. Increasingly diverse societies with greater immigration to developed countries, intercultural marriages and changing borders lead to a greater need to be culturally aware. Culturally competent care has been defined as:

> Care that takes into account issues related to diversity, marginalisation and vulnerability due to culture, race, gender and sexual orientation . . . It is also care that is provided within the historical and 'dailiness' context of clients. (*Meleis 1996*.)

Campinha-Bacote (1994) proposes a culturally competent model of care which involves cultural awareness, cultural knowledge, cultural skill and cultural encounter. Cultural awareness is the process of becoming sensitive to interactions with other cultures. The nurse practitioner must be aware of bias and prejudice and must refrain from imposing his or her own beliefs on others. Cultural knowledge relates to the educational foundation that the nurse acquires. Cultural skill allows the nurse to assess a person's beliefs and practices without relying on written information or stereotyping about cultures. The cultural encounter is a further process whereby the nurse directly engages in cross-cultural inter-actions with clients of varied cultural backgrounds.

Two assessment tools that might be useful in providing a culturally sensitive structure for history-taking are the framework of Kleinman *et al.* (1978) and Leininger's (1978) transcultural framework.

Kleinman *et al.* (1978) developed a framework for cultural assessment and suggested that the following series of open-ended questions would be useful during the history-taking process:

- What do you think has caused your problem?
- Why do you think it started when it did?
- What do you think your sickness does to you?
- How severe is your sickness?
- What kind of treatment do you think you should receive?
- What are the most important results you hope to achieve from these treatments?
- What are the chief problems your sickness has caused?
- What do you fear most about your sickness?

Leininger (1978) developed a theory of trans-cultural care: one of her main underlying assumptions was that clients who show signs of cultural conflict, non-compliance, stresses and ethical or moral concerns need nursing care that is culturally based (Reynolds and Leininger 1993). The theory identifies nine domains to consider during cultural assessment:

1   Patterns of lifestyle
2   Specific cultural values and norms
3   Cultural taboos and myths
4   World view and ethnocentric tendencies
5   General features that the person thinks are different or similar to other cultures
6   Health and life care rituals and rites of passage to maintain health
7   Degree of cultural change
8   Caring behaviours
9   Folk and professional health–illness systems used

People of varying cultures are not only of varying ethnicity but also have differing sexual preferences, live in different parts of the country, are of varying gender type or are of different ages. Cultural sensitivity is essential in history-taking with all people. In the last 20 years there has been a cultural shift to more openness about lifestyles. Gay, lesbian, bisexual and transgender groups have become more outspoken, pointing out the heterosexual bias of society and health-care professionals. Morrisey (1996) points out that stereotyping or stigmatizing may interfere with care and, if nurses are to provide quality care, they must examine any homophobic feelings they may harbour.

It is important to demonstrate respect for people as unique individuals – culture is only one component that makes them who they are. Recognizing that there is diversity, being open to learn about different cultures and taking an open attitude without stereotyping is a beginning towards cultural competency. Nursing research has also turned to anthropology to explore culture. By studying culture we have to explain it in relation to ourselves and therefore gain insight into human life. Caring acts and rituals are found in all cultures and by appreciating culture we understand and appreciate ourselves better.

Alcohol and other recreational drug use

Alcoholism is a stigmatizing illness (Hennessey 1992) which causes a multitude of health problems for both men and women. An association exists between alcoholism and several obstetric and gynaecological problems such as infertility, sexual dysfunction, miscarriage and breast cancer and therefore women are particularly at risk of the detrimental effects of alcohol. Alcohol is part of the British culture – the 'pub' is a central place in many communities. Often people understate the amount they drink because they may feel judged as deviant or are embarrassed to admit to their full alcohol consumption. The person who has an alcohol problem often denies the amount consumed or may try to rationalize consumption by stating that last week was an exception. Despite these difficulties it is important to establish an average alcohol intake without judging or offending the patient. If alcohol-related questions are included in the main body of the history-taking process it can appear to be part of the routine interviewing and data collection that contribute to the whole health assessment, and therefore reduces the stigma associated with the question. Hennessey (1992) suggests that helpful qualities in the clinician include self-examination, self-acceptance, empathy, respect, honesty, support, warmth and genuineness. The clinician needs to be self-aware in order to be able to establish an alliance with patients, gain trust and help with their difficulties.

General screening questions include:

- Do you drink alcohol?
- How much do you drink?
- When was your last drink?
- What do you like to drink?

A valid screening tool is the CAGE framework. If the person answers yes to any of these questions it indicates that there is a problem (Mayfield *et al.* 1974):

- **Cutdown:**   ever felt the need to cut down ?
- **Annoyed:**   ever felt annoyed by criticism of your drinking?

- **Guilty:**   ever had guilty feelings about drinking?
- **Eye-opener:** ever felt the need for a morning drink (eye-opener)?

Following on from screening questions about alcohol it may be necessary to ask about the use of other recreational drugs or the possible misuse of prescription drugs. It is useful to integrate the questions into the routine history after a rapport has been established. Most experts recommend a non-judgemental approach, which means not apologizing for asking such questions, as an apology may imply that stigma or embarrassment is attached.

An example of an introductory question might be: 'I have asked you about smoking and drinking alcohol, now I would like to ask you if you use any recreational drugs.' If the person says 'no', it is worth following up by asking if he or she has ever used drugs in the past. Depending on the response, other questions may include:

- What is your drug of choice and how often do you use it?
- Have you had any bad reactions?
- Have you ever got into trouble or had family problems because of your use?
- Ever tried to quit?

More detailed history for alcohol or substance abuse

1 Normal use or pattern
2 Date and time of last drink (or drug use)
3 Substances used (type of alcohol or drug)
4 Quantity
5 Past history of blackouts, tremors, hallucinations
6 Past history of abstinence
7 Normal pattern of eating
8 Legal problems
9 Family problems
10 Occupational problems
11 Family history of alcoholism
12 Other drugs/medications used

Sexual problems

A sexual history provides the nurse with information about the person's lifestyle and may highlight areas of need for risk assessment. We live surrounded by sexual messages in our music, literature, films and television. Nudity and titillating articles appear daily in the tabloid press and yet many nurses find it difficult to ask questions about sexual issues. Although part of a holistic assessment, it is usually an area which is left to another time – which never comes.

There are many barriers to taking a sexual history. The nurse practitioner can feel that it is none of his/her business, that the patient did not want to talk about it or that you may be protecting the patient in some way by not addressing the subject. These are often excuses, however, which only serve to cover up personal discomfort with this subject. It is important to recognize whether it is your own discomfort rather than the patient's that is preventing you from asking questions. Looking at your own feelings, attitudes and values about sexuality may help to identify any personal defences that stand in the way of making a thorough assessment.

It is useful to start with a general question that sets up a safe, comfortable environment for the patient. Your choice of question depends on your personal style and the context of the situation, but the following are a selection that might be useful:

- Many of the people who come to this clinic have concerns about sexual health. Is there anything you would like to ask?
- People with your symptoms (illness) often experience other problems, sometimes in the area of sexual functioning. How has this affected your life?
- Many people around this time have questions about sexual activity. Do you have any concerns?

If the patient has concerns you may want to use more focused questions. Often people talk about the genitalia or sexual issues using euphemisms which are intentionally vague to avoid embarrassment. It is important for the interviewer to gain an accurate understanding and therefore it is useful to ask specific questions to clarify the situation.

Many people are eager to ask questions once the subject of sexual health has been introduced. By introducing the subject in a non-judgemental way you let the patient know it is permissible to discuss this subject with you. This may also enable the patient to return to the issue at a later time.

Domestic violence

Health professionals are not very good at asking questions about this topic. Domestic violence is so prevalent, however, that it is now being viewed as a public health issue. A strategy to deal with the problem effectively should include health professionals and should be a multidisciplinary approach. The nurse practitioner needs to be familiar with community resources in order that she or he may refer appropriately.

Often health professionals have difficulties dealing with patients who suffer domestic violence and either ignore symptoms or label the person 'difficult'. When a woman continues to stay in a violent situation, health professionals may get frustrated and feel that intervention is futile. The patient may be caught in an emotional double-bind with little control over her life. Choosing to leave the environment with which she is familiar but which may contain the only support she knows is a difficult decision. Empowering a woman to make such major changes can take a long time. It is still worth trying to get the real story and obtain any information that may help an intervention rather than ignoring the issue. A useful way in might be: 'Many patients have told me they have been hurt or abused at home. How is it at home for you?' Domestic violence includes child abuse. You may therefore include a question such as: 'Most parents get upset when their baby cries a lot. What do you do when your baby won't stop crying?' or, more directly, 'Are you afraid you might hurt your child?'

Record-keeping

The problem-oriented record is one of the commonest ways of recording medical information. The initial collection of data should be made as significant and complete as possible. The only limitations should be the discomfort and expense to the patient. The reason for discussing this in a history-taking chapter is that the processes of obtaining and recording data are intrinsically linked and often force us to gather our information in a problem-oriented way. For the nurse practitioner it is important to create a format that allows a health-oriented approach. One frequently used format for recording notes in the medical record is SOAPIER (Eggland and Heinemann 1994). The acronym SOAPIER stands for subjective data, objective data, assessment, planning, intervention, evaluation and review. This has been shortened to SOAP, SOAPIE or even PIE (problem, intervention and evaluation). The method chosen will depend on the norms of the nurse practitioner's area of practice. It is essential that the notes allow health-care professionals to communicate effectively with each other.

Closure of history-taking and transition to physical examination

During the history-taking process, it helps the patient if you can give him or her a sense of structure by summarizing at the end of each section or using a simple phrase to indicate you are moving to another section. For example, 'I've asked you about your past history, now I'd like to ask about your family history.' At the end of the interview you should offer a simple summary of the main points to make absolutely sure that the patient is in agreement with your perception of the story. Always conclude by asking: 'Is there anything more that you would like

to add?' You are now ready to move to the examination.

In practice, clinicians will often ask questions as they perform an examination. However, once the physical examination starts, the clinician is in a more directing position and the patient may feel vulnerable and therefore wary about answering sensitive questions fully. This has obvious implications for the type of questions asked. For the beginner it is also essential to separate history-taking from physical examination as it is easy for the inexperienced to get muddled and lose a sense of order.

History-taking is an important skill and is often the key to diagnosis. Keeping a logical order can help the nurse practitioner cover a lot of ground and discover extensive information. The art is to be thorough without being too interrogative and to listen to patients' responses and encourage them with verbal and non-verbal signals to tell their story.

Nurse practitioners struggling to master the art of asking difficult questions can take heed from studies in doctor–patient communication. Simpson et al. (1991) reviewed the literature and found communication problems were common: most patient complaints could be linked with poor communication. The skills needed in an interview were identified as data-gathering, forming and maintaining relationships and being able to deal with difficult issues such as sexual history-taking or breaking bad news. These are skills that can be learned but need continual development. Reflection on practice, peer review and continuing education are important to develop the art of questioning so that history-taking is appropriate and relevant to culture and context.

References

Benner P., Wrubel J. (1989) *The Primacy of Caring*, California, Addison Wesley.

Burnard P. (1992) *Know Yourself! Self Awareness Activities for Nurses*, London, Scutari Press.

Campinha-Bacote J. (1994) Cultural competence in psychiatric mental health nursing: a conceptual model, *Nursing Clinics of North America*, **29**(1), pp. 1–9.

DeGowin, E. (1987) DeGowin & DeGrowin's *Bedside Diagnostic Examination*, 5th edn., New York, Macmillan.

Eggland E.T., Heinemann D.S. (1994) *Nursing Documentation: Charting Recording and Reporting*, Philadelphia, JB Lippincott.

Hennessey M.B. (1992) Identifying the woman with alcohol problems, *Nursing Clinics of North America*, **27**(4), pp. 917–924.

Kleinman A., Eisenburg L., Good B. (1978) *Culture illness and care*, Annals of Internal Medicine, **88**(251). Cited in: Campinha-Bacote J. (1994) Cultural competence in psychiatric mental health nursing: a conceptual model, *Nursing Clinics of North America*, **29**(1), pp. 1–9.

Leininger M. (1978) *Transcultural Nursing: Concepts, Theories and Practices*, New York, John Wiley.

Mayfield D., McLead G., Hall P. (1974) The CAGE questionnaire, *American Journal of Psychiatry* **131**(1121).

McCaffery M., Beebe A., Latham J. (eds). (1994) *Pain Clinical Manual for Nursing Practice* London, Mosby.

Meleis A. (1996) Culturally competent scholarship: substance and rigor, *Advances in Nursing Science,* **19**(2) pp. 1–16.

Morrisey M. (1996) Attitudes of practitioners to lesbian, gay and bisexual clients, *British Journal of Nursing*, **5**(16), pp. 980–982.

Morton P. G. (1993) *Health Assessment in Nursing*, 2nd edn., Philadelphia, FA Davis.

Nightingale F. (1859) *Notes on Nursing,* London, Harrison.

Neighbour R. (1987). *The Inner Consultation*, Lancaster, MTP Press.

Pendleton P., Schofield T., Tate P., Havelock P. (1987) *The Consultation: An Approach to Learning and Teaching*, Oxford, Medical Publications.

Reynolds C., Leininger M. (1993) *Madeleine Leininger: Cultural Care, Diversity and Universality Theory*, London, Sage.

Simpson M., Buckman R., Stewart M., *et al.* (1991) Doctor patient communication: the Toronto consensus statement, *British Medical Journal*, **303**(6814), November 1991, pp. 1385–1387.

Suzuki S. (1986) *Zen Mind, Beginner's Mind*, New York, John Weatherhill.

CHAPTER 3

Disorders of the skin

Mike Walsh

Introduction

Dermatological conditions account for a substantial proportion of the primary health care nurse practitioner's work, many systemic diseases also produce significant alterations in the skin and its appearance. No consideration of the skin would be complete without adding to these two groups of patients those who have suffered traumatic wounds. The external nature of the skin means that any lesion or disorder is more readily apparent to the individual than a problem affecting many of the internal organs. The effect on the patient's perception of his or her appearance may also be profound. The nurse practitioner is therefore likely to see many patients whose presenting condition will involve a skin disorder of one sort or another. This chapter will cover the more common presenting conditions but the nurse practitioner wishing to know more, particularly about the rarer conditions, should consult a dermatology textbook.

Pathophysiology

Definitions of frequently used terms

The following terms are frequently used in describing skin disorders, therefore some simple definitions will be given here to avoid confusion.

- Macule: a small, flat, clearly delineated area of altered colour such as a freckle or spot
- Papule: a small elevated and therefore palpable solid mass up to 5 mm across
- Nodule: as for a papule but greater than 5 mm across
- Vesicle: a superficial, fluid-filled elevation of the skin. The cavity is filled with serous fluid but less than 5 mm across, e.g. lesions of herpes simplex
- Bulla: a vesicle but greater than 5 mm across, e.g. a burn blister
- Pustule: similar to a vesicle but filled with pus, e.g. acne.

Figure 3.1 shows a cross-section through normal skin.

Common conditions primarily affecting the skin

Inflammatory disorders

Eczema refers to a pattern of inflammatory skin reaction which may be caused by outside (exogenous) or internal (endogenous) agents. In some individuals both factors may be present, producing a mixed picture. The term dermatitis is synonymous with eczema (Graham-Brown and Burns 1996) and it can be used to indicate any inflammation of the skin. Although there are different forms of eczema, all involve both the dermis and epidermis and feature the formation of vesicles; the patient experiences dry, itchy, scaling skin. Eczema may be either acute or chronic and may spread from the site of the initial appearance.

Outside agents may have a chronic irritant effect upon the skin and eczema develops as a result of an accumulation of exposure (e.g. a trainee hairdresser exposed to large quantities of shampoo) or as a result of exposure to a substance leading to an immediate irritant or allergic reaction (e.g. nickel or certain plants such as primulas). This latter situation is called contact dermatitis as the rash occurs at the point of contact.

Atopic eczema is a common example of endogenous eczema and frequently affects children. There is a genetic predisposition towards developing eczema but other environmental and emotional influences are involved. The disorder often appears before the age of 2 and, while initially it may be generalized, subsequently tends most frequently to affect skin around joints such as the wrists, elbows and knees. Itching leads to the child scratching, which exacerbates the formation of skin lesions (erythema, vesicles and crusts) and therefore leads to more itching (Singleton 1997). Other forms of eczema are known but poorly understood, such as stasis eczema associated with varicose veins and seborrhoeic

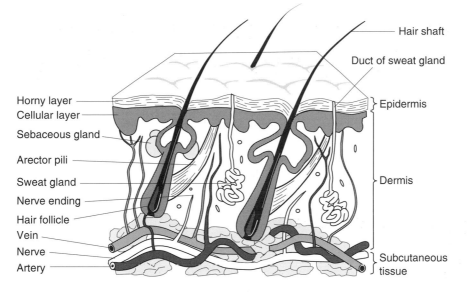

Figure 3.1   A cross-section of dermis and epidermis

eczema which may affect the scalp and face of infants in the first few months of life or the scalp, face and upper torso of adults.

Psoriasis is one of the commonest inflammatory skin disorders which usually presents as patches of red scaly plaque which, if removed, may expose bleeding tissue. The scalp, knees and elbows are common sites but anywhere on the body may be affected. The condition is not usually itchy. The cause is unknown but a genetic predisposition is suspected in many cases and trigger factors include trauma and infection.

Acne is a common and distressing problem, particularly amongst adolescents. Although in most people the problem resolves over a 2–3-year period, it may persist into adult life in a small number of cases. The number of spots varies over time but is often worse at stressful periods. Although the face, neck and upper trunk are most affected, other parts of the body may be involved. The person first becomes aware that the skin and scalp have become more greasy (due to increased secretion of sebum) before spots erupt. The nurse practitioner will usually notice that the spots are at different stages of development. The so-called blackhead is a blocked hair follicle and these lesions are characteristic of acne. Other lesions are found, such as papules and pustules, and scarring may also be present. The psychological distress caused by acne to adolescents when they are at such a vulnerable stage in their development cannot be overemphasized.

Acne is sometimes confused with rosacea, which is a chronic, inflammatory, cutaneous vascular disorder of unknown origin. Although men may be affected, this condition most commonly affects women, typically around the menopause, and produces a picture of facial flushing, erythema, oedema, telangiectasia (fine irregular red lines due to capillary dilatation), papules and pustules (Chalmers 1997). The central part of the face is most affected, from the chin up to the forehead. In men, the nose is affected and becomes large, bulbous and puffy with connective tissue hypertrophy. This is known as rhinophyma and Chalmers (1997) points out that the familiar face of the great early Hollywood star, W.C. Fields, was a classic example of this condition!

Skin cancer

Although malignant lesions of the skin are much less common than non-malignant ones, they are potentially serious and are best classified as melanoma and non-melanoma skin cancer (Schofield and Kneebone 1996). The key difference is that melanoma is much more aggressive and more likely to metastasize rapidly if not treated promptly, although it occurs far less frequently than other forms of skin cancer. The ultraviolet component of sunlight is implicated as the major causative factor in skin cancer and people of Celtic origin with skin that burns easily are most at risk.

Schofield and Kneebone (1996) estimate that although the incidence of melanoma has doubled in the last 10 years, the average general practice will see only one case every 10 years. Melanoma tends to affect younger adults and is commonly found on the legs in women and trunk in men, particularly in those whose skin type predisposes them to burn rather than tan in the sun, such as red-haired individuals or those of Celtic descent. The common presentation is the appearance of a new mole or an existing mole that has recently changed in appearance. It can present in elderly people on the face in a premalignant form known as a lentigo maligna. This is a darkened flat area of tissue that may have been present for many years before beginning to change, indicating malignancy (Taylor and Roberts 1997). Examination reveals a superficial, pigmented and spreading lesion more than 7 mm across. The prognosis is good if detected promptly and if the lesion is excised while less than 1.5 mm thick, but poor if detected late.

The principal non-melanoma skin cancers are basal cell carcinoma (rodent ulcer) and squamous cell carcinoma (epithelioma). Rodent ulcers are by far the most common of the skin cancers and, although they do not usually metastasize, they can be very invasive. They occur most commonly in older people on those parts of the head and neck most exposed to the sun. They may be nodular or pigmented in appearance. Squamous cell carcinoma also affects mostly older people and involves sun-damaged skin. Unlike a rodent ulcer, it may metastasize and may also arise from an existing diseased area of skin. The initial appearance may be a nodule or plaque but it usually progresses to a non-healing, irregular ulcer.

There are some other skin lesions which may be described as premalignant. Bowen's disease will progress to epithelioma and others, such as solar keratoses (red scaly patches which come and go over time), also have the potential to become malignant. Prolonged exposure to the sun in fair-skinned people of advanced years is a common feature of solar keratoses.

Infectious diseases

The varicella-zoster virus causes both chickenpox and herpes zoster (shingles). Shingles occurs most frequently in those over 50 and is thought to be due to the virus being reactivated after lying dormant for many years after an earlier attack of chickenpox (Reifsneider 1997). Pain or a burning sensation may precede the appearance of any lesions by 3–5 days and is localized to a single dermatome. Tissue is erythematous – a group of vesicles marks the affected area. The skin lesions clear after approximately 2 weeks but may leave some scarring. Pain may persist after the attack has resolved.

Herpes simplex type II (genital herpes) is considered in more detail in Chapter 10. Type I virus produces itchy, uncomfortable cold sores commonly affecting the lips. This may be a recurrent pheno-menon as groups of vesicles coalesce, burst and resolve in 2 weeks or so. Attacks may be brought on by fever or exposure to strong sunlight.

Warts are benign lesions which are viral in origin. The human papillomavirus (HPV) group is usually the culprit: different strains produce different types of wart. The term verruca refers to a wart on the sole of the foot. Warts are not usually painful; this distinguishes them from a whitlow, which is a painful lesion on the finger produced by the herpes simplex virus. Although warts are usually self-limiting with no long-term consequences for health, warts in the genital area have been linked to cancers affecting the genitalia of both sexes (Graham-Brown and Burns 1996).

Individuals working in agriculture are prone to contract orf, a viral disease which normally affects sheep and goats but which can be transmitted to humans, usually producing a single lesion on a finger. This develops into a domed haemorrhagic pustule which may rupture, leaving a nodular ulcer which will usually resolve within 2 months.

Infection of the skin with *Streptococcus pyogenes*, usually after a small wound, can lead to cellulitis. This is most common in the lower limb, especially in oedematous tissue, and the elderly are most at risk. This is often associated with leg ulcers. The tissue is red, feels hot and appears swollen. Tissue necrosis may occur along with systemic effects such as pyrexia, generally feeling unwell and even a confusional state in older patients.

Localized staphylococcal infections give rise to furunculosis or boils. Usually a hair follicle becomes infected. The boil matures and then discharges its central contents. A group of adjacent hair follicles may become infected, giving rise to a rounded lesion, typically on the neck, known as a carbuncle. This ruptures and discharges pus after a few days, similar to a single boil.

Fungal infections of the skin, such as tinea pedis or athlete's foot, are common. Itchiness gives way to soreness as skin in the toe webs becomes scaly and broken. Athlete's foot is usually contracted as a result of cross-infection in areas such as swimming pools and sports changing rooms. Tinea pedis is an example of a type of fungus known as a dermato-phyte, and different varieties affect other areas of the body. It is perhaps best to use the general term ringworm to label these infections, followed by the area of the body involved (Graham-Brown and Burns 1996), rather than enter into the complicated nomen-clature of the dermatologist. Common presentation is as an erythematous spreading margin with the central area becoming clear, although toe and fingernails may be involved.

Candidiasis (thrush) is caused by infection of the skin and mucous membranes by *Candida albicans*. This yeast fungus normally occurs in the gastro-intestinal tract and vagina without causing disease. If there is a change in the local environment, however, such as reduced resistance in immunocompromised individuals (for example, those with diabetes), it can become invasive and cause disease. Other trigger factors include antibiotic therapy and endocrine disorders such as diabetes. Common sites for disease include the mouth, vagina, beneath the breasts and in the groin, while balanitis may develop in the uncircumcized male. Persistent oral infections may be the first sign of AIDS. Intertrigo describes the occurrence of macerated skin, possibly colonized by *Candida*, where two skin surfaces meet, such as under the breasts.

The skin is also vulnerable to attack from parasitic organisms. The mite *Sarcoptes scabiei* gives rise to scabies, which is passed from one person to another through close physical contact. Children and young adults are most at risk, as the female mite burrows into the skin to lay her eggs, giving rise to itchiness and small linear skin lesions. Itchiness is also associated with head lice, which are frequently a problem in schools as the wingless insects can only be transmitted by direct hair-to-hair contact. Head lice feed on blood in the scalp and lay their eggs at the base of the hairs. Nits are the empty egg cases and are most frequently found in the occipital region of the scalp and above the ears. Body lice are usually associated with a person wearing the same clothes for prolonged periods of time as they only move on to the body to feed. They are most likely to be found on vagrants and rough sleepers who live in one set of clothes. Despite common belief, crabs or pubic lice are not contracted from toilet seats. They are transmitted by direct physical contact and may live in hair other than the pubic region, such as the axilla or beard. Itchiness is usually the symptom that makes the infected person aware of the problem and the lice are clearly visible to the naked eye on inspection.

Systemic disease and the skin

Systemic diseases may produce significant changes in the skin. It is therefore worth briefly summarizing some of the main diseases which produce signs that the nurse practitioner may find when examining the patient's skin.

Infectious diseases of childhood

Measles has an incubation period of 7–14 days, followed by a prodromal period of 2–4 days when the patient is most infectious. This is accompanied by the appearance of symptoms such as a cough, runny nose, loss of appetite and pyrexia. Measles is accompanied by a characteristic rash consisting of pink macules which first appear behind the ears, before spreading over the face to the trunk and limbs. The rash consists of irregular spots which may join together to form larger, dark red areas on the trunk and limbs. The classical picture of measles is completed by the finding of Koplik's spots, which are very small bluish-white spots on the buccal mucosa towards the end of the prodrome period.

Rubella produces a characteristic rash consisting of separate pink macules which appear on the face and trunk, lasting for only 1–3 days. Adults tend to have been unwell for several days before the rash appears, whereas children are much less affected.

Chickenpox occurs most often in winter and usually affects children under the age of 10. Unlike measles, the rash may be the first sign that something is wrong, as prodromal symptoms often do not occur in children, although adults are usually unwell for 2–3 days before the characteristic rash appears. The rash usually starts on the scalp and as it spreads tends to be more concentrated on the trunk; spots appear in waves over several days. The rash consists initially of small superficial macules which progress through a papular phase before becoming vesico-pustular. The itchy nature of the rash leads to scratching, the formation of scabs and subsequently scars as the scabs drop off.

Parents of young children with a rash may be concerned about the risk of meningitis. Young children who develop acute meningococcal meningitis due to infection with *Neisseria meningitidis* may become seriously ill in a matter of hours with septicaemia, septic shock and disseminated intravascular coagulation in addition to the other signs of meningitis. The condition is associated with the rapid appearance of a petechial or purpuric rash due to disorder of the normal clotting mechanism.

Endocrine disorders

The increased risk of *Candida* infections in patients with diabetes has already been referred to. Amongst other effects are the formation of neuropathic ulcers on the soles of the feet and the development of fat hypertrophy at frequently used injection sites.

Hypothyroidism produces characteristic changes in the skin: it becomes thickened, dry and may take on a yellowish tinge due to the deposition of carotenes. Swelling may develop around the eyes while the hair becomes thinner and more brittle. Excess thyroid activity leads to warm moist skin and redness of the palms as well as rare conditions such as thyroid acropachy – a form of finger clubbing.

Other diseases which affect the skin include Cushing's syndrome (thinning of the skin, purple striae on the trunk, hair loss and easy bruising) and Addison's disease (hyperpigmentation).

Trauma

Wounds

Although various wound classification systems have been developed, the most practical approach is probably to classify wounds according to the characteristics that relate directly to their treatment. The following points are therefore important:

- The age of the wound – this determines the method of closure and the risk of infection

- Whether there has been any tissue loss, as this also affects wound closure
- The presence of contamination and/or devitalized tissue—this increases the risk of infection and can delay healing. Infection with *Clostridium tetani* is particularly of concern. This anaerobic organism, whose activity is encouraged by the presence of devitalized tissue in the wound, can have a devastating impact. The neurotoxin it produces —tetanospasmin—blocks the sympathetic nervous system and the normal inhibition of motor reflexes, leading to severe muscle spasm and disruption of the autonomic nervous system. The results are potentially fatal, despite all the resources of modern intensive care
- The risk of damage, to other structures, ranging from superficial nerves and tendons to internal organs such as the spleen or bowel in deep penetrating wounds.

Burns

Damage to the respiratory system and the possible toxic effects of the inhalation of smoke and fumes represent the most immediate threat to life in victims of a fire. Oedema and swelling may obstruct the airway, while most household furnishings are capable of releasing a lethal cocktail of toxic fumes when burnt. Carbon monoxide poisoning and the development of pulmonary oedema are other possible and rapidly fatal outcomes.

Burn injuries from whatever cause remove the normal protective outer layer of skin, exposing the individual to risk of infection. The depth of the burn injury is extremely important as this determines the possibility of regrowth of normal dermis and epidermis (Figure 3.2). A superficial burn involves only the surface epithelium (e.g. sunburn). Blisters are rare and the tissue is erythematous. If deeper layers of the epidermis are involved, this is known as a superficial partial-thickness burn. Localized fluid loss from damaged capillaries and the consequent formation of blisters occur in partial thickness burns. Healing occurs by regeneration of new epidermis from surviving tissue. A deeper partial-thickness burn which has destroyed the epidermis and part of the dermis, leaving only islands of epidermis deep within hair follicles and glands, will take considerably longer to heal (3–4 weeks) as new epidermis has to be generated from these surviving fragments. The quality of the new skin will be much poorer than the original. All these types of burn injury are extremely painful and often accompanied by a great deal of psychological distress, as the person fears being scarred for life.

A full-thickness burn which reaches down to the underlying fat and muscle will only heal very slowly after the formation of much granulation tissue and

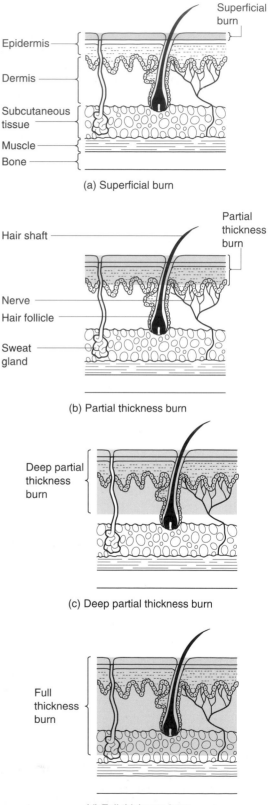

(a) Superficial burn

(b) Partial thickness burn

(c) Deep partial thickness burn

(d) Full thickness burn

Figure 3.2   The depth of burn injuries from (a) superficial to (d) full-thickness

consequent scarring. Blistering and oedema are common but the burn is characterized by leathery devitalized tissue which may be slate-grey or black in colour. This tough, leathery eschar tissue formed at the time of the injury is inelastic and may create a tourniquet around the limb (or even chest) in the case of circumferential burns, leading to gangrene. A full-thickness burn also destroys nerve endings and, although the most severe form of burn, may be less painful than a more partial-thickness or superficial burn, where the nerve endings survive. The picture is usually complicated as the patient often presents with a mixture of full- and partial-thickness burns. Surgical intervention and grafting is the only solution for such a deep burn.

The fluid loss from damaged tissue can rapidly cause hypovolaemic shock, which is exacerbated by the effects of pain and toxin release in burns of larger areas. The composition of the burn fluid closely resembles that of plasma. Shock is likely in 10% surface area burns in children and 15% in adults (Bosworth 1997). In calculating burn area it is important to exclude superficial erythema as tissue fluid loss is negligible from these areas.

Taking a focused history

Skin disorders and wounds have a striking visual appearance which invites immediate examination. The principle of obtaining a history before examination still applies however.

The normal pattern of starting with the patient's own version of the problem should be followed. The PQRST symptom analysis is then useful as a basis for questions.

- *Provocation/palliation*: key questions relate to the possible cause of the skin problem, such as exposure to drugs, chemical agents or close contact with others. Contact with new materials may explain contact dermatitis, while extensive sun exposure over a period of years alerts the nurse practitioner to the risk of skin cancer. The nurse practitioner should also ask if anything improves the condition.
- *Quality*: the patient should be asked to describe the appearance of the skin or lesions. An accurate description of the sensations associated with the rash or lesion is essential, particularly whether it is itchy, painful, irritable or causes discomfort. Any history of bleeding, discharge or odour should also be noted.
- *Region*: it is important that the patient describes all affected regions of the body, not just the obvious currently visible areas.
- *Severity*: the impact of the disorder on the patient's everyday life should be ascertained, as this may be profound. An adolescent with acne may be

distressed at his/her physical appearance, whilst an adult who presents with a new or changed mole (naevi) may be seriously worried about skin cancer.
- *Time*: the time interval between the onset of the condition and presentation should be determined, together with any variation in appearance and sensation that has occurred over time.

The past medical history should then be checked. Key areas include previous skin disorders, known allergies, tolerance of sunlight and the presence of any systemic disorders such as diabetes or cardiovascular disease. Any other general symptoms which may be relevant should be enquired about, such as stress, fever, tiredness or general malaise.

Relevant family history should be explored, especially focusing on similar conditions and any known family history of allergy. The personal and social history is equally important; occupational or recreational exposure may provide clues to the possible disorder. The person's skin care habits should also be explored tactfully so as not to give offence. It may be important to know how frequently the person washes or shampoos, what cleansing agents and cosmetics are used and how much exposure there has been to sunlight or artificial tanning.

A detailed history is also essential if the patient presents with a wound. The exact mechanism of injury needs to be ascertained as well as the time since the accident. The nurse practitioner should enquire whether there are any other injuries apart from the obvious wound. The patient's tetanus immunization status should be determined in all cases of wounding, including burns. Relevant medical information such as known allergies (e.g. penicillin, plasters) and general health (e.g. diabetes, cardiovascular disorder) should be ascertained as this will affect treatment and healing. Social factors should be explored to determine whether the patient can continue work or how well he or she will cope at home after discharge. This is particularly important when dealing with wounds affecting the hand where an occlusive dressing may need to be kept *in situ*, clean and dry, for several days.

In cases of burn injury it is essential to find out what caused the injury. Electrical burns may cause severe deep injuries which are not immediately apparent. Burns are sometimes associated with child abuse and neglect. The history of children who present with burns should therefore be carefully checked against the injuries for consistency. The first-aid steps taken at the time should be determined as these may be helpful or harmful. Application of cold water in moderation relieves pain and limits the extent of the injury but over-enthusiastic use of cold water can lead to hypothermia, especially in children. The risk of inhalation injury should be checked.

Physical examination

A warm, well-lit but private environment is necessary for a good examination. The patient should be undressed as appropriate and any cosmetics removed. A hand lens may be helpful for detailed examination of lesions. Findings may be best recorded using predrawn blank outlines of the body.

The distribution of a skin disorder over the body is a crucial element in its correct diagnosis, so a general inspection should precede detailed examination of individual lesions. For example, if a disorder is related to sunlight, its distribution on exposed parts of the body will be apparent, while lesions distributed along a specific dermatome make the diagnosis of herpes zoster straightforward. An eruption confined to the flexor surfaces of joints such as the wrist, elbow and knee is characteristic of atopic eczema (p. 24). A generalized or symmetrical distribution usually indicates a systemic or constitutional disorder whereas fungal, bacterial or viral infections normally have a focus from which spreading may have occurred (Munro and Edwards 1995). The arrangement of lesions within a rash should also be noted. As skin disorders change and evolve over time, it may be necessary to re-examine the patient at a later date to help confirm the diagnosis and assess the impact on the patient.

A careful examination of individual lesions should follow the general overview. The terms used on p. 24 should be used when describing findings. It is also essential to note the colour, size and shape of lesions together with the nature of their margins. A useful prompt to help record the details of a lesion is to think of ABCD: A, asymmetry; B, border; C, colour; D, diameter (Young 1997).

If the patient presents with a pronounced swelling it is essential to document its position, shape and size exactly. This should be measured with a ruler as changes need to be recorded accurately. The colour and warmth of the lesion are important pointers: if it is inflammatory in origin then increased warmth and redness are to be expected, as well as pain and tenderness. Whether the lesion is mobile or fixed to underlying structures should be determined. This latter finding suggests a tumour, especially when seen in association with the familiar *peau d'orange* skin of breast cancer. The swelling should be palpated to see how hard it is or whether it is fluctuant, which would indicate a fluid-filled cyst or abscess. Palpation will also reveal whether any pulse is present within the swelling.

The patient's history (reporting pain or swelling) may indicate that the swelling is located over a lymph gland. It is therefore necessary to examine the lymph glands by palpation to check for lymphadenopathy (Figure 3.3). This may also be necessary with a range of other conditions. Lymphadenopathy can be either generalized or localized and the cause is most likely to be infective or due to malignant disease. It may

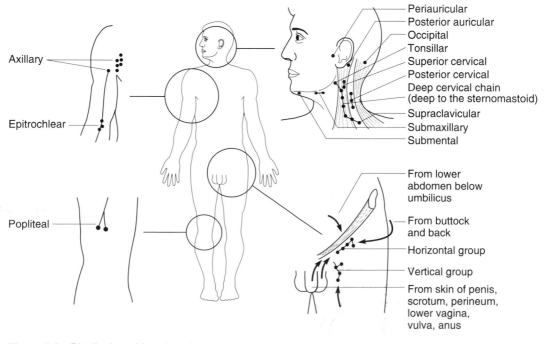

Figure 3.3   Distribution of lymph nodes

be necessary to examine the abdomen to assess the size of the liver and spleen (p. 133) while observing carefully for any evidence of clotting disorders. Examination of the glands should be assessing consistency (in Hodgkin's disease they are said to feel rubbery), tenderness (acute bacterial infection usually produces tenderness) and mobility (fixation is associated with malignant disease).

Lymph glands should always be compared immediately with the same glands on the opposite side of the body. The cervical and axillary glands should be checked with the patient sitting (Figures 3.4 and 3.5). The nurse practitioner should face the patient while examining the occipital, posterior cervical and axillary nodes but be behind the patient to examine the other cervical nodes. The abdominal, inguinal and popliteal glands should be examined with the patient lying down.

Examination of a wound should focus on the key points mentioned on p. 28 – the first point must be to check whether bleeding has actually stopped. It is necessary to clean the wound carefully before examination so that all relevant structures are visible. Universal precautions should be observed at all times due to the risk of contracting a blood-borne disease. The possibility of skin closure should be assessed in the light of any skin loss which has occurred, the site of the wound and the general condition of the patient's skin. This is particularly true in elderly patients. Evidence of contamination and devitalized tissue should be noted together with any signs of other structures such as tendons being involved. The exact site, size and shape of the wound should be recorded, using a predrawn chart if possible.

It is important not to focus only on the obvious wound, as there may be other injuries, such as a

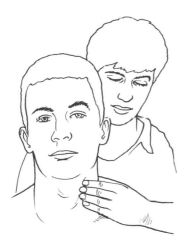

(a) Examine the glands of the anterior triangle from behind using one hand at a time

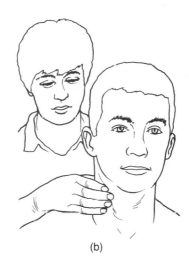

(b)

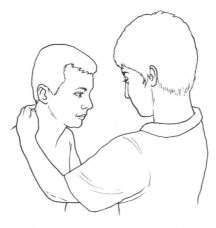

(c) Examine the posterior glands from the front

Figure 3.4   Techniques for palpation of lymph nodes

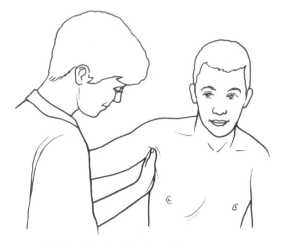

(a) Examine the glands on the right side

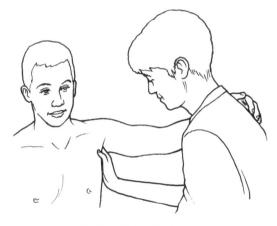

(b) Then the left side

Figure 3.5   Palpation of the axillary glands

fracture, which require examination. A small puncture wound caused by a section of bone may be the only external evidence of an open fracture. A thorough examination is especially needed for assault and more seriously injured victims as well as individuals who are drunk. In cases where the patient is brought in lying down a potentially serious error is to fail to examine the patient's back, which may show evidence of a serious penetrating wound or severe blunt trauma such as tyre marks. The amount of internal damage done by a stabbing or gunshot may bear no resemblance to the size of the wound, which may be very small. The energy and track of the penetrating object are the key determinants. The victim's clothing is potential forensic evidence in such cases and should be stored safely after removal. In serious wounding cases the patient's vital signs should be recorded as a baseline measure and repeated as necessary.

Burn victims should be immediately assessed to ensure there is no evidence of airway involvement,

as oedema affecting the airway can lead to rapid death, whilst the effects of inhaled hot gases and toxic fumes can be equally lethal. External burns should be fully assessed to determine the area and depth of burn and the amount of pain the patient is experiencing. Predrawn charts of the body are invaluable for sketching the extent of the burn, although erythema should be excluded. For a rapid assessment of area, Wallace's rule of 9 may be used (Figure 3.6), to which may be added the fact that the patient's own hand is approximately 1% of his or her own surface area. Vital sign monitoring is essential if the burn is over 10%, because of the risk of shock. Depth of burn should be estimated using the criteria mentioned on p. 28, remembering that a full-thickness burn is characterized by a loss of sensation caused by destruction of the nerve endings. Circumferential full-thickness burns are particularly significant—gangrene may develop rapidly because of the tourniquet effect. Pain levels should be continuously monitored, not only to assess the initial level but also to check the effectiveness of whatever pain relief is given.

The long-term management of burns and other wounds can be greatly assisted by careful documentation and a structured methodological approach. Polaroid photography offers an accurate way of recording findings both initially and at follow-up. Various wound assessment tools have been advocated but, as Lait and Smith (1998) note, none

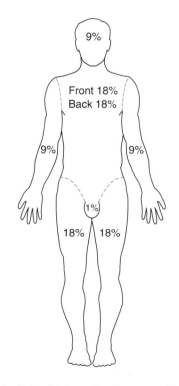

Figure 3.6   Rule of 9 for estimating area of burn

has been subjected to rigorous evaluation. Measurement with a ruler or simply tracing the outline on to an occlusive dressing is probably as good as any other method. Healing should be monitored by assessments carried out as frequently as necessary; there is no fixed time scale concerning frequency. When examining a wound the nurse practitioner needs to remember the history given by the patient to check whether the findings match the story. This is particularly true in the case of children because of the risk of abuse. Cases of violence may become the subject of police enquiry and the nurse practitioner may be required to give evidence in a court of law. Bear this in mind when carrying out an examination and documenting findings.

Investigations

The principal investigation undertaken by the nurse practitioner will consist of taking a swab from a wound or lesion suspected of being infected. All wounds will contain some bacteria; it is the presence of pathogenic organisms that is significant. The aim of taking a swab is to identify the causative organism and to determine its sensitivity to antibiotics. This requires using a sterile swab and avoiding contamination with ordinary skin flora. The swab should be carefully labelled and sent to the laboratory within 24 hours, using a transport medium where appropriate.

Dermatological clinics use a range of other techniques, such as microscopic examination of scrapings from the skin or of nails and hairs, and skin biopsy is an important investigation. These lie outside the scope of the nurse practitioner.

Treatment

Eczema

Where contact dermatitis seems a likely diagnosis the patient should be advised to avoid all contact with the suspected material. Topical steroids are a major part of the treatment of eczema, as they are for other skin disorders such as psoriasis, although they should never be used for an infective condition. The nurse practitioner should be aware that topical steroids come in different strengths and have a range of side-effects. The more severe the disorder, the stronger the steroid that may be used, ranging from mild preparations such as 1% hydrocortisone through moderately potent agents such as flurandrenolone (Haelan), potent agents such as betamethasone valerate (Betnovate) and the most potent of all, including clobetasol propionate (Dermovate).

Topical steroids produce local side-effects in proportion to the strength of the preparation used. Thinning of the skin (atrophy) is a potential problem whilst inappropriate use on the face for acne leads to periorbital dermatitis. The area around the mouth and chin becomes erythematous and erupts in papules and pustules. Application of potent steroids should be stopped and replaced with a mild topical steroid and oxytetracycline should be prescribed – initially 500 mg twice daily, reducing over a period of several weeks.

Children with atopic eczema benefit from the use of emollients to reduce the problem of dry skin. If itching is a problem an antihistamine is needed. Bathtime is a good opportunity to apply antihistamines (the temperature of the bath water should be carefully monitored to ensure it is not too hot) and a topical steroid will also be helpful. If there is a secondary infection it should be treated with antibiotics such as flucloxacillin. Replacing cow's milk with a soya preparation in the child's diet has been suggested but Graham-Brown and Burns (1996) are doubtful about the efficacy of such a step.

Seborrhoeic eczema (cradle cap) in infants is best managed initially by daily shampooing for a week. This will remove the dry scales. If this fails to improve the condition, apply an emollient such as olive oil which will soak and soften the crust, allowing later removal with shampoo. Careful education of the parents is essential to help them manage the condition (Singleton 1997). In adults, troublesome seborrhoeic eczema should be treated with a mild topical steroid and/or a topical antifungal agent such as ketoconazole cream, due to the risk of pityrosporum infection.

Psoriasis

There is a wide range of topical agents available for the treatment of psoriasis, although their use and appearance are usually unpleasant. Mild cases may only require an emollient but more severe eruptions have traditionally been treated with salicylic acid or coal-tar preparations. More recent introductions such as dithranol and calcipotriol have been used successfully; take care when using near sensitive areas such as the face. Dithranol is liable to cause severe skin irritation and if a preparation above 0.1% is to be used, skin sensitivity should first be tested (*British National Formulary* 1999). Ultraviolet light is another well-established effective treatment for psoriasis, especially when combined with other agents such as dithranol and tar.

Acne

The psychological impact of acne on immature adolescents is such that empathy and understanding are important parts of the management, together with some basic health education. A range of commonly held beliefs about the condition can be dismissed as myths. Acne is not related to fatty foods and sweets, lack of skin hygiene, hormonal problems or sexual activity (Graham-Brown and Burns 1996). In mild cases where only comedones (blackheads) are present, the application of tretinoin (an acid form of vitamin A) is recommended. Where some facial pustular lesions are also present, topical preparations of benzoyl peroxide or azelaic acid should be used (*British National Formulary* 1999). More severe cases require the addition of an oral antibiotic such as tetracycline or oxytetracycline (500 mg twice daily) to the regime. Treatment may continue for several months before there is significant improvement. Topical steroids should not be used.

Rosacea is best treated by topical metronidazole 0.75% gel (Metrogel) which should be applied twice daily after cleaning with a non-irritating agent. The skin should be washed gently with luke-warm water and patted dry before applying the metronidazole preparation. Skin care products which contain irritants such as alcohol or witch hazel should be avoided. Improvement should be noted after 3 weeks but it may take up to 9 weeks to get the maximum benefit. Oral tetracycline or erythromycin (500 mg twice daily) are also beneficial, although their effect is believed to be more anti-inflammatory than antibacterial (Chalmers 1997). Other advice includes keeping a diary to try and identify any triggers which cause flare-ups so that they can be avoided, e.g. exposure to strong winds, alcohol or spicy foods.

Skin cancer

There are numerous benign skin lesions, many of which are associated with exposure to sunlight, which may bring a patient to the health centre anxious about the risk of skin cancer. This anxiety should be recognized in the consultation. Any lesion suspected of being malignant should be referred for an immediate medical opinion.

The nurse practitioner can carry out a useful preventive function by offering health education about the harmful effects of sunlight at every opportunity, particularly with patients travelling abroad to hot climates or in general during the summer months. Individuals should be advised to avoid the strongest sunlight for 2 hours either side of noon during the summer, whilst parents should be advised of the importance of shade, T-shirts and sun hats for young children. Health education work with local primary schools is an opportunity not to be missed in the summer term, especially in view of the findings of Hurwitz (1988) that children receive three times more ultraviolet light than the average adult.

The ultraviolet radiation within sunlight is most harmful to skin, especially in the medium wavelength where it causes a range of conditions, including sunburn, premature ageing and skin cancer. This form of ultraviolet is known as UVB, as opposed to longer-wavelength ultraviolet (UVA) which, while not causing sunburn, contributes to long-term skin damage and cancer as well as problems of short-term photosensitivity. Many sunscreens are only effective against UVB; the sun protection factor (SPF) on the packaging indicates how many times more protection it gives compared to unprotected skin. Patients should therefore be advised to check the label on sunscreen products carefully and only buy a product that offers protection against both UVA and UVB. Protection against UVA is rated by a star system: a four-star preparation indicates that it gives the same protection against UVB as it does UVA, while lower ratings mean less protection. This system is controversial however (*British National Formulary* 1999). The danger exists that people may counteract the benefits of using sunscreens by simply staying in the sun longer (Taylor and Roberts 1997). The nurse practitioner should use every opportunity not to praise tanned skin and to raise issues of health in relation to sun exposure, particularly with young men who often use no sunscreen at all.

Infectious conditions

The use of antibiotics is under constant review due to the emergence of resistant strains. To be effective, conditions such as cellulitis require a systemic course of antibiotics if enough antibiotic is to reach the site of the infection via the blood stream. Local policies should always be followed concerning antibiotic therapy, especially the principle that swabs for culture and sensitivity should be taken before any course is started. Topical antibiotics should therefore only be used in certain carefully defined situations, as in many cases they are not necessary or will be ineffective. Mupirocin is however an effective topical antibacterial which is not related to any others. It is not indicated for pseudomonal infection but is recommended for treating impetigo or as a nasal ointment in a situation where a patient is found to be carrying staphylococci in the nose and suffering from recurrent boils.

Antibiotics have no part to play in the management of viral infections. Common warts are self-limiting and eventually disappear spontaneously: they may be treated by the use of salicylic acid, formaldehyde or glutaraldehyde preparations, which need to be applied for up to 3 months to be effective. Cryotherapy is the painful alternative, involving application to the lesion of a bud of cotton wool frozen in liquid nitrogen. To be fully effective it should be held against the wart until it – and at least 1 mm of surrounding skin – has turned white (Reifsnider 1997). This may need repeating at 2–3-week intervals until the lesion is fully removed. Herpes simplex infections affecting the genitals are treated with acyclovir cream, though systemic treatments may be required for vaginal infections. These treatments are usually managed by specialist clinics of genitourinary medicine. Although acyclovir will not eradicate the herpes virus, it will improve the condition. The sooner treatment is started the better, hence the importance of persuading a patient to attend a specialist clinic as soon as possible. The drug is also effective as a systemic agent in treating herpes-zoster infections, although it has a considerable range of side-effects (*British National Formulary* 1999).

Clotrimazole is effective against a wide range of fungal infections, including ringworm, and is commonly available as Canesten; nystatin is a familiar treatment for *Candida* infection but is not effective against the tinea group of fungi. The patient should be advised to keep the area clean and dry to promote healing in both candidiasis and tinea infections. If infections recur, a capillary blood glucose test should be performed to test for diabetes and the possibility of HIV infection should be considered. As transmission via sexual contact is possible in candidiasis, both partners should be treated together when a genital infection occurs.

Scabies is best treated with malathion or permethrin preparations. Application after a hot bath was traditionally the method of choice but, as the *British National Formulary* points out, this is not necessary and may reduce the effectiveness of the agent as increased peripheral blood flow following a hot bath will absorb more of the drug, diverting it away from the skin where it is needed (*British National Formulary* 1999). Lotions of malathion or carbaryl are better than shampoos for the treatment of head lice and crab lice as shampoos are often not in contact with the lice long enough to kill them.

Wounds

Nurses have a great deal of expertise in the management of chronic wounds. This section will therefore only consider trauma and will concentrate on the initial presentation. The following key principles are well-known and have been summarized by Whiteside and Moorhead (1998). They should guide the nurse practitioner when deciding how best to manage a traumatic wound.

- For healing to occur there must be adequate blood supply. Patients whose peripheral blood supply is compromised are likely to experience delays in wound healing and this must be taken into account in their management by arranging follow-up and review if needed. Pretibial flap lacerations in elderly patients are notoriously difficult to heal and should be treated by steristrip closure and a good firm dressing. If the flap is distally based (Figure 3.7), this will have an even poorer blood supply and need close follow-up. The nurse practitioner should always check that there is adequate circulation distal to any serious injury because of the risk of compromise of the arterial blood supply to the rest of the limb

- Necrotic or devitalized tissue should always be removed before wound closure. This reduces the risk of infection and contamination by foreign bodies (e.g. grit or soil). It also improves the person's defences against infection, as these are impaired by any foreign bodies in the wound. This may be done by sharp debridement with a scalpel but great care is necessary to ensure all suspect tissue has been removed while healthy tissue is not damaged. Analgesia is important as this may be a painful procedure. Bale (1997) recommends the use of lignocaine – prilocaine cream (Emla). If wound suture is planned, an injection of local anaesthetic such as lignocaine will be necessary anyway; therefore a topical cream is not likely to be needed. If there is any doubt about the viability of tissue, a medical opinion should be obtained prior to closure

- Irrigation of the wound is essential to remove contaminants and reduce the infection risk. Topical antiseptic solutions are now discredited and sterile normal saline is commonly used. Ordinary tap water of drinking quality has been shown to be sterile and is increasingly being used for wound irrigation (Riyat and Quinton 1997). Large A&E departments may save thousands of pounds a year in this way. In dirty wounds soap and water may be necessary and even a scrubbing brush may be required. Analgesia such as Entonox

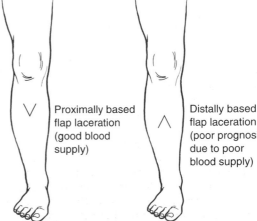

Figure 3.7 Pretibial flap lacerations

Proximally based flap laceration (good blood supply)

Distally based flap laceration (poor prognosis due to poor blood supply) should be made available to the patient if such measures are necessary

- Before closure is considered, careful exploration of the wound is necessary to ensure that no underlying structures are involved and that all contamination and necrotic tissue has been removed
- Prophylactic antibiotics are no substitute for thorough cleaning and debridement. Tetanus status must be determined and a booster given if needed
- Wound closure should only take place if the wound is clean, tidy and less than 12 hours old. Suture technique cannot be learnt from a book alone; the basic principles should be to close the wound in such a way that the skin edges are opposed (with no dead space) but not under tension (Figure 3.8). The smallest size suture should always be used. Typically, 5/0 and 6/0 are best for the face, 4/0 and 5/0 for the upper limbs and 3/0 for the lower limbs, trunk and scalp. In many cases wounds can be closed using steristrips or glue, although sites such as joints and the scalp require suture, as do deep wounds

Wound closure should not be attempted if:

- Tissue of dubious viability is present or if contamination cannot be fully removed
- Tissue loss has occurred
- The wound is a bite. Human bites are particularly infective. A common presentation is a puncture wound to the hand caused by a tooth during a fight. Such apparently trivial wounds are potentially serious and should be admitted for formal surgical debridement in theatre, due to the risk of soft tissue infection and osteomyelitis (Kelly *et al.* 1996). Diseases such as hepatitis B, hepatitis C and HIV can all be transmitted by human bites. Dog bites account for some 200 000 A&E attendances per year in the UK and carry infection rates of up to 30% (Higgins *et al.* 1997). In addition to correct wound management, the nurse practitioner also needs to think about a health education approach to reduce the risk of future bites. Indicators for antibiotic therapy in bites include a wound over 6 hours old, involvement of the hands and feet, devitalized or puncture wounds, full thickness wounds involving deep structures and the presence of alcoholism or a compromised immune system in the patient (Higgins *et al.* 1997)
- A foreign body is present in the wound. This should be removed in theatre
- There is any risk of involvement of other structures such as nerves and tendons
- The wound is ragged and may need specialist surgical closure to achieve a good cosmetic result
- Tissue oedema is present, making closure very difficult
- The wound is 24 hours old or more

In any of the above circumstances, a medical opinion should be obtained promptly.

Wound dressing is a complex area and the nurse practitioner can easily be confused by the plethora of products now on the market. It is best therefore to stick to basic principles. If a wound has been thoroughly cleaned and closed, a dressing should be applied which protects the wound, is non-adherent, thermally insulating, capable of absorbing any exudate, non-allergenic and comfortable for the patient. The dressing should also be secured in such a way as to remain in place. It should only be removed prematurely if there are localized/systemic signs of infection, or it has become soaked through by exudate or externally contaminated.

In choosing the dressing the following guide, based on the work of Bale and Jones (1997), will be useful.

Clean wounds with little exudate such as minor abrasions or wounds closed by suture/steristrip should be dressed with low-adherence dressings such as N-A Dressing or Melolin. They allow exudate to pass through and may require the addition of some extra sterile gauze backing to ensure they remain effective.

Wound beds with superficial infection benefit from the application of medicated dressings such as Inadine or Iodoflex (good for *Pseudomonas*), while Actisorb is effective against a broader range of pathogens. These dressings may need changing daily at first if the antibacterial agent is to be effective.

If the wound is exuding heavily, the alginates such as Sorbsan or Tegage should be used. They form a hydrophilic gel as they absorb the exudate, and can be used as ropes to pack deeper wounds as well as sheets for more superficial wounds. Foams such as Allevyn or Lyofoam can be used for cavities. All these dressings can stay in place for several days but should be changed once saturated.

Wounds requiring autolytic debridement are best treated with the hydrogels such as Intrasite but this requires daily dressing changes. Hydrocolloid dressings (Granuflex, Comfeel, Tegasorb) will also facilitate autolysis of devitalized tissue from the wound bed and are good for exuding wounds as they can absorb substantial amounts of exudate. They should be changed when saturated, typically every 4 days or so. An alternative is enzymatic debridement using Varidase, which should be applied directly to the wound bed. This breaks down fibrin, denatured collagen and elastin (Bale 1997).

Superficial wounds that require observation may be dressed with a semipermeable film such as Opsite or Tegaderm. These are self-adherent and can stay in place for several days but should be changed if leakage of exudate looks imminent or has occurred.

Burns

The treatment of serious burns revolves around the

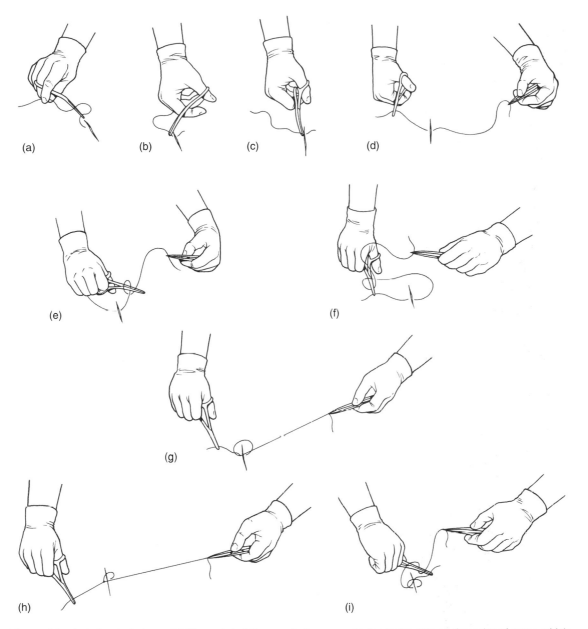

Figure 3.8 Suturing technique. (a) The point of the needle is perpendicular to the skin at the point of entry, which should be 3–4 mm from the wound. (b) The needle should be brought through and out of the wound. (c) Re-enter the needle on the opposite edge of the wound, by rotating the wrist, to bring the needle out 3–4 mm from the opposite side of the wound. (d) Pull the suture through the wound, ready to tie the knot. (e) Start tying the knot by making a loop with the needle holders. (f) Grasp the end of the suture. (g) Pull the end of the suture through the loop. (h) Pull the suture firmly but not too tightly and lay the knot to one side of the wound. (i) Repeat this method twice, looping in the opposite direction on each occasion

basic principles of airway and respiratory management, opioid analgesia, intravenous resuscitation, simple occlusive dressings and transfer to an A&E department or regional burns unit. These injuries lie outside the scope of this book; we will concentrate on minor burns in the rest of this section. It should be pointed out that such a burn may not seem minor to the patient.

Local protocols will normally determine which patients will be managed by the nurse practitioner and which should be referred for a medical opinion. The following useful principles will help in drawing up such protocols or in managing patients in the absence of local guidelines. Patients must see a doctor if:

- The burn is full- or deep partial-thickness

- Opioid analgesia is needed for pain control
- There is a risk of smoke or fume inhalation
- There is airway involvement
- Special areas such as the face, hand, perineum and ears are involved
- Surface area of burn exceeds 1%, i.e. the surface area of one hand
- Non-accidental injury is suspected
- Infection is already established in an old burn

Minor burns with none of the above characteristics are suitable for primary management by the nurse practitioner as they should heal with little or no scarring, providing they are correctly dressed. The basic principles of wound management apply to burns as they do to any other wound, particularly the need for a scrupulous aseptic technique. Irrigation with saline is essential to clean and expose the wound for careful examination. Blisters should be deroofed and devitalized tissue removed with sterile forceps and scissors to minimize the risk of infection. Blisters also prevent thorough inspection of the burn area. A fresh burn wound will exude considerable amounts of fluid for at least 24 hours. As a consequence, several layers of paraffin gauze, preferably with a low-adherence dressing, should be used in contact with the burn and it should have a thick backing layer of sterile gauze to ensure that the dressing remains patent. The dressing should be reviewed after 48 hours. Hydrocolloid dressings are recommended by Pankhurst (1997) for the long-term management of partial-thickness, epithelializing wounds after the initial exudate has subsided. Before discharge, an adequate course of analgesia should also be administered, together with advice about wound elevation to control oedema.

Silver sulphadiazine cream (Flamazine) has a broad-spectrum antibacterial effect and is useful in treating burns. Pankhurst (1997) recommends its use prophylactically in burns affecting the perineum or the ear. Serious deformity of the ear could ensue if the cartilaginous pinna is allowed to dry out, therefore after it has been applied a paraffin gauze dressing held in place with a head bandage should be used. Silver sulphadiazine is also very useful in treating burns to the hand or foot. The need to retain joint mobility precludes bulky dressings; after cleaning and debridement, silver sulphadiazine cream should be applied to the hand or foot and then it should be encased in a Gortex bag. It may also be used to treat infected burns or in the conservative management of fingertip injuries. Contraindications to the use of silver sulphadiazine are pregnancy, breast-feeding and known sensitivity to sulphonamides (*British National Formulary* 1999).

The psychosocial impact of burns should also be considered as an integral part of their long-term management. Patients may be anxious about scarring and, if asked, the only honest answer the nurse practitioner can give is to say that it is too early to say. If the patient is a child, parents may be feeling guilty and blaming themselves. Sensitivity is necessary in handling the parent who may be upset by their child's distress. In particular injuries to the hand may prevent someone from working, caring for a child or an elderly relative or from carrying out normal activities of living. These aspects should be checked before discharge to see if any help can be arranged.

There is a great potential for health education work in the field of wounds and burns, ranging from first aid to prevention. As well as displaying posters and leaflets in the waiting area, the nurse practitioner should remember that all patients (and other family members) attending with a wound or burn are potential recipients of health education, assuming they are well enough. Prevention strategies can be explored by asking how the accident occurred. This may identify unsafe working practices, such as not wearing protective clothing.

First-aid advice for burns involves copious irrigation with cold water to remove any residual heat and therefore limit burn damage. This also gives considerable pain relief; however, excessive irrigation, especially in small children, can lead to hypothermia. Patients should be advised to leave any blisters intact and not apply any lotions or creams to the burn. Tight constrictions such as rings should be removed because of the risk of swelling. If the burn can be covered with a clean dressing this should be done; cling film is especially suitable for this purpose. Before discharge, explain the need to keep the wound dressing clean and dry; point out signs that may indicate infection or that the dressing needs changing. Reinforce this information with printed leaflets or cards which the patient is given to take away and which should also include details of any follow-up appointment. Tetanus prophylaxis should also be discussed and a written record of any booster injection given to the patient in the form of a card.

Summary

The nurse practitioner plays a major role in managing a wide range of wounds and skin disorders, whether s/he works in primary care or in a minor injuries/A&E setting. It is important to retain the holistic nursing perspective and consider the psychosocial effects of the patient's condition, as this constitutes an integral part of the management strategy. The implications for work and domestic activities of the condition, together with its psychological impact, must all be talked through with the patient. Health education can prevent many disorders and first-aid teaching can limit the effects of an accident once it has happened. Every opportunity should be taken to be an active health educator, whether by displaying material in the waiting room, working with individual patients during a consultation, or engaging in community activity such as liaising with schools and sports centres. This wider approach distinguishes the nurse practitioner from the medical practitioner and constitutes the unique contribution that s/he can make as a nurse.

References

Bale S. (1997) A guide to wound debridement, *Journal of Wound Care*, **6**(4), pp. 179–82.

Bale S., Jones V. (1997) *Wound Care Nursing*, London, Baillière Tindall.

Bosworth C. (1997) *Burns Trauma*, London, Baillière Tindall.

British National Formulary (1999), London, British Medical Association/Royal Pharmaceutical Society of Great Britain.

Chalmers D. (1997) Rosacea: recognition and management for the primary care provider, *Nurse Practitioner*, **22**(10), pp. 18–30

Graham-Brown R., Burns A. (1996) *Lecture Notes on Dermatology*, 7th edn., Oxford, Blackwell Science.

Higgins M., Evans R.C., Evans R.J. (1997) Managing animal bite wounds, *Journal of Wound Care*, **6**(8), pp. 377–380.

Hurwitz S. (1988) The sun and sunscreen protection: recommendations for children, *Journal of Dermatology, Surgery* and Oncology, **14**(6), pp. 657–660.

Kelly I., Cunney R., Smyth E., Colville J. (1996) The management of human bite injuries of the hand, *Injury*, **27**(7), pp. 481–484.

Lait M., Smith L. (1998) Wound management: a literature review, *Journal of Clinical Nursing*, **7**, pp. 11–17.

Munro J., Edwards C. (1995) *Macleod's Clinical Examination*, 9th edn., Edinburgh, Churchill-Livingstone.

Pankhurst S. (1997) Wound care. In Bosworth C. (ed) *Burns Trauma*, London, Baillière Tindall.

Reifsneider E. (1997) Common adult infectious skin conditions, *Nurse Practitioner*, **22**(11), pp. 17–33.

Riyat M., Quinton D. (1997) Tap water as a wound cleansing agent in A&E, *Journal of Accident and Emergency Medicine*, **14**, pp. 165–166.

Schofield J., Kneebone R. (1996) *Skin Lesions*, London, Chapman & Hall.

Singleton J. (1997) Paediatric dermatoses: three common skin disruptions in infancy, *Nurse Practitioner*, **22**(6), pp. 32–50.

Taylor P., Roberts D. (1997) Skin cancer prevention, *Nursing Standard*, **11**(50), pp. 42–45.

Whiteside M., Moorhead R. (1998) Management of traumatic wounds. In: Leaper D., Harding K. (eds) *Wounds; Biology and Management*, Oxford, Oxford Medical Publications.

Young T. (1997) Skin assessment and unusual presentations, *Community Nurse*, June 1997, **3**(5), pp. 33–36.

CHAPTER 4
The head and neck

Alison Crumbie

Introduction

The head and neck area involves many overlapping systems, including alimentary, respiratory, neurological, cardiovascular, musculoskeletal, ear, nose and throat (ENT). This chapter focuses on those conditions associated with the nose, ear, mouth, neck and throat which represent the most common reasons for patients seeking help from nurse practitioners. In primary health care patients will present with problems such as otitis externa, otitis media and rhinitis; in a minor injuries unit patients will present with trauma to the face, scalp or nose. It is therefore important that the nurse practitioner can carry out an appropriate assessment of the patient and has an understanding of the pathophysiology relating to the head and neck.

Pathophysiology and clinical presentations

A thorough examination of the head and neck includes the nose and sinuses, the ears, the mouth, the face, the neck and throat. The eyes are also included in the head and neck; however, ophthalmic examination will be covered in Chapter 6. It is reasonable to break the examination down into discrete sections as the nurse practitioner will choose to focus upon a particular area depending upon the patient's presenting symptoms.

The nose and sinuses

Symptoms of nasal disease include nasal obstruction, discharge and deformities (Colman 1992). Nasal obstruction is associated with nasal or sinus disease and may be due to a number of causes, including anatomical abnormality of the nose, mucous membranes or of the autonomic control of the mucosa. An anatomical abnormality may be due to a deviated nasal septum or congenital atresia of the conchae. Abnormalities of the mucosa include polyps, hypertrophy of the mucous membranes and excessive abnormal secretions. Abnormalities of the autonomic control of the mucosa include allergic disorders, including swelling of the mucous membranes and excessive production of secretions.

Nasal discharge is a common symptom of nasal and sinus disease. The discharge may be watery or thick. Watery discharge occurs with the onset of a common cold and may also be due to exposure to allergens or irritants. A thick discharge may be produced in a chronic condition of the nose or sinuses such as perennial allergic rhinitis.

Allergic rhinitis is a condition in which both nasal discharge and obstruction are present. Allergic rhinitis may be seasonal (hayfever) or perennial; both are due to the protective mechanisms of the nasal mucosa being triggered by harmless particles such as pollens. Particles trapped in the nose of people allergic to the specific allergen result in the release of mediator molecules such as histamine from the cells near the epithelial surface of the mucous membranes. Histamine directly stimulates receptors causing vasodilation, oedema and exudation of plasma. Sneezing and hypersecretion are the result of reflex activation and account for the unpleasant symptoms associated with rhinitis (Cross 1998).

If nasal discharge is excessively sticky, the normal ciliary action of the nasal lining may become impeded and mucus collection can accumulate. If infection is superimposed, the secretions may become purulent or mucopurulent. Persistent discharge of yellowy secretions or pus is indicative of sinus disease. Thick blood-stained discharge may be indicative of a tumour in the nose or sinuses. A unilateral discharge in a child may suggest a foreign body in the nose (Colman 1992).

Pain is a symptom which is often associated with sinus trouble. Colman (1992) suggests that, unless there is an acute presentation of sinus infection, the nose and sinuses are rarely the cause of the problem. If the patient complains of pain in the nose or sinus area it is worthwhile checking over the area of distribution of the trigeminal nerve to check for trigeminal neuralgia. Alternatively, dental problems may be the cause of referred pain.

A direct blow to the nose can result in trauma to the cartilage or bones. Injury to the nose may result in cartilaginous destruction, resulting in a flattened bridge and an alteration in shape. Diseases such as cancer, tuberculosis or syphilis may result in severe nasal deformities which require the specialist care of an ENT consultant.

The nasal sinuses are air spaces in the bones of the skull which communicate with the nasal cavity. There are two groups of sinuses: the anterior group is made up of the frontal air sinus, maxillary air sinus and ethmoidal air cells and the posterior group comprises the posterior ethmoidal cells and the sphenoidal sinus (Figure 4.1).

Sinusitis is an inflammatory condition of the mucous membrane lining of the sinuses and often progresses to pus formation. Any condition which tends to obstruct the drainage of the sinuses will predispose the patient to sinusitis. Deflection of the septum, nasal allergy, foreign bodies and tumours all predispose to sinusitis. The mucous membranes of the sinuses pass through the usual stages of infection, including increased secretions, oedema of the membranes, and increased ciliary activity, followed by a decrease in ciliary activity. The infection may be in one sinus or it may spread to all of the sinuses, this condition is known as pansinusitis.

Differential diagnosis in disorders of the nose and sinus

When nurse practitioners are presented with a patient who complains of the vague symptoms of the common cold or a stuffy nose it is important to consider the differential diagnoses of these symptoms so that the patient can be appropriately reassured and appropriate self-management advice can be provided. It is important to differentiate between allergic rhinitis, sinusitis and the common cold by taking a thorough history and carrying out an examination of the head, neck and respiratory tract. A patient with a fever of greater than 39°C is unlikely to be suffering from a simple upper respiratory tract infection and should be assessed for pharyngitis, otitis media, sinusitis, meningitis or bacterial pneumonia. A patient who complains of malaise, chills and shivering may be suffering from flu and patients who complain of pain over the sinuses which is exacerbated by coughing are likely to have sinusitis.

The ears

There are several conditions associated with the ears that may cause the patient to seek help from the nurse practitioner. These include earache, discharge, deafness, tinnitus and vertigo or dizziness. It is useful to consider clinical conditions of the ears in three categories – the external ear, the middle ear and the inner ear. Figure 4.2 is a diagrammatic representation of the ear.

The external ear

In children it may be possible to detect congenital abnormalities of the external ear, including bilateral protruding pinnae or atresia of the pinna. Often the cause may not be determined; however, there are links to the teratogenic effects of medications in early pregnancy and genetic defects (Colman 1992). The pinnae of any patient can become inflamed due to acute dermatitis, perichondritis or infections such as herpes-zoster oticus (Ramsay Hunt syndrome). Acute dermatitis may occur due to an extension of otitis externa or to a sensitivity to topical treatment; this in turn may develop into perichondritis. This is inflammation of the covering of the cartilage which may be caused by ear piercing, trauma to the ear or extending otitis externa, as described above. This condition may be extremely destructive, causing the patient great pain and discomfort. On inspection the pinna appears red and shiny. Herpes-zoster oticus may involve the seventh and eighth cranial nerves. Symptoms may include facial paralysis, giddiness, nystagmus and hearing loss in addition to the herpes-zoster lesions and herpetic pain.

The pinna of the ear is frequently omitted when people apply sunscreen to protect themselves against the damaging effects of the sun. For this reason it is not uncommon to observe squamous cell and basal cell carcinomas on the edge of the pinna. On close

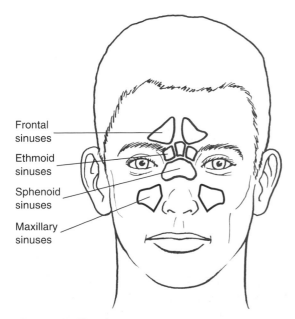

Frontal sinuses
Ethmoid sinuses
Sphenoid sinuses
Maxillary sinuses

Figure 4.1   The sinuses

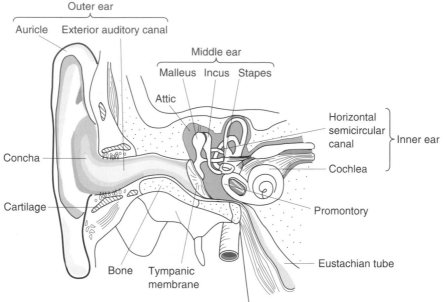

Figure 4.2   The ear

inspection of the pinna it is possible to discover areas of hyperkeratosis and small lesions which may be early carcinomas. Biopsy is necessary to determine the histology of the lesion.

Diseases of the external meatus include infections and blockages. Infections may result from furunculosis which is an infection of a hair follicle and otitis externa, which is a generalized infection of the whole skin of the external canal. Furunculosis is usually caused by *Staphylococcus* and the pain has been reported to be as severe as that of renal colic (Bull 1996). Otitis externa can be fungal or bacterial; and the irritation of the meatus is accompanied by desquamation and scanty discharge. The conditions which predispose to otitis externa include hot humid climates, swimming baths, dusty environments and traumatized skin following scratching of the ears or the presence of eczema. There are many organisms which have been linked to otitis externa, including *Staphylococcus pyogenes*, *Pseudomonas pyocyanea*, *Escherichia coli* and others (Bull 1996). Otitis externa is most commonly bilateral; unilateral otitis externa is so uncommon that an underlying middle-ear infection should be considered as a possible cause of the problem. Furunculosis and otitis externa; can both lead to an impairment in hearing; indeed, anything which causes an obstruction in the external auditory meatus can cause deafness.

One of the commonest causes of impaired hearing is the presence of wax in the ear. Wax or cerumen is a completely normal finding in examination of the ear. Impacted wax may cause irritation and can occasionally cause tinnitus if the wax presses on the eardrum. Pieces of Lego, beads, insects and cotton buds are not normal findings in the examination of the external meatus! The presence of a foreign body is not an uncommon occurrence in children and in adults foreign bodies tend to be those associated with cleaning the ears, such as matchsticks and cotton buds.

A further fairly common abnormal finding on examination of the external auditory meatus is exostosis or osteomata. An exostosis is a bony outgrowth from the wall of the external auditory meatus and it is associated with people who have engaged in a lot of swimming in cold water, although the cause is unknown. Patients are often unaware of the presence of the exostosis, which only becomes apparent when the meatus is finally closed due to the collection of wax or the presence of other inflammatory conditions.

Middle ear

The tympanic membrane can be damaged by trauma or by the infection of otitis media or other problems with the ear. Trauma to the ear can be direct, e.g. from attempts to clean the ears with matchsticks, or indirect, such as a slap to the ear or a blast from a shotgun. The patient will complain of acute pain at the time of the rupture, may report hearing loss and may occasionally complain of tinnitus and vertigo. There may be bleeding from the ear and a visible tear in the eardrum. The message in the management of traumatic perforation is to leave the ear alone. In virtually all cases the membrane will repair rapidly and all that is required is a protective dressing and prophylactic antibiotics.

Perforations of the eardrum may also be caused by infection. In general, if an ear discharges and there are no signs of external otitis, there must be a perforation. There are three main types of perforation – central, marginal and attic, depending on location (Figure 4.3). Marginal and attic perforations are characteristic of progressive disease and are associated with bone destruction. This is a potentially dangerous situation which requires referral to prevent further hearing loss.

Otitis media

Otitis media may be acute or chronic. Acute otitis media is an inflammation of the lining of the middle ear; if this fails to resolve a mixed infection may persist which can lead to further damage to the middle-ear structures and greater potential for conductive deafness.

Acute otitis media

Acute otitis media is common in children and often follows an acute upper respiratory tract infection. Without a culture of discharge from the ear it is impossible to differentiate between viral and bacterial causes of the condition. Organisms invade the mucous membrane of the middle ear via the eustachian tube or occasionally via the external auditory meatus, causing inflammation, oedema, exudate and, later, pus. The swelling causes closure of the eustachian tube which prevents aeration and drainage. Pressure from the pus rises, causing the tympanic membrane to bulge; necrosis of the tympanic membrane results in perforation and the

ear drains until the infection resolves (Bull 1996). The patient may complain of earache which may be slight or severe and often there will be a history of resolution of the pain if the tympanic membrane perforates. Deafness always accompanies acute otitis media and may be the presenting complaint in adults. There may be pyrexia and a child can appear quite flushed and ill. Pain, impaired hearing and discharge are the cardinal signs of acute otitis media.

Chronic otitis media

Chronic otitis media may be caused by late or inadequate treatment of acute otitis media, upper airway infection, immunosuppression and particularly virulent diseases such as measles. There are two major types – mucosal disease and bony disease. In mucosal infection the ear often discharges copious amounts of mucoid fluid. The ear may improve from time to time and the perforation may heal spontaneously. In bony disease there may be scanty discharge with aural polyps which may fill the meatus, granulations and cholesteatoma. Cholesteatoma is formed by squamous epithelium and results in the accumulation of keratotic debris which may be visible through the perforation and may be smelly. This can lead to intracranial complications if left untreated and requires referral to assess the extent of the disease and possible surgical intervention.

Glue ear

Mucous otitis is otherwise known as glue ear. This is a common condition in childhood and involves the accumulation of fluid in the middle ear in the absence of acute inflammation. The fluid may be thin and serous or even partially solid. The condition is most often bilateral and the child's hearing will be impaired. The cause of glue ear is debated, although it is probably linked to poor eustachian tube function and low-grade infection (Colman 1992). Bull (1996) states that other causes include parental smoking, allergic rhinitis, untreated acute otitis media and barotrauma, such as descent in an aircraft when suffering from a cold. The eardrum will appear dull, may have visible vessels and a yellow/orange or a blue-grey tinge and will be retracted. In long-standing cases the eardrum may become atrophic and even collapse. The eardrum will be immobile on testing for mobility. As impaired hearing and the presence of fluid in the ear may cause permanent conductive hearing loss and impaired development, it is essential that children who have mucous otitis are treated appropriately. Referral to an ENT specialist should be considered if the problem does not resolve.

Complications of otitis media include acute mastoiditis, meningitis, extradural abscess, brain abscess, subdural abscess, labyrinthitis, lateral sinus thrombosis, facial nerve paralysis and, rarely,

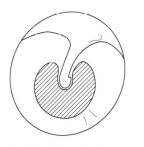

(a) Central perforation

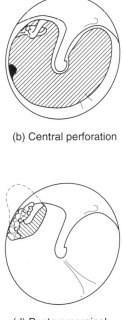

(b) Central perforation

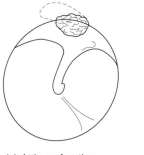

(c) Attic perforation

(d) Posteromarginal perforation

Figure 4.3 The main types of perforation

petrositis affecting the sixth cranial nerve, resulting in diplopia and trigeminal pain. These are serious and in some cases life-threatening illnesses – this emphasizes the importance of making an accurate diagnosis and correctly treating diseases of the ear.

The inner ear

The inner ear includes the cochlea, vestibule and the semicircular canals and is often termed the labyrinth. Labyrinthitis is a complication of acute or chronic otitis media and may be the precursor to meningitis. The usual symptoms of middle-ear disease – loss of balance, giddiness, vomiting, hearing loss and nystagmus – are seen. If the disease progresses, all hearing ability will be lost and the labyrinth may fill with bone.

Differential diagnoses of ear disorders

Patients who present to the nurse practitioner are most likely to complain of the symptoms of disorders of the ear. The major symptoms include earache, hearing loss, tinnitus, dizziness and vertigo. The following section will consider each of these complaints and possible differential diagnoses.

Earache

Seller (1993) states that most earaches are caused by acute infections of the middle ear or external auditory meatus. If examination does not reveal the cause, then referred pain should be considered. The possibilities are listed in Table 4.1.

Bull (1996) points out that malignant disease of the posterior tongue, vallecula, tonsils, larynx or pharynx will produce earache. This earache tends to be intractable. The nurse practitioner should examine the cervical lymph nodes and assess the

Table 4.1 Differential diagnoses of earache

Otitis media	Tends to occur in children with unilateral severe pain
Serous otitis media	Occurs in children and some adults; unilateral; less painful
Otitis externa	Tends to be bilateral and occurs in people who are diabetic, swimmers and people who have eczema
Trauma	History of a traumatic event
Mastoiditis	Presents as pain in and behind the ear
Foreign body/wax	Tends to cause vague discomfort and may impair hearing
Referred pain	Such as dental abscess or temporomandibular joint dysfunction; in adults tumours occur more frequently with advancing age

patient for dysphagia, entertaining a high suspicion of malignancy until proven otherwise.

Coley and Kay (1992) differentiate between the earache of viral otitis media and bacterial otitis media by highlighting the possible variations in findings on otoscopy. In viral otitis media the handle of malleus is flush, bubbles are sometimes seen behind the tympanic membrane and the membrane appears dull or may have no light reflex. In bacterial otitis media the tympanic membrane may appear red and bulging, with evidence of haemorrhagic areas. A central perforation may be present, associated with a discharge of pus. During the history-taking process the nurse practitioner might find that a viral otitis media is secondary to a recent upper respiratory tract infection, is of recent onset with a mild pyrexia and may be present in one or both ears. In bacterial otitis media there may be a history of tonsillitis with marked pyrexia. The bacterial otitis media is more often unilateral. A history of purulent and bloody discharge from a spontaneous perforation associated with pain relief is a sign of bacterial otitis media.

Hearing loss

It is important to understand that there are three classifications of deafness: conductive deafness, sensorineural, and mixed conductive and sensorineural deafness. Conductive deafness results from the mechanical obstruction of the sound waves in the outer or middle ear, preventing the stimulation from reaching the cochlear fluid of the inner ear. Figure 4.4 shows the area of the ear which, if blocked for some reason, may result in conductive hearing loss.

Sensorineural deafness results from the defective functioning of the cochlea or auditory nerve and this prevents neural impulses from travelling to the auditory cortex of the brain. Mixed deafness is a combination of conductive and sensorineural deficits. Table 4.2 lists the most common causes of hearing loss.

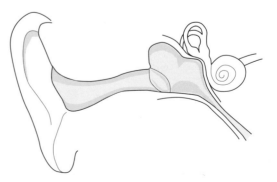

Figure 4.4 Conductive deafness is caused by an abnormality of the external auditory canal in the outer or middle ear

Table 4.2   Causes of hearing loss

Conductive	Sensorineural
Cerumen, foreign body	Presbycusis (deafness of old age)
Acute or chronic otitis media	Noise-induced (occupation)
Otitis media with effusion (glue ear)	Congenital
Trauma to the tympanic membrane	Ménière's disease
Otitis externa	Drug-induced
	Infections

Hearing loss has a variety of causes and a thorough history and examination are necessary to determine an accurate diagnosis.

Tinnitus

Tinnitus is a common condition which can cause a great deal of suffering for patients. It is the constant or intermittent perception of noises in the ears and has been described as a swarm of bees, whistling, a diesel lorry ticking over or a cistern filling with water (Fisher 1998). Tinnitus is a symptom which is often a feature of general ill health and it has several causes. Table 4.3 lists the potential causes of tinnitus.

Table 4.3   Causes of tinnitus

Damage to the ear	Other general causes
Blockage in the ear	Fever
Presbycusis	Cardiovascular disease
Ménière's disease	Anaemia
Impacted wisdom teeth	Multiple sclerosis
Otosclerosis	Alcohol abuse
Ototoxic medications	Tiredness and anxiety
Tumour (glomus jugulare/ acoustic neuroma)	Head injury
Aneurysm (intracranial)	

When the history and physical examination reveal normal findings for the ear, the other general causes of tinnitus should be considered. The management of tinnitus will be discussed later in this chapter and, regardless of the cause of the problem, patients must be taken seriously and referred to self-help groups for support and information.

Dizziness and vertigo

Seller (1993) states that most instances of vertigo and dizziness are not caused by ear problems. The history taking process is particularly important in these patients to differentiate between true vertigo and dizziness. Vertigo is the illusion that one's surroundings are moving or, with eyes closed, that one's body or head is moving in space. Nystagmus is the objective sign of vertigo. Dizziness is a sensation of syncope which is not followed by a faint. The accompanying symptoms of the dizziness or vertigo help to differentiate between diagnoses and clearly the origin or cause of the problem depends on the underlying pathology. It is important to determine the timing and persistency of the episodes, aural symptoms and neurological symptoms. The instances of vertigo which are associated with ear problems are summarized in Table 4.4.

Table 4.4   Vertigo associated with ear problems

Episodic	Constant
Ménière's disease	Ototoxicity
	Acoustic neuroma
Solitary attack	Chronic otitis media with
Vestibular neuronitis	labyrinthine fistula
Labyrinthine fistula	

Other cases of vertigo include migraine, cardiac arrhythmias, cervical spondylosis, multiple sclerosis, hyperventilation and alcoholism. A solitary attack may be caused by head injury, vascular occlusion or a vasovagal faint.

The mouth

A variety of lesions can occur around the mouth and lips. Nurse practitioners may be faced with patient's concerns about infection, lesions, loss of taste, bleeding around the gums or discomfort of the tongue. A few of the commoner conditions will be considered here.

Ulceration

This is the most common disease to affect the oral mucosa: 20% of the population will suffer from ulcers at some time. There are several different forms of ulcers and diverse aetiological factors have been implicated in the pathogenesis. Nutrition, hormones, psychological causes, infection and trauma are all potential causes of ulcers and in the case of persistent ulceration it is important to consider the possibility of HIV infection, which is commonly linked to disorders of the mouth. Ulcers can occur in isolation or in crops which may disappear for weeks and then return. In the case of herpes-zoster there may be hundreds of tiny ulcers which cause the patient considerable discomfort and suffering.

Leucoplakia

Leucoplakia is associated with people who have AIDS. It appears as whitish patches of irregular size, often in several sites in the mouth and it is considered to be premalignant – careful observation and biopsy are necessary to monitor the condition. Smoking, spirits, syphilis and sharp teeth are other pre-disposing factors.

Moniliasis

Moniliasis (thrush) most commonly occurs in the mouths of immunosuppressed patients, people on antibiotic therapy or chemotherapy in malignant disease, debilitated elderly patients and sick children. The lesions appear as creamy-white curdy patches over the soft palate and may extend to the tongue. Monilia has even been noted on dentures and an essential part of the patient's treatment is a thorough cleaning of false teeth.

Raw red tongue

A raw red tongue suggests possible deficiency syndromes such as iron-deficiency anaemia, mal-absorption and pellagra. Further investigation and examination of the patient are required to determine the cause.

Gingivitis

The state of the gums and the teeth gives a good indication of the patient's general health and well-being. Swelling and redness of the margins of the gums are often the result of irritative calculus forma-tion. This may progress to peridontitis which is an inflammation of the deeper tissues around the teeth and is a common cause of the loss of teeth in adults. Gross hypertrophy of the gums with infection, bleed-ing and necrosis may be a sign of acute leukaemia.

Salivary disorders

The parotid, submandibular and minor salivary glands can be affected by acute or chronic inflam-mation, cysts, calculi and tumours. Mumps is the most common acute inflammatory condition of the salivary glands which causes swelling in the parotid glands, resulting in great pain and discomfort for the patient. Chronic inflammation is usually due to sialectasis (duct dilatation leading to stasis and infection). The gland becomes thickened and the patient complains of pain. Salivary retention cysts occur most often in the floor of the mouth and can become very large, expanding to involve the loose tissues. The saliva produced from the submandibular gland is mucoid and this results in the development of calculi in some patients.

As salivary glands contain lymph nodes within their structure, they may become the site of meta-stases from a primary site or from blood dyscrasias such as leukaemia. A solid parotid tumour in a child under the age of 16 is more likely than not to be malignant (Bull 1996).

Cancer

Cancer can occur anywhere in the mucosa of the lips, mouth, tongue and palate. Smoking, chewing tobacco, drinking spirits and poor oral hygiene may all play a role. The most common presentation is on the edge of the tongue as an ulcer. The ulcer will bleed easily and has a typical rolled edge. Occasionally a tumour may present as a lump beneath the surface of the tongue or as a fissure. Urgent biopsy is required in all of these cases.

Carcinoma of the lip

A localized chronic ulceration of the lips may be due to a carcinoma. The lower lip is the commonest site. Predisposing factors include pipe smoking and exposure to sunlight.

Loss of taste

Loss of taste is a problem which may not necessarily be linked to the function of the tongue. The ability to taste relies upon tactile, gustatory, thermal and olfactory sensations. If there are blockages in the nose due to polyps, a head cold or the inflammatory responses due to sinusitis, the patient will not be able to taste properly. If there is no abnormality to be found in the nose, the problem may be caused by viral injury, head injury or concussion.

Tonsillitis

Tonsillitis is common in children but can occur at any age. In children over 3 years of age tonsillitis is most commonly associated with *Streptococcus pyogenes* (Bull 1996). The patient will present with pyrexia and enlarged tonsils which are red and may exude pus; the pharyngeal mucosa will be inflamed and cervical lymph nodes may be enlarged. Tonsillitis may develop into acute otitis media or peritonsillar abscess (otherwise know as quinsy). Other complica-tions include acute nephritis, acute rheumatism and pulmonary infections.

Pharyngitis

Pharyngitis is common and may be caused by simple irritants such as exposure to cold, fumes, certain fruits or viral infection. Infective pharyngitis is most often caused by streptococcal infection. In simple acute pharyngitis the patient will be dysphagic and the mucosa of the pharynx will be hyperaemic. Infective pharyngitis leads to more severe dysphagia, pain and malaise.

If the soreness of the throat is persistent, the patient may have developed chronic pharyngitis. Predis-posing factors include smoking, drinking spirits, mouth-breathing, chronic sinusitis, chronic periodontal disease, use of antiseptic throat lozenges and repeated exposure to industrial fumes.

Differential diagnoses of sore throat

Seller (1993) differentiates between pharyngitis with ulcers and pharyngitis without ulcers when considering the differential diagnoses of sore throat. Most commonly the causes will be bacterial or viral pharyngitis; other causes are considered in Table 4.5.

Table 4.5 Differential diagnoses of pharyngitis

Without pharyngeal ulcers	With pharyngeal ulcers
Viral	Herpangina
Infectious mononucleosis	Candidiasis
Streptococcal pharyngitis	Herpes simplex
Gonococcal pharyngitis	
Allergic pharyngitis	

The face

A general review of the face can provide vital information for the nurse practitioner. A patient's face will reflect a variety of systemic diseases, including Cushing's syndrome, acromegaly, myxoedema, Parkinson's disease and Down's syndrome. In more localized conditions it may be possible to detect the swelling of the parotid glands in salivary gland disorders or the slightly gaping mouth of a patient who is unable to breathe effectively through the nose, for example in perennial allergic rhinitis. More specifically associated with the structure of the face is facial nerve paralysis.

Facial nerve paralysis

The causes of facial nerve paralysis are numerous and are listed in Table 4.6.

Table 4.6 Causes of facial nerve paralysis

Cerebral vascular lesions	Suppuration (otitis media)
Poliomyelitis	Multiple sclerosis
Cerebral tumours	Guillain-Barré syndrome
Bell's palsy	Sarcoidosis
Trauma	Herpes-zoster oticus
Tumours	

The patient will present with weakness of the facial muscles, causing an asymmetry which is accentuated on smiling or attempting to close the eyes. It is essential to be aware of the innervation of cranial nerve VII and the different findings you might expect for each of the differential diagnoses. In supranuclear lesions such as cerebral vascular lesions or cerebral tumours, for example, movements of the upper part of the face are likely to be unaffected as the forehead muscles have bilateral cortical representation.

Bell's palsy

The aetiology of Bell's palsy is unknown. However, the symptoms result from an acute inflammatory response which causes swelling in the facial nerve. Swelling within the myelin sheath of the nerve results in ischaemia in the axon. It usually has an acute onset and slowly progresses over 7–10 days. Patients often complain of pain behind the ear and may also complain of tinnitus, fever or a mild hearing deficit. Voluntary and involuntary movements of the face will be affected in varying degrees.

Bell's palsy is a diagnosis of exclusion and a high degree of suspicion of tumour must be maintained in the presence of associated tics or spasms, slow onset of paralysis and paralysis of isolated branches of the facial nerve. A thorough physical examination is essential to determine the exact location of the neural deficit.

The neck

The neck contains a vast number of structures, any number of which can be the source of ill health in a patient. This section will focus on the commonest complaints associated with the neck. For neck pain associated with the cervical vertebrae, see Chapter 12.

Neck swellings

Swellings in the neck may result from thyroid swellings, an acute abscess, cysts or metastatic nodes due to malignant involvement of a lymph node. A thyroid swelling may be a solitary nodule or a diffuse goitre which moves on swallowing.

Laryngitis

Laryngitis is commonest in the winter months and is usually caused by the common cold or influenza. The patient will present with dysphonia or aphonia and the larynx will appear red and dry with stringy mucus between the cords. Laryngitis is commonest in the winter months and is usually caused by the common cold or influenza. Predisposing factors include shouting, smoking and the consumption of spirits.

Acute laryngitis in children can lead to airway obstruction. The child will be unwell, have a harsh cough and a hoarse voice or aphonia. Acute epiglottitis is an emergency in children. Infection of the epiglottis by *Haemophilus influenzae* causes severe swelling which obstructs the laryngeal inlet. The child will have a quack-like cough and will prefer to sit up, leaning forward slightly.

History-taking

As with all history-taking, it is essential to be thorough and include the patient's past medical history, family history, social history, a systems review and a full analysis of the presenting symptoms. The following are examples of history-taking for the various components of the head and neck, with a specific focus on the main problems associated with each area. In exploring the history of a problem within the head or neck it is important that the nurse practitioner considers not only the presenting problem but also the surrounding structures.

Nose and sinuses

The blocked nose
Nasal obstruction may or may not be associated with nasal discharge. This history and initial assessment are particularly important when the patient complains of a blocked nose because they provide clues as to whether the problem is due to a functional abnormality or a mechanical obstruction (Solomons 1995). Nasal obstruction in children is most likely to be caused by a foreign body rather than a polyp, which is rare in a child. In adults the opposite is true and therefore the patient's age is an important factor in the assessment process for a blocked nose.

Rhinorrhoea
In nasal discharge it is important to assess the chronology of the illness. Is it seasonal, intermittent or continuous? Does the patient feel that the nose is blocked or irritable? Is it unilateral or bilateral? Unilateral rhinorrhoea requires careful consideration as the cause may be a deviated nasal septum, foreign body or tumour. Is it associated with any other symptoms, such as sneezing, watery eyes, facial pain, headache, fever or sore throat? It is important to enquire about medications as certain drugs, such as oral contraceptives, are related to a stuffy nose.

Rhinitis
A careful history charting the chronological history of rhinitis is essential to discover potential allergens and triggers of the condition. The nurse practitioner should be searching for clues relating to seasonal or diurnal variations or obvious exacerbating factors such as the work place (Scadding 1997). Personal and family history are also important when the patient presents with this problem, as a history of atopy makes the diagnosis of rhinitis more likely.

The ears
If the patient complains of ear pain, local causes are most likely in children. In adults it has been estimated that half of all ear pain is due to secondary causes (La Rosa 1998). The incidence of referred pain certainly increases with age (Seller 1993) and a thorough history is important to explore all possible causes of the problem.

The external ear
The history relating to otitis externa should focus on hearing loss, location of pain, facial twitching, paralysis, dizziness and trauma. It is also important to explore the patient's occupation, swimming habits, methods of cleaning the ears and any problems with the mouth, sinuses, nose or throat. Recent ear-piercing is an important clue in perichondritis and a history of atopy is useful in determining whether the patient may have eczematous ear canals.

Ask the patient to describe the drainage from the ear. A milky or bloody drainage may be linked with otitis externa but, more specifically, a cheesy green-blue/grey discharge may result from *Pseudomonas* infection, and clear drainage suggests eczematous weeping (La Rosa 1998).

The middle ear
It is important to explore drainage from the infection of the middle ear. Timing of drainage linked to the patient's report of pain will assist the nurse practitioner in determining whether there may be a perforation of the tympanic membrane and will therefore help guide the physical examination.

The inner ear
It is important to encourage the patient to describe the sensations associated with dizziness or vertigo. It is possible to differentiate between true vertigo and dizziness (p. 45). If the patient states that tinnitus is present in association with vertigo, the nurse practitioner should have a high suspicion of Ménière's disease, as tinnitus will be absent in benign postural vertigo. Nausea and vomiting may be present in all cases of dizziness or vertigo; unilateral weakness, diplopia, numbness or tingling may be due to brainstem disease. The duration and timing of the symptoms are important, as in positional vertigo the symptoms last from minutes to hours, in Ménière's disease from hours to days and in brainstem disease from days to weeks. In all conditions of the ear it is useful to know the patient's occupation to determine exposure to irritants such as dust and any recent trauma to the ear such as close proximation to a gunshot, barotrauma or air travel.

The mouth
Many of the disorders associated with the mouth

have a systemic component and it is important to ask the patient about general health and other illnesses. There is a close link between lesions of the mouth and HIV infection and therefore issues of HIV status should be explored with the patient. Treatments in malignant disease such as radiotherapy and chemotherapy will predispose the patient to candida of the mouth; information on current illnesses and medications should be elicited.

As there is a close link between smoking and carcinomas of the lips and mucosa of the mouth, the patient's smoking history should be explored. The type of tobacco used is important, as pipe smoking is a predisposing factor of carcinomas of the lip and chewing tobacco is a predisposing factor for cancers of the mouth. Alcohol consumption is also important here, with particular reference to the quantity of spirits consumed.

The face

Important questions in the focused history of a patient with unilateral facial palsy include determining whether the weakness is unilateral, if postauricular pain is present and if there is ipsilateral lacrimation. These three signs are strong indicators of Bell's palsy (Biullue 1997). Other important questions include whether the onset was acute or slow, duration of symptoms, history of chronic disease, drooling, altered taste, skin lesions, asymmetrical facial expressions, history of a tick bite and pregnancy. Herpes simplex, HIV, Lyme disease, pregnancy, tumours, infectious processes, diabetes mellitus, hypothyroidism and demyelinating disease are all differential diagnoses of Bell's palsy and should be considered during the history-taking process.

The neck

A swelling in the neck may be due to a variety of causes and can be related to systemic diseases as well as local causes. Focusing on the patient's general health to explore level of energy and family history to consider thyroid disorders will assist in the subsequent physical examination and further investigations.

Physical examination

As with all examinations, physical examination of the patient who presents with a problem in the region of the head or neck should commence with observation. The examination will be focused on the problem area, however, it is important to look beyond the presenting symptom and consider these surrounding structures and potential links between these structures. Palpation of the affected area follows observation. Percussion and auscultation are generally not required in an examination of the head and neck.

The nose and sinuses

A general inspection of the external nose is necessary to note any deformity, swelling or erythema. Observe for signs of the allergic crease, which is a small wrinkle which develops just above the tip of the nose and is due to the constant rubbing associated with allergic rhinitis. This is known as the allergic salute. The inspection is continued by placing gentle pressure on the tip of the nose to widen the nostrils. A penlight or otoscope is necessary to provide a view of the nasal vestibule. The nasal septum can be observed for signs of deviation, which is not uncommon and rarely obstructs airflow.

The inside of the nose can be inspected as Bates (1993) suggests, using a large ear speculum with an otoscope or, as Colman (1992) suggests, using a nasal speculum and a bull's-eye lamp and head mirror. Whichever approach is used, the speculum must be inserted gently. The nasal mucosa is sensitive and the patient will automatically withdraw and tilt the head away from the examiner. It is important to view the nasal septum, inferior and middle turbinates in a systematic way, focusing on the mucosa for signs of swelling, bleeding or exudate and the septum for deviation, perforation or inflammation. Observe for any abnormalities such as ulcers and polyps.

Palpation of the sinuses should be carried out with care and consideration: the patient may be experiencing discomfort and pain from infection and inflammation of the mucous membranes. Palpate for areas of local tenderness by pressing up on the maxillary sinuses (just below the cheekbones) and over the frontal sinuses (just below the eyebrows).

The ears

Observation of the ears commences with an inspection of each auricle and the surrounding tissues, noting any lumps, skin lesions, deformities, discharge from the ear and areas of erythema. Otoscopic examination of the ear canal should be carried out with the largest ear speculum that the canal will accommodate. It may be necessary to straighten the ear canal by grasping the auricle and pulling it upwards, backwards and slightly away from the head. This movement may be painful for the patient and may be a sign of acute otitis externa. It is essential to ensure that the otoscope is held in a firm and secure manner by anchoring the instrument with the examiner's hand placed firmly against the patient's head. This prevents any injury should the patient move and is particularly valuable in the examination of a child.

The ear canal should be observed for cerumen, foreign bodies or any discharge or oedema and the skin of the ear canal should be inspected for signs of inflammation.

The eardrum should be shiny with a clear cone of light and the handle and short process of the malleus should be visible. Abnormalities of the eardrum may be present, including perforations, red bulging drums, the amber colour of a serous effusion or chalky white patches of tympanosclerosis. It may not always be easy to achieve a full view of the eardrum and the examiner will have to move the otoscope around gently to gain as full a view as possible.

If the patient has complained of poor hearing or the examiner suspects that the hearing has been impaired, a gross hearing test can be carried out during the examination. Auditory acuity is tested by standing 30–60 cm away, exhaling and then whispering softly towards one ear while the second ear is occluded. This process should be repeated for the second ear and the results of the two sides compared. Weber's test for lateralization can be utilized to assess for unilateral conductive hearing loss. A 512 or 1024 Hz tuning fork is placed on the top of the patient's head and the patient states whether the sound can be heard equally on both sides or if it can be heard more easily on one side. In unilateral conductive hearing loss the sound is heard in the impaired ear. In unilateral sensorineural hearing loss the sound is heard in the good ear.

Air and bone conduction can be compared by carrying out the Rinne test. The tuning fork is struck and then placed on the mastoid bone behind the ear and level with the ear canal. Normally, sound conducted by air is louder than sound conducted by bone. Therefore if the patient is asked to compare the loudness of the sound in this position with that produced by holding the vibrating ends of the fork by the ear, an abnormal result would be to say that the sound heard with the fork on the mastoid process is louder. Further information can be obtained after placing the fork on the mastoid and asking the patient to state when the vibrations can no longer be heard, noting the time interval involved. The tuning fork is then quickly moved to be placed just at the entrance of the ear canal and the length of time the patient can still hear the sound is also noted. Normally, air conduction will be longer than bone conduction and the record in the patient's notes is AC > BC (positive Rinne). If bone conduction is longer than air conduction there may be conductive hearing loss – a foreign body or cerumen in the ear canal, for example. If air conduction is longer than bone conduction, this may be a normal finding or the patient may have sensorineural loss. Table 4.6 provides a summary of the interpretation of Rinne and Weber tests.

Table 4.6   Interpretation of Rinne and Weber tests

Right ear	Left ear	Interpretation
Rinne positive (AC > BC) Weber central	Rinne positive (AC > BC)	Normal or Mild/moderate or severe bilateral sensorineural loss
Rinne positive (AC > BC) Weber → left	Rinne negative (AC < BC)	Left conductive or mixed hearing loss
Rinne negative (AC < BC) Weber central	Rinne negative (AC < BC)	Bilateral mixed or conductive loss

Source: Adapted from Toghill (1995).

The diagnostic decision is based on the rest of the patient's history and physical examination.

The mouth

Examination of the mouth should begin with the lips to observe for colour, ulcers, cracking or discoloration. The corners of the mouth should particularly be checked for cracking as this may be a sign of iron deficiency. It is useful to wear gloves and to use a tongue depressor to examine the oral mucosa. With a good light the roof of the mouth, the gums and teeth and the underside of the tongue should be inspected carefully for lesions and signs of infection.

Ask the patient to put out his or her tongue. An assessment of cranial nerve XII can be made depending on whether the protruding tongue is symmetrical or asymmetrical. The condition of the tongue, its hydration and the turgor of the skin reflect the degree of hydration.

There are several unusual but normal findings in examination of the tongue. The geographic tongue has a map-like appearance due to areas of epithelium which are denuded of papillae. This can be a normal part of advancing age. A black hairy tongue results from the elongation of the filiform papillae on the dorsal surface and again, in the absence of antibiotic therapy, this can be a normal finding.

With the patient's mouth open and the tongue not protruded, the pharynx can be inspected by asking the patient to say 'ah'. This also checks the movement of the soft palate and pharynx and includes an assessment of cranial nerve X. In Xth nerve paralysis the soft palate fails to rise and the uvula deviates to one side. The soft palate, pharynx, uvula and tonsils can be inspected for swelling, erythema, exudate or white spots.

The face

A general inspection of the face provides the nurse practitioner with an overall idea of systemic illness, for example, enlargement of the bones in acromegaly or a fixed expression of Parkinson's disease. Facial pain or paralysis requires a more detailed examination of the facial cranial nerve (cranial nerve VII). All branches of the facial cranial nerve must be assessed, as involvement of just one branch may indicate a tumour. If the forehead is intact, a more central aetiology can be suspected. Ask the patient to puff out the cheeks, grimace, clamp the eyes together and wrinkle the brow. Test taste sensation on the anterior two-thirds of the tongue. A careful examination of the skin includes checking for herpes-zoster and the ear canal should also be checked for the vesicular lesions of herpes.

The neck

The neck should be inspected for symmetry, signs of swelling and any visible lymph nodes. The patient must be relaxed for palpation of the lymph nodes and the examiner should follow a structured pattern to cover all 10 areas. Lymph nodes should be noted for size, shape, mobility and tenderness and it should be possible to roll a node in two directions. An enlarged supraclavicular node is highly suggestive of metastatic disease, any hard or fixed nodes suggest malignancy and tender nodes suggest inflammation. Table 4.7 provides an overview of the lymph nodes and a systematic method of examination. See also Figure 4.5 for a diagrammatic representation of the lymph nodes.

Continuing on the external surface of the neck, the trachea and thyroid gland should be inspected

Table 4.7   Examination of the lymph nodes

1	Periauricular
2	Posterior auricular
3	Occipital
4	Tonsillar
5	Submandibular
6	Submental
7	Superficial cervical
8	Posterior cervical
9	Deep cervical chain
10	Supraclavicular

for symmetry and any signs of swelling. It should be possible to place your finger between the trachea and the sternomastoid and the space should be equal on both sides. By asking the patient to swallow, the thyroid cartilage, thyroid gland and cricoid cartilage will all rise and it should be possible to note the symmetry of the movement. The same assessment is carried out during palpation. The patient is examined from behind and the examiner places the fingers of both hands on the patient's neck so that the index fingers are just below the cricoid. By asking the patient to swallow, it may be possible to palpate the glandular tissue as it rises and then falls back to the resting position. Benign and malignant nodules may be palpated and the patient may report tenderness in thyroiditis. If the thyroid gland is enlarged, listen over the lateral lobes with a stethoscope for bruits. A bruit over the thyroid may suggest hyperthyroidism.

Bull (1996) suggests that indirect laryngoscopy can be carried out to visualize the vocal cords,

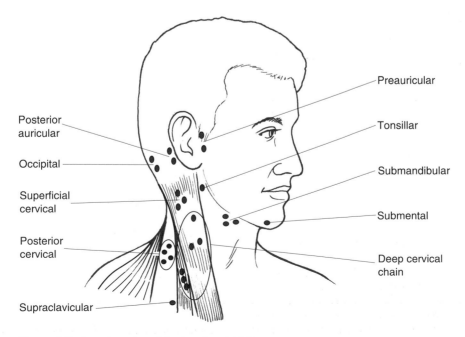

Figure 4.5   Lymph nodes of the head and neck

epiglottis and larynx. This takes instruction and practice and requires the use of a laryngeal mirror. This is one method of viewing the larynx, although if examination is essential in the diagnostic process, it might be necessary to refer for fibreoptic laryngoscopy or direct laryngoscopy under general anaesthesia.

Management and patient education

The management of disorders of the head and neck will vary according to diagnosis, patient choice, local protocols and referral procedures. The following suggestions may be particularly useful in practice.

Instillation of nasal drops

The management of sinusitis or rhinitis will be with nasal drops. Patients require instruction on the use of nasal drops as they frequently administer them in an upright position and most of the medication runs down into the oesophagous or runs straight back down the nose and on to the patient's handkerchief. The success of treatment depends upon the medication reaching the right place and remaining there. Colman (1992) suggests that the patient adopts the head-back or Mecca position (Figure 4.6). The Mecca position is particularly effective and the patient should hold the position for a few minutes after administration of the drops.

Instillation of ear drops

Ear drops are used in the management of otitis externa and, like the nasal drops, the administration of the medication depends upon correct technique and patient understanding. The patient should be instructed to lie down on the side that is not infected (if there is bilateral involvement, the patient has to do one ear at a time with adequate rest in between). The drops are then dropped into the ear one at a time. The patient may need to move the pinna gently to help the drops move down into the canal. The patient must remain lying in the same position for 2–3 minutes. Before returning to the upright position it is useful to place a piece of cotton wool which has been soaked in a few of the drops in the outer part of the ear. The cotton wool prevents the drops from running out of the ear and can be removed after an hour or so (La Rosa 1998).

Tinnitus

Often little can be done to relieve the suffering of tinnitus. Patients may become depressed, fearful and anxious and will search for a cure. Bull (1996)

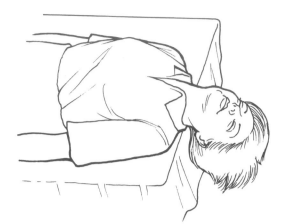

(a) The patient lies prone on the bed with head hanging over the side

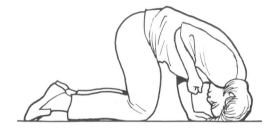

(b) The Mecca position

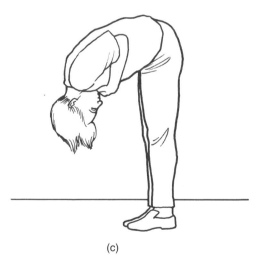

(c)

Figure 4.6   Recommended positions for using nasal drops

suggests that there are several points which are helpful in the management of tinnitus:

- Take the patient seriously
- Treat any abnormalities of the ear
- When appropriate, reassure the patient that the condition is benign
- Examine the patient thoroughly

- Be honest with the patient
- Sedatives and tranquillizers may help in some situations
- Treat depression thoroughly and expertly
- A hearing aid may help if the patient also has hearing loss
- Tinnitus maskers are available to produce 'white noise'
- Playing a radio at night may help the patient to sleep
- Relaxation techniques may help some patients
- Refer to self-help groups and other sources of information.

Rhinitis

Some helpful tips for people who suffer from seasonal allergic rhinitis have been suggested by Scadding (1997). These tips can form the basis of a self-management plan and are specifically aimed at reducing the risk of exposure to allergens.

- Listen to the pollen forecast and plan your day accordingly
- Wear wrap-around sunglasses
- Rub petroleum jelly (Vaseline) into the inside of your nose
- Avoid irritants such as paint or cigarette smoke
- Bring in the washing and close bedroom windows before the evening as pollen grains descend as the air cools
- Keep car windows closed and consider buying a car filter
- Avoid walking through or cutting grass
- Avoid picnics and camping
- If you go out in the countryside, shower and wash your hair when you return
- Take an intranasal spray regularly if prescribed.

Otitis externa

Patients can be instructed on the prevention of otitis externa: one of the golden rules is never to place anything smaller than your elbow in your ear! Patients should be encouraged not to clean their ears with hair grips or cotton tips and should also be advised to wear ear plugs when swimming. Patients can be advised to mix equal parts of vinegar and water and place 2–3 drops in each ear after swimming. This helps prevent any infection from developing. If patients develop otitis externa they should be advised not to swim for 7–10 days. Petroleum jelly (Vaseline) can be used to provide a simple yet effective barrier to water when showering and the patient should be encouraged to dry both ears thoroughly if they do get wet (La Rosa 1998).

As with all regimes of management and treatment, the likelihood of success relies heavily on the accuracy of the initial diagnosis and the knowledge and cooperation of the patient. Nurse practitioners who spend time listening to their patient's concerns and helping them to understand their illness and treatment will have a greater success in the management of disorders of the head and neck.

References

Bates, B. (1995) A Guide to Physical Examination and History Taking, 6th edn., Philadelphia, JB Lippincott.

Biullue J.S. (1997) Bell's palsy: an update on idiopathic facial paralysis, Nurse Practitioner, 22(8), pp. 88–105.

Bull P.D. (1996) Diseases of the Ear, Nose and Throat, 8th edn., Oxford, Blackwell Science.

Coley A.N., Kay N. J. (1992) ENT Practice for the GP Surgery, Edinburgh, Churchill Livingstone.

Colman B.H. (1992) Hall and Colman's Diseases of the Nose, Throat and Ear, and Head and Neck, Edinburgh, Churchill Livingstone.

Cross S. (1998) Perennial allergic rhinitis, Practice Nursing, 9(11), pp. 34–38.

Fisher P. (1998) Tinnitus, Practice Nursing, 9(3), pp. 33–36.

La Rosa S. (1998) Primary care management of otitis externa, Nurse Practitioner, 23(6), pp. 125–133.

Scadding G.K. (1997) Rhinitis explained, Asthma Journal, 2(1), pp. 11–17.

Seller R. (1993) Differential Diagnosis of Common Complaints, 2nd edn. Philadelphia, W B Saunders.

Solomons N.B. (1995) Practical Introduction to ENT Disease, London, Springer-Verlag.

Toghill P. (1995) Examining Patients: An Introduction to Clinical Medicine, 2nd edn., London, Edward Arnold.

CHAPTER 5

The nervous system

Mike Walsh

Introduction

The importance of the nervous system, and in particular the central nervous system (CNS), cannot be overestimated as it is this system which makes us essentially human. The higher cerebral functions distinguish us from the rest of the animal kingdom and give us the power to think and reason. Without such an advanced CNS and the special sense of vision, you would not be able to read this book, neither would we have been able to write it.

The nurse practitioner is likely to meet patients in everyday practice whose primary presenting problem relates to alterations in consciousness, other aspects of the CNS or peripheral nerve problems. Patients with migraines and headaches, minor head injuries, faints, fits, dizziness and collapses will be encountered frequently in primary health care and minor injury settings. The nurse practitioner may also see patients with early signs of more serious disorders such as Alzheimer's disease, parkinsonism or a cerebral tumour, whilst peripheral nerve problems such as carpal tunnel syndrome may also present. It is important therefore to be able to recognize signs and symptoms suggestive of more serious disease which require medical management and differentiate these patients from others with less serious conditions that the nurse practitioner can manage.

Pathophysiology

Headache

A headache is a symptom of an underlying disorder rather than a disease in itself. The underlying problem is usually minor, although the headache itself may be causing considerable distress; in a small number of cases there may be serious pathology such as meningitis.

The two most common presentations are tension headache and migraine. The exact process involved in a tension headache is unclear but it typically presents as a generalized aching sensation which may become localized to the rear of the head or around the temporal region. It may be brought on by any activity which requires sustained concentration, such as driving, and is often associated with anxiety and high stress levels. The patient usually complains of recurrent headaches over a substantial period of time which can be relieved by mild analgesics such as paracetamol.

Migraines are more serious and debilitating. They are caused by arterial dilatation inside or outside the skull. The pain is usually localized to one or more specific areas; it is severe and persistent and may be associated with nausea and vomiting. The onset may be associated with visual disturbances and may be provoked by certain foods. Mild analgesics alone often do not relieve the pain which may last for hours or even days in severe cases.

Other causes of headache include visual problems in a patient who needs glasses. S/he may be unaware of this fact and has been attempting to compensate for loss of vision by prolonged contraction of the extraocular muscles. The pain is a steady dull ache localized around the eyes and a visual acuity test will quickly reveal the cause of the problem. Sinusitis may also lead the patient to attend, complaining of frontal headaches across the forehead and cheeks. Trigeminal neuralgia, another potential cause of presentation, causes severe, stabbing facial pains, typically of only a few seconds duration but recurring frequently. The pain follows the path of the second and/or third divisions of the trigeminal nerve (see p. 60), though involvement of both sides of the face is rare (Rees and Williams 1995). Its cause is unknown, though specific triggers such as shaving or touch may be identified by the patient.

Meningitis, subarachnoid haemorrhage and brain tumours are the commonest serious disorders producing severe, generalized headaches. Each has its own pattern of associated signs and symptoms. The pain is typically constant and severe and is not relieved by over-the-counter analgesics. Onset is usually rapid with meningitis and subarachnoid haemorrhage, and associated with neck stiffness and photophobia as a result of meningeal irritation. Pain associated with a tumour has a more gradual onset and neurological symptoms vary depending on the site of the tumour.

Trauma

The management of severe head injuries clearly lies well outside the remit of the nurse practitioner. However, minor head injuries with no loss of consciousness or with only a brief interruption to consciousness may present frequently. Bullock and Teasdale (1991) estimated that head-injured patients accounted for 10% of the workload of the A&E service. Most patients have simple concussion where the brain impacts against the internal surface of the skull, leading to a brief interruption of the reticular activating system and consequent loss of consciousness (less than 5 minutes) and a short period of amnesia (Walsh 1996). Alternatively the patient may be dazed and suffer a decreased level of consciousness for a few minutes without actually being unconscious. These may be thought of as primary brain injuries which are diffuse in nature. Injuries involving higher energy levels may produce a primary focal injury localized to the point of impact (or directly opposite), such as contusion of the brain which leads to a more prolonged period of unconsciousness. Skull fracture may occur whilst severe injuries involve ruptured blood vessels and haematoma formation. There may also be widespread primary diffuse brain tissue damage. Delayed secondary brain damage may occur in severe head injuries due to cerebral hypoxia, ischaemia or brainstem herniation due to raised intracranial pressure (Sinclair 1991). The nurse practitioner should be aware that occasionally patients present with a lucid interval when they have regained consciousness, but then as intracranial pressure rises (usually due to haematoma formation), the level of consciousness deteriorates into coma.

Convulsions and collapses

It is important to differentiate between convulsions, simple faints and other causes of loss of consciousness such as transient ischaemic attacks. The nurse practitioner usually has to rely upon a second-hand account of the incident, or it may even be unwitnessed, so diagnosis is difficult. A good grasp of the pathology involved assists in making sense of the presenting clinical signs and reaching a differential diagnosis.

Convulsions or seizures are classified by Bates (1995) into those that commence with focal manifestations (partial seizures) and those that affect the whole body, producing bilateral convulsions and/or loss of consciousness. Partial seizures may be subdivided according to whether the patient remains conscious (simple) or loses consciousness (complex). Partial seizures are usually caused by a localized lesion within the cerebral cortex such as a tumour or an area of scarring. Partial seizures may be of the Jacksonian type, where motor activity dominates, leading to localized tonic/clonic movements, although consciousness is retained throughout.

Generalized seizures (the term grand mal describes a generalized seizure involving tonic and clonic activity) indicate a bilateral cortical cause which is frequently idiopathic in origin and manifestations usually appear in childhood. However, if the onset is in later life the cause may be a cerebral lesion such as a tumour, scarring from an old head injury or withdrawal from alcohol sedative drugs when there is dependence. The seizure may be metabolic in origin and disorders such as uraemia, hypoglycaemia, hyperglycaemia and water intoxication are likely. The effects of flashing lights cannot be ruled out in inducing generalized seizures. The term petit mal was used to describe a transient loss of awareness, but not consciousness. This is now known as an absence seizure (Hilton 1997).

After initial collapse and loss of consciousness, the person passes through a tonic phase of muscle rigidity and cyanosis, followed by the clonic phase of generalized convulsions during which significant head injury may occur. A period of unconsciousness follows associated with profound muscle relaxation which may lead to incontinence before the patient passes through a confused, drowsy period. This postictal phase may be characterized by an elevated temperature associated with the clonic muscular activity. A positive Babinski response is commonly found (p. 63) postictally and the patient will have no recollection of events surrounding the seizure.

Collapse due to a sudden reduction in blood reaching the brain is known as syncope. Simple fainting (vasovagal syncope) is due to a sudden fall in blood pressure caused by peripheral vasodilatation with no compensatory rise in cardiac output. A syncope attack is often associated with some form of generalized motor activity, hence it is often confused with a fit (Hilton 1997). The cause is usually a major emotional disturbance such as fear or pain and predisposing factors include hunger, tiredness and a hot stuffy atmosphere. If someone stands up suddenly he or she may faint as a result of postural hypotension if there is an insufficient reflex response to increase cardiac output and blood pressure. This may be caused by antihypertensive medication or a disorder of the autonomic nervous system. As soon as the person reaches the horizontal position, the brain receives adequate blood flow and consciousness is regained, although there may be a short period of confusion immediately afterwards. Cardiac arrhythmias may also cause a sudden collapse as they may lead to inadequate cardiac output (p. 97). This may be associated with tachycardia or bradycardia. More seriously, ventricular fibrillation may have occurred, in which case there is no effective cardiac output and immediate resuscitation is required. In an elderly patient, it is always worth checking whether s/he is on a pacemaker as a failure in the pacemaker can lead to profound bradycardia.

The nurse practitioner should be aware of the possibility that the collapse may have been caused by a hypoglycaemic state. In this case the classic picture of increasing confusion, sweating and tremor before collapse, in a known diabetic, coupled with a low capillary blood sugar reading, makes the diagnosis simple. Some individuals with disordered personality may also collapse. This is usually hysterical behaviour and is accompanied by normal vital signs and no obviously abnormal signs. Hysterical overbreathing will produce signs of tetany (carpopedal spasm) due to imbalance in blood gases as carbon dioxide levels fall, inducing respiratory alkalosis. Drug abuse should always be suspected in cases of collapse – recent rises in heroin abuse and fatal reactions to Ecstasy are salient warnings.

The possibility of a transient ischaemic attack due to temporary cerebral ischaemia should also be borne in mind. Problems may be associated with emboli in the internal carotid artery which often present with a mild or transient hemiparesis and/or transient blindness, whilst vertebrobasilar ischaemia can produce a sensation of vertigo leading to unsteadiness, nausea and vomiting.

A presentation which may lead patients to worry that they have had a stroke is the unilateral facial paralysis of Bell's palsy. This is due to inflammation of the facial nerve. The inflamed nerve is compressed on its passage through the temporal bone, leading to muscle paralysis developing over 7–10 days. Recovery begins after 3 weeks and for 85% of patients is complete within 6 months. Some are not so lucky and may be left with a permanent facial deformity (Billue 1997).

There is a grey area between a collapse and a fall. Elderly patients in particular may present with a vague history of falling and it is important to try and establish whether the person did fall accidentally as a result of tripping or loss of balance, or whether s/he collapsed as a result of a medical reason such as syncope or transient ischaemic attack. Eye-witness accounts are crucial in deciding between these two possibilities. How much the person can recall of the event is also a valuable guide: if s/he cannot recall hitting the ground, this suggests s/he lost consciousness first and then fell, which makes an accidental fall, unlikely.

Degenerative brain disease (Alzheimer's disease)

A consultation with a person aged 45–70 may take place for many reasons. In the process of the consultation the nurse practitioner may easily miss the early signs and symptoms of Alzheimer's disease. Behaviour which may be dismissed as inattentiveness or carelessness may be the first warning signs before the disease progresses to more advanced stages where there is recent and long-term memory loss, personality changes, apathy, loss of initiative, neglect of personal hygiene and appearance, disorientation followed by motor aphasia (inability to recall words even though the person wishes to say them) and speech-slurring. In the later stages there is complete disintegration of the person with total loss of recognition of family and friends, disorientation, inability to perform simple cognitive tasks such as writing your own name and loss of motor function, including the ability to walk. Finally the person loses all language skills, becoming doubly incontinent and immobile. Although at present there is no cure, early detection by an alert nurse practitioner could lead to better management of the disorder, whilst there is hope that in the future treatments may become available to slow down the progress of the disease and may be one day lead to a cure.

Other neurological disorders

Many disorders of the CNS have signs and symptoms of problems with balance, walking and coordination. It is possible that a consultation with the nurse practitioner may be the first point of contact with the NHS for a patient in the early stages of such a disorder. It is therefore essential to recognize abnormal signs or suggestive features in a history so that the patient may be speedily referred on to a medical practitioner. It is beyond the scope of this book to go into a detailed account of such neurological disorders; however, we will briefly mention some of the more common neurological diseases.

Many patients who present with problems associated with balance or gait are suffering from disease of the CNS. Parkinson's disease (paralytic agitans) is one such disease which affects one person in every 100 in the 60–70-year age group. The disease is a complex clinical syndrome which stems from a lack of dopamine which usually exerts an inhibitory effect on movement by opposing or inhibiting the effects of the neurotransmitter acetylcholine. Lack of dopamine induces tremor, rigidity, difficulty in voluntary movement and slowness, but the person's higher mental faculties may escape damage for many years. The nurse practitioner will be familiar with the classical shuffling gait of Parkinson's disease where the person appears to be about to fall forwards, the loss of facial expression and also the characteristic tremor of the upper limb which is maximal at rest and produces a pill-rolling movement as the thumb moves back and forth across the fingertips. It is possible that the nurse practitioner will encounter the patient in the early stages of the disease before such a classical picture has developed and s/he will have to be alert for early signs of stiffness and slight tremor.

Multiple sclerosis commonly presents in young adults: 60% of patients have their first attack aged between 20 and 40. The disease affects 40–60 people per 100 000 in the UK and women are twice as likely as men to be affected (Rees and Williams 1995). This chronic, progressive disease leads to patchy demyelination of the brain and spinal cord and its early signs and symptoms can be variable, depending on the exact location of the damage. Symptoms such as bladder or bowel dysfunction, fatigue, muscle weakness, visual disturbance, transient tingling sensations or numbness (paraesthesia) are all associated with multiple sclerosis. Unlike parkinsonism, tremor is pronounced when the person is trying to do something (intention tremor) rather than at rest. Relatives may report personality changes and increased emotional lability.

The nurse practitioner needs to be aware of the signs of raised intracranial pressure: not only is it crucial to detect this in cases of head injury, but signs are also present in someone developing a brain tumour, although the onset is much more insidious with a tumour (weeks and months rather than minutes). Rising intracranial pressure leads to a reduction in perfusion of cerebral tissue and cerebral hypoxia. A key early sign in response to a cerebral tumour is papilloedema (p. 79), while later signs of rising intracranial pressure include decreasing level of consciousness, unreactive dilated pupils (only one pupil may be affected if the lesion is localized), raised blood pressure and bradycardia. The history may reveal complaints of headaches and nausea. Neurological deficits may also be observed depending on the area of the brain affected, whilst convulsions and changes in mental capacity may also occur.

The term polyneuropathy describes a symmetrical disorder of the peripheral nerves that usually involves both sensory and motor tracts. The disease process involves either demyelination or damage to the axon itself. The patient tends to complain of altered sensation and weakness in varying degrees depending on which sort of nerve tracts are attacked. The longest nerves are affected first, hence symptoms tend to start at the feet and work upwards, affecting the hands later. There are a wide range of causes such as Guillain–Barré syndrome, vitamin B_{12}

deficiency, diabetes, systemic lupus erythematosus, vasculitis and alcohol abuse. Peripheral nerve problems associated with trauma and compression are discussed in Chapter 12, with particular reference to the upper limb and the lumbar spine.

The CNS may be attacked by pathogens and acute bacterial meningitis has recently received a great deal of publicity. Various organisms may cause this infection, giving rise to meningeal inflammation, raised intracranial pressure, disturbance of cerebrospinal fluid circulation and cerebral ischaemia. This pathology manifests as pyrexia, headache, photophobia, neck stiffness, vomiting and reduced level of consciousness. The most serious form of the illness involves *Neisseria meningitidis*, possibly leading to septicaemia, a petechial or purpuric rash, disseminated intravascular coagulation, septic shock and death within a few hours.

Taking a focused history

The nurse practitioner should remember that neurological disorders may produce no obvious signs at the time of the examination. Arriving at a likely diagnosis depends on taking a good history. The picture is complicated by the fact that neurological symptoms may be induced by stress alone (Munroe and Edwards 1995).

Headaches

The PQRST mnemonic may be used to explore the main symptoms. If the main complaint is headaches, start by asking what brings them on (*provocation*); possible causes include sleeping, posture, reading or other activities involving concentration. What relieves the headaches (*palliation*)? Ask the patient to describe the pain in his or her own words (*quality*); it may be a dull ache, tight, boring, burning, pressing. It is important to describe where the pain is and whether it radiates (*region*), together with how intense it is (*severity*) using a three- or five-point scale. Finally, duration of episodes needs to be discovered together with any particular time of day or month (*time*). A good description of headaches obtained in this structured way should permit a safe conclusion about their probable cause.

Impaired function and abnormal sensation

The same approach can be applied to other presenting complaints. Problems with gait, coordination, weakness or unusual sensations can be explored attempting to discover what brings the problem on and whether rest relieves the problem (P). Patients' own description of their feelings and perceptions together with an account of how the problem affects them should be explored (Q). The areas of the body affected should be ascertained (R). It is important to know how severe and disabling the symptoms are (S). Speed of onset and variation of symptoms with time should be checked (T). Problems such as numbness and paraesthesia (tingling or other abnormal sensation) affecting the sensory nervous system should be assessed in the same way.

Level of consciousness and orientation

In dealing with a head injury, collapse or convulsion, it is important to discover how much the patient can remember. If there is a gap in memory this indicates that the patient was probably unconscious. Eye-witness reports are invaluable and should be checked against the classic stages in a grand mal convulsion to see if the story matches. Alternatively the person may have fallen and recovered consciousness quickly with no evidence of tonic/clonic phases, indicating that a syncope (simple faint) is the most likely explanation. The presence of any odd feelings or sensations immediately before the collapse should be checked, such as dizziness, palpitations or an epileptic aura. It is important to know if this has happened before and, if so, whether the person is taking antiepileptic medication or whether there is a pattern to these episodes.

Patients' orientation in time and space should be ascertained to ensure they have fully recovered and for their own safety. (Where are you? What time is it?) The first sign of deterioration in a head-injured patient will be a decreasing level of consciousness, related to rising intracranial pressure. If the patient presents in a confused condition, it is important to ascertain from relatives or friends the normal level of mental functioning and whether this has changed significantly recently, as well as any change in personality. For non-trauma patients, it is possible to check orientation and memory tactfully in the guise of confirming information held in their notes, but not by asking closed questions which have a yes/no answer, where the patient can guess the correct answer. Questions such as When did you last see us? What is your address? Who do you live with? What day is it today? can easily be asked in a manner which will not cause offence to the fully alert, oriented person.

If the patient has had a generalized seizure (grand mal) s/he will remain confused and disoriented (postictal) for up to an hour afterwards, whereas in a simple syncope attack the person will be oriented and able to answer questions within 2–3 minutes. This is a useful aid to making a differential diagnosis between these two possibilities.

Other symptoms

In addition to the three main features discussed above, patients should be asked whether they have noticed any other unusual symptoms recently. This open-ended question may reveal important information. Visual disturbances should be noted together with any complaints of dizziness. Nausea and vomiting are key indicators of raised intracranial pressure and should be included in the history. Only when these key areas have been explored should the nurse practitioner move on to other aspects of the history.

Previous medical history

It is important to ask about previous medical history in all cases, especially in an individual who has collapsed. Key indicators include whether the person suffers from diabetes, epilepsy or Ménière's disease, is under treatment for hypertension or cardiac arrhythmias or has a history of transient ischaemic attacks. In some cases of neurological disorder, the causative event may have happened many years previously, a careful medical history should include questions about childhood and early adult life. Significant aspects of the previous medical history include recent infections, head or spinal injury, congenital abnormalities, birth trauma, meningitis or any previous cerebrovascular accident. The nurse practitioner should enquire tactfully about any previous mental health problems which may be relevant.

Medication

It is important to enquire about medication as this will give important clues about relevant factors in the medical history, such as cardiovascular disease, diabetes or epilepsy. It is also necessary to ask about recreational drugs as they all act upon the CNS. Withdrawal from drug use may be the problem. A timely reminder is necessary here to the nurse practitioner not to stereotype patients and make assumptions about illegal drug use. This is now a widespread phenomenon across all sections of society, particularly with the young, and it is not restricted to deprived urban areas. In dealing with persons who collapse, questions about drug use should always be asked, especially with younger individuals.

Family history

The history should also bring in family history, as many neurological disorders involve a genetic predisposition. Epilepsy, multiple sclerosis and migraine are cited by Munro and Edwards (1995) as common examples, while other rarer diseases such as muscular dystrophy and Huntington's chorea are known to be genetic disorders.

Personal and social history

The personal and social history is important as stress or occupation could be contributing to the disorder. Symptoms such as headaches and migraines can be brought on by stressors such as divorce, bereavement, other domestic problems, moving house or changing jobs while these factors may also be associated with exacerbations of multiple sclerosis or epilepsy. Occupational factors include prolonged concentration on VDUs leading to headaches, exposure to dangerous chemicals such as organophosphates in farming and recurrent overuse of certain joints such as the wrist which may lead to carpal tunnel syndrome. Drug use is a key area of social history which has been dealt with above. Alcohol intake is particularly important as it may be contributing to the problems of diabetes or epilepsy.

The history should also explore whether there have been any recent changes in memory or behaviour, particularly focusing on the ability to care for self (dressing, hygiene, toileting) as deterioration in self-care and memory are early signs of dementia. Sleeping patterns should be explored together with factors which may have increased stress recently, such as financial worries. The patient's general educational level and understanding may be usefully ascertained whilst taking a history.

The possibility of having acquired HIV infection should be explored as a large number of patients with AIDS develop neurological disorders, ranging from vascular myopathy which leads to degeneration of the spinal cord, ataxia, loss of sensation in the feet and paraplegia through to full-blown AIDS encephalopathy and dementia. A range of psychiatric disorders are also possible, including depression and various psychotic states mimicking schizophrenia and manic depression.

History-taking which focuses on mental health problems such as anxiety or depression is dealt with in Chapter 18.

Physical examination

The physical exam follows a logical structure, starting with observing how patients walk into the room and sit down, looking at their general appearance and demeanour before focusing on the cranial nerves, motor and sensory nervous systems and finishing with an assessment of higher cerebral functioning.

Gait and general mobility

Close observation of how patients walk across the consulting room and sit down by your desk, how mobile they are and how easily they can undress will yield important information. Check the patient's gait and look for any abnormality such as an obvious hemiparesis. Parkinsonism produces a characteristic gait involving difficulty in starting, small steps which become more rapid and inability to swing the arms in the normal way when walking. Alternatively, the patient may show signs of footdrop, including pronounced hip flexion on the affected side while walking and the foot being noisily stamped on the ground. Ataxia is demonstrated by walking with the feet an abnormally wide distance apart and difficulty in remaining upright, grabbing at objects for support. This usually indicates disorder of the cerebellum. A range of other abnormal walks is possible and the nurse practitioner should be able to describe the gait accurately using the correct medical terminology, in his/her notes, for possible discussion with a medical practitioner later. Note factors such as whether there is adduction or abduction, length and rate of stride, balance, width of gait and whether feet are picked up cleanly.

Normally a person maintains balance through several mechanisms, some of which do not involve vision. The semicircular canals in the inner ear play a key role in maintaining balance via the vestibular nerve fibres, various structures in the brainstem, the cerebellum and ultimately nerves which innervate skeletal muscle. If you close your eyes, you cannot depend on visual information to maintain balance and you have to rely on the vestibular system together with proprioceptors. The effectiveness of this system may be assessed by Romberg's test: patient stands with feet together and closes his/her eyes for 20 seconds. The nurse practitioner observes how well the patient maintains balance. Stand immediately behind the patient to steady him/her if he/she loses balance. Instruct the patient to open the eyes immediately if he/she, loses balance – this is a positive Romberg's test and failure of the vestibular system. In cerebellar ataxia the person has difficulty standing with feet together even with eyes open.

The nurse practitioner should examine the neck and spine before moving on to the nervous system, as degenerative changes are commonly associated with neurological complaints in older persons. Check passive movements of the neck (rotation from side to side and flexion–extension) to ensure there is no restriction or pain on movement. Observe how readily the patient can undress and take off a shirt or blouse.

If the meninges become inflamed due to bleeding (subarachnoid haemorrhage) or infection (meningitis), this produces a reflex muscle spasm and consequent neck stiffness (nuchal rigidity) so that it is impossible to touch the chin to the chest even with a passive movement. This test should be carried out gently, with the patient lying on the back (supine) and the occipital region of the head supported by both hands. Kernig's sign is another related sign:

this is caused by meningeal irritation in the lumbar region. The resultant spasm means that passive flexion of the hip and knee in the same leg followed by passive extension of the knee with the hip still flexed produces pain and resistance. This procedure is carried out with the patient lying supine and a positive result indicates meningeal irritation.

Auscultation for cranial and cervical bruits should be routinely carried out as vascular disease is a common cause of brain dysfunction in the late middle-aged and elderly (Munro and Edwards 1995).

Cranial nerves

This section will focus on testing the cranial nerves during a basic physical examination. Abnormal findings usually indicate local nerve damage, a lesion in the cerebral hemisphere or the effects of trauma. Students should refresh their knowledge of the anatomy and physiology of the 12 cranial nerves so that examination technique is underpinned by the necessary knowledge to make an accurate differential diagnosis.

Olfactory nerve (I)

The absence of a sense of smell is known as anosmia and is most frequently due to obstruction of the nasal passages, although it may be caused by an old head injury damaging the olfactory nerve. Vials of various substances can be used to test the sense of smell and should be administered with the patient's eyes closed via one nostril at a time, while the patient occludes the other by pressing with a finger.

Optic nerve (II)

Detailed examination of the optic nerve is covered on p. 78.

Oculomotor, trochlear and abducens nerves (III, IV and VI)

These nerves are considered on p. 78; their functions are closely interrelated, controlling pupil size and eye movement.

Trigeminal nerve (V)

This has both motor and sensory components. The motor fibres innervate the muscles responsible for chewing, movements of the jaw and swallowing. Muscle wasting may be observed best above the zygomatic arch; the patient should be asked to clench the teeth tightly while the nurse practitioner tests muscle tone over the jaw. It should be symmetrical and free from fasciculation. Muscular wasting or weakness may be found in myasthenia gravis or various myopathies.

The sensory fibres transmit sensation from the face and frontal part of the scalp. The three sensory divisions of the trigeminal nerve are the ophthalmic, maxillary and mandibular branches; the names broadly indicate the areas of the face served by these fibres. Examination of pinprick and light touch sensation should be carried out with the patient's eyes closed and working in an unpredictable pattern over all areas of the face. The sensations reported on the left side of the face should be compared with the right; normally they will be the same. The end of a needle and cotton wool may be used to test for sensation and moist cotton wool should also be used to test the corneal reflex (ophthalmic branch). A light touch on the cornea should produce an immediate bilateral blink reflex.

Unilateral impaired function is a serious finding and commonly indicates a tumour affecting the fifth cranial nerve or higher sensory pathways, although a patchy deficit may be due to trauma damaging some peripheral branches of the nerve.

Facial nerve (VII)

Many facial movements are innervated by the motor branch of the facial nerve whilst it provides sensation to the frontal portion of the tongue. It is also involved in the corneal blink reflex and the production of tears and saliva.

The motor branch can be tested by first checking for any obvious asymmetry in the patient's facial appearance and then asking him/her to perform the following manoeuvres and examining for asymmetry or weakness:

- Raise both eyebrows
- Frown and then smile
- Close both eyes and keep them closed while you try to open them
- Show both upper and lower sets of teeth
- Blow out both cheeks

Upper motor neuron lesions tend to have a minimal effect on the upper part of the face (e.g. the eye can still be closed) but cause significant paresis in the lower facial muscles, with drooping of the corner of the mouth and dribbling of saliva. Tumours and vascular lesions occurring in the brainstem may cause abnormal seventh nerve signs, whilst this nerve is the most commonly affected cranial nerve in Guillain–Barré syndrome.

If the lower motor neuron is involved this causes a unilateral weakness of all the facial muscles. An acute onset is commonly seen in Bell's palsy, though the exact cause is unknown. There may also be a loss of taste over the frontal two-thirds of the tongue in Bell's palsy, indicating sensory involvement. The eye should be thoroughly examined if Bell's palsy is suspected as the corneal reflex is diminished and blindness may develop. A visual acuity test is recommended by Billue (1997) as a baseline measurement. Abnormal lacrimation may also be noted.

Vestibulocochlear nerve (VIII)

The eighth nerve has two branches: the vestibular, which is concerned with balance and posture and the cochlear, which is concerned with hearing. Assessing the patient's hearing is dealt with in Chapter 4, whilst testing the vestibular branch is normally the preserve of hospital medical specialists.

Glossopharyngeal and vagus nerves (IX and X)

These nerves are usually considered together because of their close anatomical relationship. Hoarseness may indicate vocal cord paralysis whilst a nasal tone may be produced if the palate is functioning abnormally. Observing the patient saying 'ah' will reveal any abnormality in movement of the uvula or palate. Deviation of the uvula indicates a tenth nerve lesion (such as a meningioma or fractured base of skull) on the opposite side and will usually be seen with asymmetrical elevation of the soft palate. The gag reflex should also be tested (after warning the patient first) by touching either the tonsil or pharynx on each side. If the reflex is absent on one side this indicates a lesion affecting either the ninth or tenth cranial nerve.

Accessory nerve (XI)

This important motor nerve innervates the intrinsic muscles of the larynx, the sternomastoid muscles and part of the trapezius. The patient is best examined from behind to check for any paralysis of the trapezius, shown by drooping of the shoulder and downward lateral displacement of the scapula. S/he should then be asked to shrug the shoulders and maintain that position against downward pressure from the nurse practitioner to check for any weakness which would be indicative of a peripheral nerve disorder.

The sternomastoid muscles should be inspected and palpated for any signs of atrophy. Test their strength by asking the patient to rotate his/her head whilst the nurse practitioner resists with firm pressure to the opposite side of the face. The contraction of the sternomastoid should also be noted during this procedure. If there is bilateral wasting of the sternomastoids, the patient will have difficulty raising the head from the pillow while lying in the supine position. Isolated lesions of this nerve are rare, but findings indicative of a myopathy may be noted.

Hypoglossal nerve (XII)

The XIIth nerve is the motor nerve responsible for innervating the muscles of the tongue. When the patient's tongue is protruded it should lie symmetrically in the midline with no fasciculations or atrophy. If there is a unilateral lesion the protruded tongue deviates towards the affected, weaker side. The patient should be able to move the tongue equally well to either side of the mouth and in the vertical plane as if to lick the chin or the tip of the nose.

Unilateral abnormalities are often due to cranial tumours or vascular lesions, although they may also be traumatic in origin. Diseases such as myasthenia gravis result in abnormal findings such as dysarthria and dysphagia whilst a cerebrovascular accident may cause deviation of the protruded tongue in the acute phase.

Motor system

This section should be read in conjunction with Chapter 12. Examination of the motor system begins as the patient walks into the room and sits down as problems of gait and balance may be immediately obvious (p. 59). In a detailed examination, the nurse practitioner needs to be competent in testing for normal coordination, deep tendon reflexes and plantar responses, together with assessment of muscular tone and power. Abnormalities can indicate whether the problem is an upper or lower motor neuron disorder or whether it involves the muscles. The exam can only be carried out properly with the patient undressed to underwear, therefore a warm and private environment is essential.

Coordination and balance

Proprioception and cerebellar function are essential for coordination and balance. In a simple test the patient carries out rapid alternating movements such as touching each finger of the right hand with the right thumb in sequence and then reversing the sequence before repeating the movements with the other hand. Alternatively ask the patient to hold out the right hand palm upwards and repeatedly touch the upwards-facing fingertips with the front and back of the fingers of the left hand, rapidly rotating the left hand to accomplish the manoeuvre. Repeat with the other hand. The patient should be able to carry out these movements smoothly and rhythmically; jerky, slow or irregular movements are abnormal.

Accuracy of movement may be tested using the finger-to-finger test. The nurse practitioner should hold his/her index finger about 45 cm in front of the patient and ask the person to touch his or her nose tip and the nurse practitioner's finger alternating between the two. The patient should have the eyes open and the nurse practitioner should hold the finger in several different positions during this test. Both hands should be tested. The patient should be able to perform this test smoothly and accurately but if the finger repeatedly goes past the nurse practitioner's finger this may indicate cerebellar disease. In a variation of this test the patient closes the eyes and repeatedly touches the tip of his/her own nose with the index finger of each hand. A further test for accuracy involves asking the patient to lie down and then to run the heel up and down the shin of the opposite leg in a straight line.

Abnormalities in these tests indicate disorder of the cerebellum. Cerebrovascular disease, multiple sclerosis, alcoholism and degenerative disease are the most likely competing explanations.

Romberg's test for balance has already been described (p. 59): in a further test the person stands on one foot for 5 seconds with the eyes closed and then hops on to the other foot, holding that position for a further 5 seconds.

Deep tendon reflexes

The effect of a reflex arc is to produce an involuntary response when the appropriate stimulus is provided. The involuntary nature of the response provides the examiner with objective information about the nerve pathways involved, if only the appropriate tendon is stimulated by the tendon hammer.

When testing reflexes it is important that the patient should be relaxed and comfortable. The hammer should be held between the thumb and index finger: a flick of the wrist provides a sharp tap on the tendon. The major tendon reflexes should be tested systematically (see below), comparing responses on opposite sides of the body. Results may be recorded on a stick figure using the following standard notation:

- +++ Hyperactive
- ++   Normal
- +   Sluggish
- –   Absent

Considerable experience is needed before the nurse practitioner will feel confident about using such a scoring system.

- *Biceps jerk* (reflex arc involves spinal segment C5 and C6): the patient's elbow is flexed at 45° the elbow is held with the fingers over the biceps muscle and the thumb on the biceps tendon (Figure 5.1) and the thumb (not the tendon) is struck. The reflex jerk should produce visible or palpable flexion of the elbow.
- *Supinator jerk* (reflex arc involves spinal segment C5 and C6): the patient's arm rests on the nurse practitioner's arm with the elbow flexed at 45° and the arm slightly pronated (Figure 5.2). The aim is to strike the patient's brachioradial tendon some 4 cm above the wrist: this should produce pronation of the forearm and flexion of the elbow.

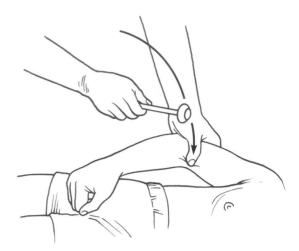

Figure 5.1   Testing biceps jerk

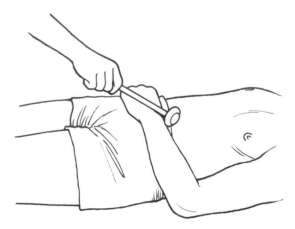

Figure 5.2   Testing supinator jerk

- *Triceps jerk* (reflex arc involving spinal segments C6 and C7): the individual's elbow is flexed to 90° with the arm resting against the side of the body (Figure 5.3). The aiming point is the triceps tendon just above the elbow. This should produce

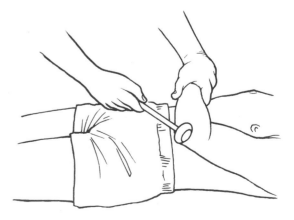

Figure 5.3   Testing triceps jerk

contraction of the triceps muscle which will cause visible or palpable contraction of the elbow.
- *Knee jerk* (reflex arc involving spinal segments L3 and L4): the patient sits with the lower limb hanging loosely and the knee flexed at 90°. The upper leg should be supported by the nurse practitioner (Figure 5.4) and the patella tendon is struck just below the patella. The lower leg should extend in response to contraction of the quadriceps muscle.
- *Ankle jerk* (reflex arc involving spinal segment S1): this is most readily tested with the patient kneeling on a chair, toes pointing towards the floor, although it may be tested with the patient lying recumbent (Figure 5.5). The Achilles tendon is struck at the level of the malleoli. This should produce contraction of the gastrocnemius muscle and therefore plantar flexion of the foot.

If reflexes are difficult to elicit or absent, the nurse practitioner should use reinforcement to make them easier to observe. For the lower limb the patient interlocks the flexed fingers and attempts to pull them apart just as the tendon is about to be struck, while for the upper limb, the patient squeezes the knees together immediately before testing. If reinforcement has been used to elicit a reflex, it is recorded as ±.

Hyperactive reflexes usually indicate upper motor neuron disease. Muscles may show some loss of strength but little evidence of atrophy in upper motor neuron disease. If reflexes appear to be brisk or hyperactive it is worth testing for clonus. The knee should be supported in a partly flexed position and the foot briskly dorsiflexed: if rhythmical tremors in the foot are felt, clonus is said to be present. If there is a symmetrical loss of reflex this may indicate generalized peripheral neuropathy, whereas a single lost reflex suggests a localized problem. Absent or diminished reflexes are found in lower motor neuron disorders which are usually associated with loss of muscle tone and muscle wasting. A delayed reflex suggests hypothyroidism.

Simulation of the lateral border of the sole of the foot leads to plantar flexion (toes curl downwards). Dorsiflexion of the big toe (Babinski response) indicates an upper motor neuron lesion or may be found after an epileptic seizure.

The sensory system

The patient may present with a history of reduced sensation (hypoaesthesia) or altered sensation (paraesthesia). It is important to test sensitivity to light touch, pressure and temperature with the patient's eyes closed and to map the results carefully in order to build up an accurate picture of sensory disturbance. The nurse practitioner needs to know the distribution of the major peripheral nerves and dermatomes in order to interpret areas of altered sensation (Figure 5.6). Normally, sensation should be distributed symmetrically about the body and the person should be able to describe correctly the stimulus (sharp/dull) and differentiate between sites (proximal/distal) in successive stimuli.

Superficial touch can be tested with light strokes of a piece of cotton wool. Superficial pain can be tested with a pin. Hypodermic needles should be avoided because they are too sharp and may accidentally puncture the patient's skin. A disposable pin should be used to avoid any risk of transmitting

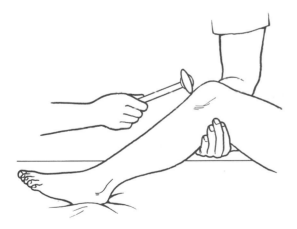

Figure 5.4 Testing for knee jerk

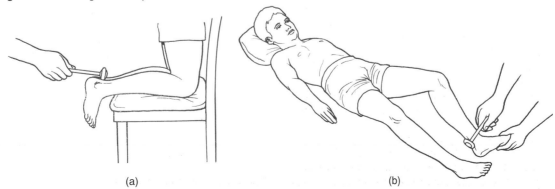

(a) (b)

Figure 5.5 Testing for ankle jerk of (a) kneeling patient and (b) recumbent patient

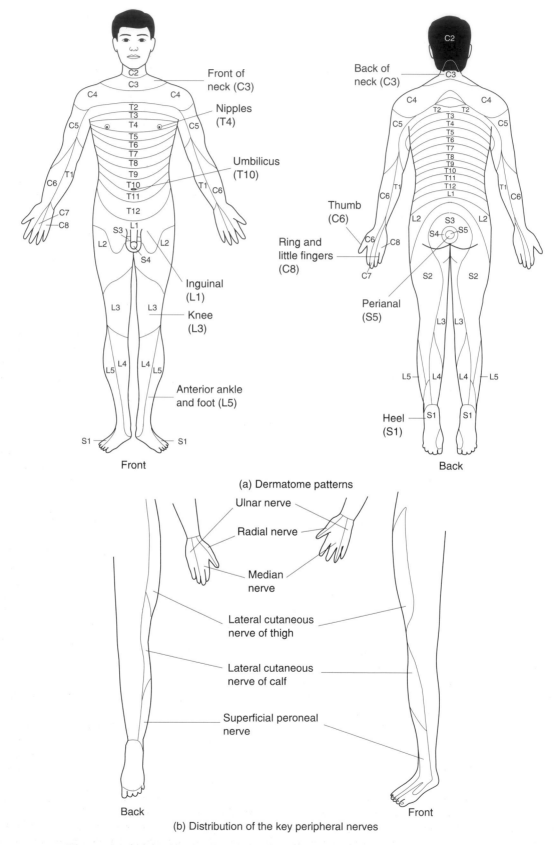

(a) Dermatome patterns

(b) Distribution of the key peripheral nerves

Figure 5.6   The distribution of (a) dermatomes and (b) key peripheral nerves

a blood-borne disease. The patient can be asked to differentiate between sharp and dull sensation (use the side of the needle). Only if superficial pain sensation is abnormal should temperature be tested, using sample bottles of warm and cold water which can be pressed against the skin. Great care should be taken to ensure that the water is not too hot. Deep sensation can be tested by squeezing muscle between finger and thumb.

Vibration can be tested with the aid of a tuning fork held against various bony prominences (e.g. sternum, shoulder, wrist) whilst joint position is tested by holding a distal phalanx laterally and moving it up or down and asking patients (still with their eyes closed) which direction the movement takes in a short series of random movements. If the patient is unable to identify correctly the direction of movement, the nurse practitioner should work proximally along the limb, repeating the test.

Two-point discrimination can be tested with an unfolded paper clip. Either one or both ends are applied to the skin at random on the pulp of both index fingers and thumbs. The distance between the two ends can be varied to ascertain the minimum separation that the patient can identify. Again the patient must have the eyes closed. A normal person can distinguish between two points 3–5 mm apart on the pulp of the index finger.

Disorders affecting specific single peripheral nerves (mononeuropathy) normally give rise to reduction in all sensations and/or a feeling of numbness in nerve distribution. Common examples include carpal tunnel syndrome (median nerve, usually affecting the dominant hand first) and damage to the sciatic nerve producing footdrop, absent Achilles tendon reflex and anaesthesia over the foot. The radial and ulnar nerves may suffer from compression or direct trauma in arm injuries. Peripheral neuropathies and spinal injuries are associated with disorders of touch, pain and temperature perception together with joint position and two-point discrimination. If the pattern of sensory loss is symmetrical, this suggests a poly-neuropathy. Such disorders affect the peripheries of the longest nerves first and progress proximally. The feet are therefore commonly affected first. Patchy sensory disorder suggests a spinal cord problem rather than a polyneuropathy which tends to be uniform in its distribution. Complex patterns of sensory disturbance may present with various cerebral lesions which are often vascular.

Cortical function and the sensory system

A lesion in the posterior (ascending) columns of the spinal cord or in the sensory cortex may be demonstrated by testing the patient's ability to interpret and discriminate between sensory inputs.

The following simple tests may be performed, all with the patient's eyes closed:

- Stereognosis: can the patient identify by touch alone common objects such as a coin?
- Extinction: touch both hands simultaneously with a pin and ask whether the patient is being touched on the left, right or both hands.
- Graphesthaesia: draw a number on the patient's palm and ask what it is.
- Point location: touch the patient's skin and ask him/her to point to the area touched.
- Subtraction skills: ask the patient to take away 7 from 100, and for example, continue subtracting from the result.

Stereogenesis is impaired by posterior column disease, while lesions of the sensory cortex lead to a failure in the other tests described above (Bates 1995). It is important in these tests to check that the patient's touch and position sense are normal, or only slightly impaired, as these parts of the sensory nervous system must be functioning to carry out valid tests on the sensory cortex. If touch and position sense are normal but the patient has an abnormal two-point touch test result (see above) of >5 mm when the finger pad is tested, this indicates probable disease of the posterior columns in the spinal cord.

The unconscious patient

Nurses are familiar with the care of the unconscious patient in the traditional nursing role. It is unlikely that a nurse practitioner will be required to make an initial health assessment and commence a programme of care for an unconscious patient, therefore we will present only a brief outline of the physical examination required.

The primary assessment must follow the well-known ABCD format, checking for patent airway (A), effective breathing (B), cardiac output (C) and evidence of disability (D) associated with a spinal injury. It is crucial that a history be obtained from anybody who witnessed the incident to find out whether the patient has suffered a head injury, fit or collapse, is likely to have taken drugs or alcohol or whether there is no known history.

It is necessary to have an objective measure of the patient's level of consciousness and this is provided by the well-known Glasgow Coma Scale (GCS; Figure 5.7) which should be recorded initially and at regular intervals thereafter (15 minutes while unconscious, more frequently if the patient's level of consciousness is fluctuating). The patient is in coma if s/he does not open the eyes in response to painful stimulus (nailbed pressure), utters no sounds and fails to respond to any command (GCS = 3).

Vital signs should be monitored at 15-minute intervals. If the intracranial pressure is seriously

Frequency of recordings																																		Date
																																			Time
C o m a s c a l e	Eyes open	Spontaneously																																Eyes closed by swelling -C
		To speech																																
		To pain																																
		None																																
	Best verbal response	Orientated																																Endotracheal tube or tracheostomy -T
		Confused																																
		Inappropriate words																																
		Incomprehensible sounds																																
		None																																
	Best motor response	Obey command																																Usually record the best arm response
		Localize pain																																
		Flexion to pain																																
		Extension to pain																																
		None																																

Figure 5.7 Glasgow coma scale chart

elevated after head injury, this produces a reflex slowing of the pulse as blood pressure rises in an attempt to increase brain perfusion. On the other hand, unsuspected internal injuries may lead to the rapid development of hypovolaemic shock.

Pupil size and reaction should also be closely monitored. Pressure on the third cranial nerve will lead to a sluggish pupil response and to a fixed dilated pupil on the affected side. This may be due to an expanding haematoma in head injury. Bilateral fixed dilated pupils in head-injured patients indicate major brain swelling and hence damage as both branches of the third cranial nerve are affected. Early observations are essential as developing periorbital haematoma may soon make it impossible to open a patient's eyes sufficiently to observe the pupils. Overdose of tricyclic antidepressants may also produce bilateral dilated pupils due to their anticholinergic effect. Pinpoint pupils suggest opioid drug use as the most likely cause of coma. In the absence of head injury, a capillary blood glucose reading should be taken to eliminate hypoglycaemic coma.

Motor function should be checked bilaterally as part of the GCS together with reflexes. This may provide crucial information about spinal cord involvement.

Head-injured patients should also be examined for cerebrospinal fluid leakage or bleeding from within the ear, indicating a basal skull fracture. Bruising over the mastoid process is known as Battle's sign and indicates a fracture through the middle fossa. The scalp should be carefully examined for lacerations; as well as exacerbating the risk of hypovolaemic shock due to other injuries, scalp wounds may indicate the possibility of an open and/ or depressed skull fracture with the risk of meningitis from contamination of the meninges.

If the nurse practitioner has to assess and manage an unconscious patient without access to immediate medical assistance it is important that s/he remembers that maintenance of a patent airway and effective breathing at all times is essential for the patient's survival. In undressing and examining the patient, the nurse practitioner should also assume there is spinal injury until proven otherwise.

Differential diagnosis

The patient's history is the single most important factor in arriving at a differential diagnosis. It also guides the physical examination. The following common presenting complaints are analysed to illustrate the steps to follow in arriving at a differential diagnosis of the patient's health problem.

Headache

The likely alternatives are migraine or a tension

headache. The PQRST mnemonic should elicit sufficient information to differentiate between the two: migraine has a characteristically rapid onset and is often associated with known provocative factors; relief is obtained by lying down in a darkened room; unlike a tension headache, ordinary mild analgesics fail to relieve the severe pain of migraine. Associated symptoms of nausea and vomiting or flashing lights help distinguish this from a tension headache. The nurse practitioner should also consider sinusitis or eye strain as possible causes of a generalized headache; facial pain distribution and a story of rapid stabbing and severe pains suggest trigeminal neuralgia.

More serious pathology such as meningitis or subarachnoid haemorrhage are suggested by cerebral irritation and impaired consciousness. A patient complaining of headaches should always have a blood pressure check to eliminate hypertension.

Collapse

An eyewitness account is essential to differentiate between causes such as a simple vasovagal syncope or a convulsion. If the person has had a generalized seizure s/he will be in a confused and disoriented (postictal) state for up to an hour afterwards, unlike syncope where orientation is quickly regained. If a convulsion is ruled out, it is necessary to eliminate the possibility of a cardiac arrhythmia (perform ECG, check history) or in the case of an elderly person a simple fall (check history). A capillary blood glucose test will eliminate the possibility of a hypoglycaemic attack. If the patient is found in a collapsed state, the smell of alcohol or evidence of other drug use (e.g. intravenous needle marks, respiratory depression) point towards alcohol or drug abuse as a likely cause; nevertheless, the nurse practitioner should also carry out a careful exam to eliminate the possibility of a coexisting head injury. Abnormal neurological findings indicate the possibility of a cerebrovascular accident.

Other neurological problems

There are many circumstances where the nurse practitioner might observe a significant neurological sign and it is essential therefore that s/he is able to develop an early line of clinical thinking with a differential diagnosis, record findings accurately and consult or refer appropriately. A useful approach suggested by Munro and Edwards (1995) is to ask what is disturbed, where and why? This requires an accurate record of the observed abnormality, its location and a suggestion as to its cause. The following simplified table (Table 5.1) indicates specific signs which can be attributed to lesions in the nervous system.

Table 5.1 Attribution of signs to probable lesions in the nervous system

Sign	Region of nervous system
Weakness or paralysis of movement Increased tendon reflexes Extensor plantar response	Upper motor neuron
Wasting, weakness or paralysis of muscles Diminished tendon reflexes Reduction in tone	Lower motor neuron
Ataxia of gait Disordered coordination and fine movements Intention tremor	Cerebellar lesions
Reduced superficial sensation in peripheries Wasting and weakness of distal musculature Early loss of tendon reflexes	Generalized neuropathies
Impaired position sense (positive Romberg test) Decreased appreciation of vibration Ataxia of gait	Sensory tracts, dorsal columns
Muscle wasting and weakness, usually proximal Reduced reflexes with marked muscle wasting	Muscles
Amnesia and cognitive disorders Dysphasia Right/left disorientation Hemiparesis Apraxia Visual field defects	Cerebral cortex dysfunction

Source: Adapted from Munro and Edwards (1995).

Management and patient education

This final section of the chapter will focus on the management of common neurological conditions.

Headaches

Migraine

The patient with a history of migraines may be distressed because of the debilitating nature of the attacks and the disruption they cause to everyday life. This may lead to time off work, disruption of study for a student or serious problems for a mother bringing up a young family, particularly if she is a lone parent. The person may also be anxious, interpreting the migraines as a symptom of a more serious disorder such as a brain tumour.

A key step in managing migraine is to try and identify any precipitating factors which the patient may be able to avoid. The patient may find it useful to keep a diary over a period of time recording the frequency of attacks and associated symptoms, the presence of an aura, and what s/he was doing immediately before the attack. This may lead to the discovery that attacks coincide with the menstrual cycle. It may be possible to identify certain foodstuffs which seem to be provoking episodes, such as cheese, chocolate, red wine or caffeine, which can then be avoided. The contraceptive pill aggravates migraine and if an increase in frequency of attacks coincides with a woman starting oral contraception, she should be advised to use alternative methods. A recurring aura is also grounds for suggesting alternative contraception (Rees and Williams 1995).

Periods of stress and anxiety may be associated with an increased frequency of migraine. The nurse practitioner may therefore explore stress reduction strategies with the patient as a means of lessening the incidence of migraines. If the patient is caring for young children, s/he may need to work through some coping strategies with the nurse practitioner which may include identifying helpful relatives or friends who can look after the children while s/he recovers.

Simple analgesics such as aspirin or paracetamol frequently have little effect against migraine as during the attack peristalsis is reduced, leading to impaired absorption. Soluble or effervescent preparations should be used to deal with a migraine (*British National Formulary* 1999). Even more effective is a combination of an analgesic and an antiemetic such as metoclopramide which, in addition to preventing nausea and vomiting promotes gastric emptying. Paramax is one such PoM medication (paracetamol 500 mg and metoclopramide 5 mg) and Migravess another (aspirin 325 mg and metoclopramide 5 mg); both are available in effervescent form.

More severe attacks may be relieved with ergotamine if unresponsive to analgesics. However, many side-effects limit the usefulness of this approach. These include nausea and vomiting, abdominal pain, muscular cramps and the danger of peripheral vasospasm. Consequently ergotamine should always be accompanied by an antiemetic and should never be taken by someone with a history of vascular disease. The nurse practitioner must stress to the patient who has been prescribed ergotamine that s/he should never take more than the prescribed dose, should not repeat the dose within 4 days and should never take the drug prophylactically. These are important patient education points that should be explained carefully.

An alternative drug for the treatment of severe, unresponsive migraine is sumatriptan, which is a 5-hydroxytryptamine antagonist. It may be given orally (100 mg) or administered by subcutaneous injection (6 mg). Autoinjectors are available for this route. The drug has potentially serious side-effects and should not be taken by patients with a history of coronary artery disease. It must not be taken with ergotamine. At least 24 hours should elapse between taking an ergotamine preparation and taking sumatriptan, to avoid complications. The nurse practitioner is referred to the *British National Formulary* (1999) for a detailed discussion of interactions between sumatriptan and other drugs.

If migraine is seriously affecting the patient, there are three types of drugs that can prevent attacks – pizotifen, beta-blockers and tricyclic antidepressants. The side-effects of these medications are such that their use for more than 6 months is not recommended. Concentrate on working with the patient to address various lifestyle issues which may successfully reduce the frequency of attacks. A medical prescription for such prophylactic agents is a last resort and even then, only a temporary solution.

Tension headache

When the nurse practitioner is reasonably confident that the patient is having tension headaches, it is necessary to explore the causes of stress and anxiety before looking at what measures can be taken to reduce these factors. A diary may be helpful to identify particular situations which lead to headaches so that they can be avoided. This can be reviewed at a follow-up appointment together with progress on stress reduction strategies. Positive reinforcement is important for the patient.

The consultation is a good opportunity to educate the patient about the dangers of paracetamol which may be consumed in significant quantities as the patient tries to deal with the symptom (headaches) rather than the cause of the problem (stress). Many people do not realize that paracetamol may cause serious liver damage and is therefore contraindicated in those with liver disease, including those with a history of alcohol abuse. Twenty paracetamol tablets (10 g) is a potentially fatal overdose (*British National Formulary* 1999). It is important to stress that if the patient is taking paracetamol to relieve headache the *maximum daily dose is 4 g or eight tablets*. Tactful enquiry should also be made about alcohol intake.

Other causes of headache

If a Snellen test has revealed eyesight problems, the patient should be referred to an optician. If sinusitis is the cause of the patient's pain, a 2-week course of amoxycillin, doxycycline or erythromycin is the recommended antibiotic therapy.

If the nurse practitioner suspects trigeminal neuralgia the patient should be referred to the GP.

Carbamazepine is effective at reducing the severity and frequency of attacks although side-effects include rashes, dizziness, nausea and vomiting. The usual approach is to start the patient on 300 mg/day in divided doses and gradually increase the dose until it is effective without problems from side-effects. The nurse practitioner needs to educate patients about side-effects and encourage them to return if they become problematic. As a last resort it is possible to destroy the trigeminal nerve to relieve pain, but this leaves the patient without any sensation on the side of the face and at risk of corneal ulceration.

The nurse practitioner may receive a phone call from a patient complaining of headache, anxious that it may be something serious such as meningitis. The following key features are suggested by Briggs (1997) as indicators for calling an emergency ambulance and should be checked over the phone:

- Pyrexia and a stiff neck, especially in a child, shown by difficulty in bending the head forwards
- Rapid appearance of a rash
- Confusion and a marked decrease in level of consciousness
- Sudden onset of weakness or numbness on one side of the body
- Difficulty speaking
- Sudden severe pain which is worse than anything the person has ever had before

Collapse

Generalized seizure (grand mal fit)

If the nurse practitioner witnesses the fit, s/he should not interfere with the patient during the tonic and clonic stages. Any hard objects which may cause injury should be removed from the immediate vicinity and if it is possible to place a blanket or something similar under the patient's head as a means of protection, this should be done. Once the clonic stage is over, the individual will remain deeply unconscious and may occasionally have a further fit. S/he should therefore be placed in the recovery position to protect the airway and, if suction is available, this should be used to remove secretions from the oral cavity. The profound muscle relaxation which accompanies this stage may lead to urinary incontinence if the individual's bladder contained significant amounts of urine. This should be checked and if possible wet clothing removed to prevent embarrassment when consciousness is recovered. Recovery proceeds through the postictal stage, during which time the patient slowly regains consciousness but may be confused and disoriented; s/he should be kept under observation until fully oriented.

It is possible that the fit happened elsewhere and the patient has been brought to the nurse practitioner

(e.g. in a minor injuries unit of a community hospital). The nurse practitioner should try and obtain a reliable eye-witness account in order to assess the probability of a generalized seizure. By the time the patient arrives at the unit s/he will usually be in the postictal phase if this is the case.

The nurse practitioner should first check the ABCD and then carry out a careful neurological examination (including checking for evidence of head injury) and obtain a history of the event. In the immediate postictal period, observation and regular assessment of level of consciousness are essential and it is important to ascertain whether the individual has a history of epilepsy. If this is positive, local protocols may allow the patient home with a responsible adult and notification of the GP. If the patient has no history of epilepsy, s/he should be carefully followed up by a medical practitioner – epilepsy is not a disease in itself, rather it is a sign of some possibly serious underlying pathology.

If the person has a history of epilepsy, the nurse practitioner may make a follow-up appointment to discuss medication and lifestyle. Good control is essential if chronic accumulative brain damage from repeated fits is to be prevented. Patients should be advised about the need to take medication regularly to maintain effective plasma concentrations. Compliance is often poor because there are no obvious effects if a single dose is missed. It is estimated that up to 50% of patients with epilepsy do not comply with their medication regimes (Hilton 1997). If the person suddenly ceases medication altogether, this can produce rebound seizures. Many antiepileptic drugs can interact with other drugs. A particular problem occurs with drugs that reduce hepatic enzyme activity, as this leads to a considerable reduction in the efficacy of combined and pro-gestogen-only oral contraceptives (*British National Formulary* 1999). Examples include phenytoin, carbamazepine and phenobarbitone.

Patients will be particularly concerned if they drive as epilepsy will lead to the loss of their driving licence. They may be reassured that a single attack will not cost them their licence, providing their EEG is normal. Subsequent seizures or an abnormal EEG will lead to the loss of a licence and the individual has to be fit-free for at least 2 years to recover the licence. The regulations concerning heavy goods vehicle and public service vehicle licences are much stricter; losing such a licence may lead to losing a job. The nurse practitioner must be aware that such a patient will be very concerned and will need considerable support in coming to terms with possible loss of livelihood.

Syncope

Laying the person flat allows sufficient blood to reach the brain for him/her to regain consciousness rapidly. It is important to have made a differential diagnosis that rules out possibilities such as hypoglycaemia, transient ischaemic attack or cardiac arrhythmia. The examination should also have ruled out any possibility of head injury incurred secondary to collapse. Under these circumstances, the patient should be allowed to leave when well enough, preferably in the company of a responsible adult.

Alcohol or other drugs

Individuals may be brought to the minor injuries unit in a comatose or drowsy state as a result of alcohol and/or other drug abuse. It is essential to carry out a thorough examination so that head trauma or other injury is not missed. Assuming that there are no other injuries, the intoxicated individual is best placed in the recovery position to safeguard the airway, and allowed to sleep it off under observation. The floor is the safest place to lay such individuals as they have a habit of falling off trolleys, even if cot sides are in place.

If opioid drug use is suspected, careful observation must be maintained, watching out for respiratory depression and possible respiratory arrest. Oxygen saturation should be continually monitored with a pulse oximeter. The specific antidote, naloxone, should be readily available if the person is comatose or there is doubt concerning respiratory function. It is given intravenously in small amounts (1–2 mg at 2-minute intervals) up to a maximum of 10 mg and is quick-acting in reversing the effects of opioids. Naloxone has a short half-life and its effects soon wear off. This latter point is important as on regaining consciousness, many individuals wish to leave quickly. The risk of lapsing into coma shortly afterwards should be explained and if possible the person kept for observation to ensure this does not happen. If such a patient insists on leaving the minor injuries unit s/he should be allowed to go, but if possible someone else known to the individual who could keep him or her under observation should be apprised of the risks. At this point it is appropriate to remind the nurse practitioner of the importance of observing universal precautions *at all times* as a protection against HIV and other blood-borne infections.

The use of Ecstasy is not confined to large city centres, and young adults collapsing after taking this drug may be brought to a minor injuries unit in rural areas. The nurse practitioner needs to be aware of this as a possible cause of collapse in a previously fit young adult brought from a party or nightclub. The presenting picture is one of dilated pupils, hypotension, tachycardia and hyperpyrexia and the history will include collapse and possibly convulsions. This is a serious medical emergency as death from the rapid onset of respiratory failure and associated disseminated intravascular coagula-tion may follow. Urgent transfer to medical care and an intensive treatment unit is essential (Walsh 1996). Steps to cool the patient in order to reduce the risk of hyperpyrexia should be taken whilst waiting for an ambulance (Jones 1993).

Other causes of collapse

If examination reveals neurological deficits suggestive of a stroke or other CNS pathology or if there are signs consistent with syncope due to a cardiac problem, the patient should be referred for an immediate consultation with a medical practitioner, in accordance with local protocols.

Head injury

In dealing with an acute head injury, the nurse practitioner will frequently have local protocols to follow. Where there has been no loss of consciousness and there are no abnormal neurological signs, medical referral is usually unnecessary and the patient may be sent home. Some minor injuries unit protocols may insist on a skull X-ray. Any one telephoning for advice who mentions changes in level of consciousness, visual disturbances, persistent vomiting or headache, changes in behaviour, bruising around the ears or eyes developing after head injury or blood or other fluid draining from the ears or nose should be advised to attend immediately (Briggs 1997).

It is important to educate the patient about the risk of dizziness, poor memory and loss of concentration which may last for days after a minor head injury. Objective support for the risk of significant post-head injury symptoms comes from Lowden *et al.* (1989) who found that 90% of a sample of 114 adults discharged from A&E after minor head injuries reported these symptoms for up to 2 weeks subsequently. The nurse practitioner should emphasize that, while mild symptoms are normal for a short while, if they worsen or persist, the patient should return. A medical referral at this stage is essential.

Where there has been a loss of consciousness or cerebrospinal fluid leakage, bleeding from the ears or any abnormal neurological signs, the patient should be referred to a medical practitioner. An accurate GCS is an essential part of the referral process, as deterioration in the GCS will probably be the first sign that the patient has significant intracranial trauma. It is worth noting that Morris (1993) reported that, of 100 consecutive referrals to a regional neurosurgical unit, the referring medical staff had incorrectly used the GCS in 70% of cases and that 18% of the doctors in question were completely unable to use the GCS. Nurse practitioners must aim for 100% accuracy with this vital tool to provide objective data about the patient's level of consciousness.

Other neurological problems

As we have seen in the history-taking and physical examinations sections, the nurse practitioner may elicit evidence suggestive of a range of more serious neurological disorders than those covered in this section. Such disorders clearly fall within the remit of the GP and hospital consultant and it is essential that there are well-defined nurse practitioner referral mechanisms to ensure prompt medical attention.

Summary

The nurse practitioner may encounter neurological disorders whether s/he works in primary health care, a minor injuries unit or within the hospital environment. Often nothing is found on physical examination and the nurse practitioner will have to be guided by the history provided by the patient or witnesses. Many patients with headaches, minor head injuries or who have momentarily collapsed due to a faint can be successfully managed by the nurse practitioner. The first signs of more serious disorder which need medical management may be noticed by an observant nurse practitioner. It is possible that the nurse practitioner in primary health care may be involved in the long-term management of these individuals; clinical nurse specialists such as continence nurses and those specializing in palliative care may also be involved.

In conclusion, although the nurse practitioner may at first be intimidated by the complexity of the nervous system, it is essential that s/he can take a thorough focused history and perform a systematic baseline neurological examination if s/he is to refer appropriately and collaborate in the management of patients.

References

Bates B. (1995) *A Guide to Physical Examination and History Taking*, Philadelphia. JB Lippincott.

Billue J. (1997) Bell's palsy: an update on idiopathic facial paralysis, *Nurse Practitioner*, **22**(8), pp. 88–105.

Briggs J. (1997) *Telephone Triage Protocols for Nurses*, Philadelphia, Lippincott.

British National Formulary (1999) London, British Medical Association/Royal Pharmaceutical Society of Great Britain.

Bullock R., Teasdale G. (1991) Head injuries. In: Driscoll P., Skinner D., Earlam R. (eds) *ABC of Major Trauma*, London, *British Medical Journal.*

Hilton G. (1997) Seizure disorders in adults: evaluation and management of new onset seizures, *Nurse Practitioner*, **22**(9), pp. 42–59.

Jones C. (1993) MDMA: the doubts surrounding ecstasy and the response of the emergency nurse, *Accident and Emergency Nursing* **1**, pp. 193–198.

Lowden I., Briggs M., Cockin J. (1989) Head injury, *Injury*, **20**(4), pp. 193–194.

Morris K. (1993) Assessment and communication of conscious level: an audit of neurosurgical referrals, *Injury*, **24**(6), pp. 369–372.

Munro J., Edwards C. (1995) *Macleod's Clinical Examination*, 9th edn., Edinburgh, Churchill Livingstone.

Rees P., Williams D. (1995) *Principles of Clinical Medicine*, London, Edward Arnold.

Sinclair M. (1991) *Nursing the Neurological Patient*, Oxford, Butterworth-Heinemann.

Walsh M. (1996) *A & E Nursing: A New Approach*, 3rd edn., Oxford, Butterworth-Heinemann.

CHAPTER 6

Vision and the eye

Mike Walsh

Introduction

The nurse practitioner in primary care or working in a minor injuries unit will be likely to encounter patients on a regular basis complaining of 'something in my eye' or 'my eye is all red and sore'. Acute problems caused by a foreign body or an inflammatory response are likely to be seen frequently. The patient may present with a story of visual disturbance which requires careful assessment in order to distinguish between those patients with minor problems and those with a more significant problem that needs referral to a medical practitioner or optician. A full physical examination by the nurse practitioner involves an assessment of vision and examination of the eye, with an ophthalmoscope. The nurse practitioner should be alert for signs of serious visual problems, such as glaucoma; other systemic disorders such as hypertension and diabetes also produce telltale signs which may be detected with an ophthalmoscope. Taking a focused history and carrying out a careful assessment of vision is an essential part of nurse practitioner practice in both hospital and primary health care.

Pathophysiology

A logical approach is to start at the outside and work inwards. The basic structure of the eye is shown in Figure 6.1. The optic nerve, extraocular muscles and nerve supply will therefore be considered first. Complaints of visual impairment or diplopia (double vision) are the most likely clinical presentation indicating that there may be a problem in this area. The eye itself will then be considered, again working inwards from the exterior.

Cranial nerves and the eye

Optic nerve (II)

Lesions affecting the optic nerve, such as neoplasms, usually lead to loss of vision. Figure 6.2 shows the complicated nature of the visual fields as the nerves from the eyes join at the optic chiasma before proceeding separately to the primary visual cortex. A lesion at (a) will cause total blindess in the affected eye whereas a lesion affecting the optic chiasma (such as a pituitary tumour) at (b) causes bitemporal hemianopia. The term hemianopia means defective vision or blindness in half of the visual field. If the lesion occurs at point (c), this causes a homonymous hemianopia involving nerve tracts arising from the same side of each eye, therefore the visual defect will occur on either the left or right of both eyes. Compare this with the bitemporal hemianopia shown in (b).

The pupillary reflex depends on nerve impulses being conducted along the optic nerve from the eye that has light shone into it. The reflex response is controlled by the oculomotor nerve (III) and results in *both* pupils being constricted. A response of the eye that has not had light shone into it is known as the consensual reflex. If light is shone into it an eye and there is no direct reflex, but there is a consensual reflex when light is shone into the other eye, this logically indicates that there is a defect in the retina or optic nerve leading from the non-responsive eye. However, if the pupil is fixed and dilated and does not respond to light shone into that eye, but there is a consensual reflex in the other eye, this indicates that the lesion is affecting the oculomotor nerve supplying the unreactive eye. The ocular nerve is clearly functioning or there would not be a consensual reflex.

Oculomotor, trochlear and abducens nerves (III, IV and VI)

The close relationship between these three cranial nerves is such that they are normally considered together. The oculomotor nerve is responsible for innervation of the iris and the pupiliary reflex. It also innervates key muscles involved in eye movements, as do the trochlear and abducent nerves. These are shown in Table 6.1 working clockwise around the right eye.

The effects on the oculomotor nerve of a swelling

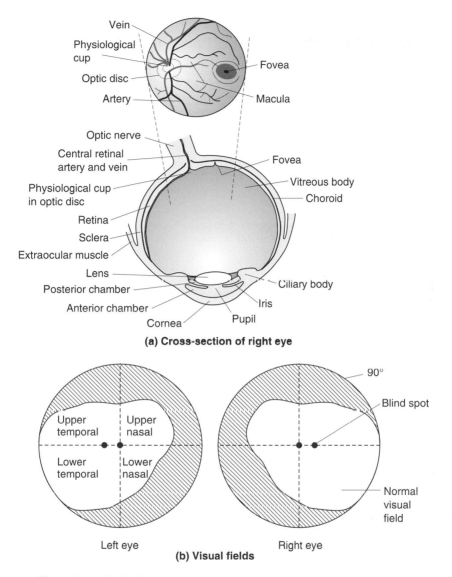

(a) Cross-section of right eye

(b) Visual fields

Figure 6.1   The basic structure of the eye

intracranial lesion after head injury are discussed in Chapter 5. A tumour may have a similar effect, producing a third cranial nerve palsy which involves ptosis (drooping of the upper eyelid) as well as a dilated and non-responsive pupil. The nerve may be compressed bilaterally by a large tumour or the problem may be due to an aneurysm compressing the nerve trunk. Lesions distorting the brainstem may affect the abducent nerve (VI) due to their anatomical closeness at the tentorium. The abducent nerve (VI) is rarely the subject of an isolated lesion, where this does occur, diabetic mononeuropathy and head injury are the main causes.

Nerve palsy produced by pressure from a tumour or aneurysm leads to diplopia or double vision. The normal eye is able to move to keep the image of the object on the macula but the affected eye, as a result of the nerve palsy, cannot track the object in the same way. The image therefore falls on the retina some way off the macula. The brain interprets the picture as a double image: the largest discrepancy between the images is in the direction where the muscle which is not functioning correctly would act. If the patient states that double vision is worse on looking sideways, then this indicates that it is a third and/or sixth cranial nerve problem (Table 6.1); if looking up and down makes the problem worse, then it is likely to be a third and/or fourth cranial nerve problem (Table 6.1). The false image from the affected eye is always the outermost one (Rees and Williams 1995); consequently, in a sixth cranial nerve lesion, as the person gazes towards the affected side the diplopia is always worse, since the lateral rectus muscle is not functioning properly on that side (Munro and Edwards 1995).

Failure of the extraocular muscles can also lead

Visual field defects

Left   *Right*

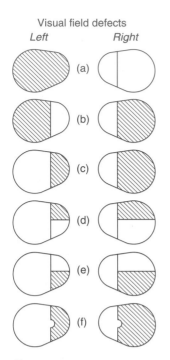

Key
(a) Total loss of vision in left eye
(b) Bitemporal hemianopia
(c) Right homonymous hemianopia
(d) Upper right quadrant hemianopia
(e) Lower quadrantic hemianopia
(f) Right homonymous hemianopia
      with sparing of the macula

Visual fields

Left   *Right*

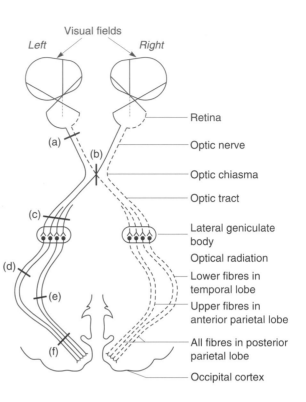

Retina

Optic nerve

Optic chiasma

Optic tract

Lateral geniculate body

Optical radiation

Lower fibres in temporal lobe

Upper fibres in anterior parietal lobe

All fibres in posterior parietal lobe

Occipital cortex

Figure 6.2 Lesions affecting the optic nerve

to a squint as the eyes fail to move in parallel. Problems with binocular vision can produce a squint. This is known as a concomitant squint and is most likely to be seen in young children. It does not produce diplopia as the child's brain corrects the image.

Table 6.1 Innervation of muscles involved in movement of the eye

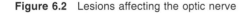

Muscle	Movement of globe	Nerve
Superior rectus	Upwards	Oculomotor (III)
Inferior oblique	Upwards	Oculomotor (III)
Medial rectus	Medially (towards the midline)	Oculomotor (III)
Superior oblique	Downwards when eyes adducted	Trochlear (IV)
Inferior rectus	Downwards	Oculomotor (III)
Lateral rectus	Laterally (away from midline)	Abducens (VI)
Levator palpebrae superioris	Opens upper eyelid (no effect on globe)	Oculomotor (III)

Extraocular problems

Many conditions affect the outside of the eye. We will only mention those which present most commonly, although those interested may read further in various ophthalmology texts.

Infection of the hair follicle of one of the eyelashes produces a painful, tender, inflamed-looking pimple, known as a stye, which is located on the lid margin. It is not to be confused with a chalazion which is an inflamed meibomian gland. This too forms a tender, inflamed-looking pimple but is usually located inside the lid rather than on the margin as in the case of a stye. In either case the eyelid may become inflamed. Other lumps include a marginal cyst developing from a sweat-secreting gland or a basal cell carcinoma (rodent ulcer), usually affecting the lower lid.

Inflammation of the eyelids is known as blepharitis and is most pronounced at the margins. It may be associated with eczema or psoriasis. Herpes simplex or herpes-zoster ophthalmicus infections present with a characteristic vesicular rash in addition to inflammation of the eyelid and may lead to herpetic ocular disease affecting various structures within the eye.

The elderly are prone to problems associated with a lid margin. It may be turned inwards (entropion), in which case the lashes irritate the conjunctiva, or the lower lid may be turned outwards (ectropion), interfering with normal drainage and leading to continual tears in the eye. Most nurses will be familiar with exophthalmos as protruding eyeballs associated with a hyperthyroid state. In may also occur in a single eyeball in the case of hyperthyroidism; this could also indicate a tumour or inflammation affecting the orbit (Bates 1995)

Trauma to structures around the eye may produce swelling and bruising which can quickly close the eye, making later inspection impossible. Lacerations which go through both surfaces of the lid or which involve structures such as the lacrimal duct may lead to complications and should therefore be referred to a medical specialist.

Perhaps the commonest cause of presentation is a foreign body in the eye which most commonly is dust, grit, a splinter of wood or metal. The foreign body will be found lodged on the cornea or the undersurface of the eyelid (subtarsal foreign body). Corneal foreign bodies can cause severe irritation, infection and, in the case of metallic objects, staining of the cornea with rust. High-energy particles can penetrate the eye with much more serious consequences and chemicals splashed in the eye can have devastating effects. Alkalis containing lime (such as wet cement) can rapidly penetrate the cornea, damaging the iris, ciliary body and lens (Walsh 1996).

It may be that no evidence of the foreign body can be found, despite the discomfort felt by the patient. This suggests that the object has led to a corneal abrasion. This painful condition is often caused by a glancing blow from something as innocent as the edge of a piece of paper.

The other common presentation is the patient complaining of a sore, red eye. The person with conjunctivitis presents with discomfort and redness of the conjunctiva. The cause is usually infective (bacterial or viral) but it may also be due to an allergic reaction. A subconjunctival haemorrhage may occur as a result of trauma or a sudden increase in venous pressure caused by coughing. It presents as a well-defined red area that fades to yellow as the red blood cells deteriorate over the next few days and finally the haemorrhage disappears. Trauma to the cornea has already been mentioned. The cornea may also become inflamed (keratitis) as a result of extension of a pre-existing conjunctivitis, the herpes simplex virus which causes dendritic ulcer formation on the cornea, exposure to ultraviolet light (careless use of sun lamps or arc welding without proper eye protection) or corneal exposure.

Intraocular problems

The cause of an inflamed red eye may lie within the eye itself. Obstruction of the outflow of aqueous humour leads to increased intraocular pressure causing visual impairment, pain and dilated blood vessels, giving the eye a reddish appearance. This is the serious condition of glaucoma which may occur as an acute emergency or as a more gradual disease process. It causes damage to the optic disc and loss of vision. Glaucoma can be primary or secondary to some other disease process such as a tumour within the eye, inflammation or infection. Painful inflammation of the iris (iritis) for example may lead to glaucoma. Inflammation of the choroid, iris or ciliary body is known as uveitis and may be due to infection or associated with collagen disorders such as rheumatoid arthritis.

Bleeding within the inner eye (vitreous haemorrhage) from retinal or ciliary vessels is a serious problem which threatens vision. It may be associated with trauma, retinal detachment, hypertension or diabetic retinopathy in which microaneurysms and atheromatous plaques develop in retinal blood vessels. Retinal detachment is a serious disorder which can cause severe visual impairment. It is usually due to degenerative changes associated with ageing or trauma such as penetrating eye injury or head injury. Needless to say, any penetrating injury to the eye can have serious consequences for vision in that eye. It may also lead to the development of sympathetic ophthalmia, a poorly understood inflammatory condition that affects the uninjured eye and that may lead to loss of vision in that eye unless promptly treated.

Opacification of the lens produces a cataract. The commonest cause by far is ageing: the person's vision in the affected eye steadily deteriorates as the cataract develops either in the centre of the lens or on the margin. Congenital cataracts are associated with children whose mother had a viral infection such as German measles in the first trimester of pregnancy or who have inherited a genetic defect leading to an inborn error of metabolism.

Taking a focused history

Patient anxiety is to be expected in any consultation, but particularly so when patients come to see the nurse practitioner concerning a problem with their eyes. Fear of blindness is an understandable cause of high levels of anxiety and the nurse practitioner should be tactful and understanding when taking a history. The following section focuses on the relevant key areas in history-taking the nurse practitioner should remember the broader holistic perspective that distinguishes nursing from medical practice whilst taking the history.

Presenting complaint

The most likely symptoms that the patient will relate

are pain or soreness, foreign body, redness of the eye or visual disturbance. In assessing pain the PQRST mnemonic is most useful, thus it is important to ascertain what brings on the pain and what relieves it (P). It may be an activity involving continual concentration such as driving, reading or working on a VDU screen, which suggests eye strain and an eyesight test is required as spectacles may be needed. Pain may also be associated with a tension headache (p. 54). If questions about the quality (Q) and severity (S) of the pain reveal that it is severe and associated with nausea and vomiting whilst questions about the region (R) indicate that it is within and around the eye (rather than the head, which would suggest migraine), this strongly suggests an intraocular inflammatory problem or glaucoma. This history may also be due to shingles affecting the trigeminal nerve (herpes zoster ophthalmicus). The time (T) of onset of pain should also be ascertained. This key fact should be established whatever the presenting complaint, including those mentioned below.

If a foreign body is the cause of the problem, the patient will usually be able to give an accurate account of the accident. It is important to try and ascertain what material is involved and whether it was a high velocity particle (e.g. from chiselling, grinding or windscreen glass in a road accident) which may have penetrated the cornea. If it is a chemical it is again important to find out what, especially whether it is alkaline, such as wet cement or mortar, given the potentially catastrophic damage that lime can inflict on the eye. First-aid measures taken at the time of the accident should also be ascertained.

The patient may complain of a sensation like having something in the eye, but cannot recall a particular incident. This sensation of grittiness and discomfort, accompanied by redness and tears, suggests damage to the cornea. Ask about pain, whether photophobia is present, whether there is any discharge from the eye and redness, checking particularly the duration of symptoms. To ask whether the person wears contact lenses, whether there has been even a trivial glancing blow to the upper face or the possibility of exposure to ultraviolet light (p. 75). The patient may be distressed and agitated, therefore a calm reassuring manner is particularly important.

If the patient is complaining of a disturbance of vision, Munro and Edwards (1995) suggest the following useful classification to help summarize the problem:

- Blurred vision: usually caused by an ocular problem interfering with the transmission of light through the eye, e.g. cataract formation or refractive errors in the lens.

- Loss of vision: check carefully whether this has occurred in one eye or both as this indicates whether the problem is anterior or posterior to the optic chiasma respectively (Figure 6.2). Sudden loss of vision suggests that the cause of the problem is vascular. Fixed blind spots within the field of vision are known as scotomas and should be distinguished from floaters (see below). The presence of a scotoma suggests damage to the retina or within the visual pathway

- Double vision: it is important to check that the patient does not interpret blurred as double vision

- Haloes and flashes of light: haloes are caused by water drops diffracting light rays as they pass through the eye and are therefore associated with corneal oedema or cataract. Flashes of light (photopsia) are caused by the vitreous tugging on the retina

- Floaters: everybody notices floating objects within their vision from time to time and this is not abnormal: however, a sudden increase in the number of floaters is abnormal and is likely to be due to a vitreous haemorrhage.

Past medical history

It is essential to find out if the person has had vision problems in the past, including whether they wear contact lenses or spectacles and if they have had any history of trauma affecting the eye or the region immediately around the eye. Asked whether the patient has had any previous problems with the herpes simplex or herpes-zoster virus. Date of the last eye test should be noted. If the person wears contact lenses, it is essential to check that s/he is following recommended good practice for care of the lenses and eyes. Previous eye surgery should be ascertained. Chronic diseases which have serious implications for vision by causing retinopathy include diabetes and hypertension, and these should be checked out with the patient.

Family history

Any family history of visual problems and disorders affecting the eye should be checked.

Personal and social history

The person's work should be discussed as this may contribute to eye strain, be responsible for allergic reactions or, in the case of a welder, directly cause inflammation of the cornea as a result of not taking proper precautions against ultraviolet light (arc eye). Exposure at work to VDU screens, high-speed machinery or hazardous sporting activity such as squash or boxing should be explored as health education may be necessary to prevent a recurrence of the problem. The precautions the person is currently taking should be discussed. Ask about any recent problems with reading or changes which suggest problems with distant vision.

Physical examination

This section will also follow the principle of working from the outside inwards, starting with assessment of the orbit, eyelids and outer eye before moving on to look at the inner eye and finally vision.

External examination

The examination starts as soon as the patient walks into the room. Eye contact is an essential part of greeting any new patient and affords an excellent opportunity for the nurse practitioner to assess for any obvious signs such as exophthalmos or a squint.

Swelling around the orbit of the eye is an abnormal finding; it may be due to allergy or in a young person such oedema could suggest renal disease. Fading bruising is evidence of a periorbital haematoma caused by a blow to the eye region. Particular attention should be paid if abuse is suspected in the case of a child or woman. A vague explanation such as 'I walked into a door' or 'I can't remember' should be treated with caution whilst the presence of a haematoma around the left eye is particularly suspicious as most punches are thrown with the right hand, making contact on the left side of the face. The human fist fits within the orbit whereas a vertical object such as a door does not, making periorbital bruising unlikely, especially when the person states that s/he *walked* into the object. At such low speeds there is unlikely to be sufficient energy in the collision to cause extensive bruising. Suspicion should not be taken too far however as one of the authors well remembers the consultant in charge of his A&E department appearing one Monday with spectacular bilateral periorbital haematomas as a result of an accident with the boom of his sailing dinghy that weekend!

The presence of orbital cellulitis is a serious sign; usually it is a result of spread of infection from the sinuses. The patient usually has orbital swelling around one eye, no history of trauma or evidence of bruising, restricted eye movements, tenderness over the sinuses and a history of feeling unwell. It is particularly serious in children where blindness is possible in a matter of hours (Elkington and Khaw 1988).

The eyelids should be checked for normal symmetrical appearance and the ability to open and close the eyes. A drooping eyelid (ptosis) suggests problems with the oculomotor nerve. It is also essential to check whether there is any inversion or eversion of the eyelashes and for the presence of any lumps or abscesses in the eyelid or at its margin (stye or chalazion). The patient should be asked to close the eyes in order to check that the lids completely cover the globe; corneal ulceration will result if this is not the case. The eye should be gently palpated and it should be possible to push the eye back into the orbit slightly without causing any discomfort. If there is resistance and the eye feels hard, this suggests glaucoma, hyperthyroidism or possibly a tumour. Only practice and experience will allow the nurse practitioner to gauge how an eye feels normally on palpation in order that raised intraocular pressure may be detected in this way.

Outer eye

The conjunctiva should be examined by pulling the lower lid downwards. Any signs of redness or sticky discharge should be noted as they are usually found in the presence of conjunctivitis. The upper tarsal conjunctiva should always be examined if the patient complains of a foreign body as this is frequently where it will be found. To do this it is necessary to evert the upper eyelid: ask the patient to look down while you gently pull the lid downwards and away from the globe of the eye. It is then possible to bend the lid backwards over a cotton wool applicator to expose the conjunctiva on the undersurface of the lid. Any foreign body can be removed, before gently replacing the lid by reversing the manoeuvre. The steps involved in this procedure should be carefully explained to the patient before commencing, as some may find this rather alarming.

The cornea can then be examined by shining a light across it tangentially. It should be perfectly clear as the cornea is avascular except for the area of the limbus where it joins the conjunctiva. A general loss of transparency is therefore abnormal and indicates oedema of the cornea or extensive epithelial damage as occurs for example in chemical injury or prolonged dryness of the cornea. Yellow fluorescein eye drops may be instilled in the eye in order to show up a localized area of epithelial damage such as that found in ulceration, abrasion or with a foreign body. The corneal reflex depends upon sensory nerve fibres in the trigeminal nerve (V) and motor nerve fibres in the facial nerve (VII). It may be tested by gently touching the cornea with a wisp of cotton wool; the result should be an immediate blinking of the eye. Loss of this protective reflex is serious as the eye is highly susceptible to trauma or infection.

Pupils

The pupils should be equal in size, regular in shape and react briskly to light both directly and consensually. However, Seidel *et al.* (1995) note that up to 20% of people have unequal pupils normally. It is important therefore to test whether any observed difference occurs as the amount of light varies.

The medical term for unequal pupils is anisocoria and this may be more pronounced in bright light as the larger pupil cannot constrict properly. In this case it does indicate disorder – usually glaucoma or oculomotor nerve paralysis. In the latter case, it is usually accompanied by ptosis and lateral deviation of the eye as the nerve damage means the lateral rectus muscle is not functioning properly. The effects of head injury and opioid drug use on pupil reaction have been discussed on p. 66. It is worth mentioning that a non-responsive pupil may be due to a realistic prosthesis!

The response of the pupils to accommodation should be examined. Ask the patient to focus on a distant object. Hold a finger 10 cm from the end of the nose; the pupils should be seen to constrict. A normal set of pupil responses may therefore be summarized as pupils equal and reacting to light and accommodation (acronym: PERLA).

If a squint has been observed, it should be remembered that in a young child it is likely to be a non-paralytic strabismus as the fault is a congenital problem in the central nervous system controlling the coordinated movement of the eyes to focus together on an object. The patient can focus with either eye separately, but not together. A paralytic strabismus presents in later life and is caused by a nerve palsy affecting the extraocular muscles. If the eye is turned medially this is known as a convergent strabismus (esotropia) while a lateral deviation is known as a divergent strabismus (exotropia). The person may or may not be complaining of diplopia, depending on whether the central nervous system adapts to viewing two separate images. A simple test involves asking the patient to look into the distance and then cover one eye. If the uncovered eye then moves to fix on the object, this is the eye with the squint.

Ophthalmoscopy

This represents a significant new area of practice for nurses moving into nurse practitioner roles. It can provide vital information about the optic disc and retina and is therefore a skill well worth mastering. The ophthalmoscope produces an upright image magnified to the power ×15 and the viewer can rotate different lenses into place to compensate for long- or short-sightedness in both the patient and the nurse practitioner. A well-dilated pupil is essential to obtain a good view and therefore the procedure is best carried out in a darkened room. Munro and Edwards (1995) recommend that in children and adults in whom diabetic retinopathy is being checked, the best views may be obtained by use of tropicamide 0.5% eye drops to dilate the pupil. These drops take 20 minutes to work and pupil reactions should always be tested *before* instillation.

The bright light may be tiresome for the patient so the nurse practitioner should allow short breaks in carrying out the exam and not prolong the proceedings unnecessarily. Hold the ophthalmoscope in the right hand if you are looking through the instrument with the right eye: use the other hand to stabilize the patient by holding his or her shoulder. Your face will be close to the patient's face for some time during this procedure, so think about what your breath smells of, particularly if you smoke.

Begin with the ophthalmoscope set to zero. Examine the right eye using your right eye and the left eye with your left eye. Ask the patient to look at a distant object and examine the eye from a distance of 30 cm. At this distance the red disc of the retina should be visible (the familiar red-eye effect produced by amateur photographers taking flash photographs). Absence of a red reflex usually indicates that the ophthalmoscope is in the wrong position, although it is also absent if there is total opacity of the pupil as a result of a cataract. Any localized opacities will be visible as dark patches against the background red glow.

Slowly approach the patient until a good view of the retina or fundus is obtained. It will not be possible to view the whole retina at once; you will only see a portion at any one time. At a distance of 3–5 cm the first blood vessels should be seen and, as these always branch away from the optic disc, this should allow visualization of this landmark. The index finger can be used to adjust the lens wheel until a sharp image is seen. Arterioles are usually slightly larger and of brighter red than venules. It is important to distinguish between them as their crossing points may reveal important information. The optic disc should have a well-defined margin, although occasionally myelinated nerve fibres are visible, creating a soft white, ill-defined edge to the disc. This is an essentially benign condition. The macula or fovea centralis may be found two optic disc diameters temporal to the optic disc but is difficult to see in an undilated pupil as the pupil reflex may obscure the view. It helps to ask the patient to look directly at the light; the macula should appear as a yellow dot surrounded by a deep pink periphery.

Description of the view is carried out systematically in a clockwise direction, viewing the retina as a clockface with the optic disc at the centre. The unit of measurement of distance is the diameter of the optic disc. Any abnormal features can be described as so many optic disc diameters from the optic disc at whatever hour it would be on a clockface.

It is important to become confident of your technique when carrying out ophthalmoscopy, and to be familiar with the normal appearance of the fundus. Only frequent practice will bring this about and this is necessary if abnormalities are to be recognized. If a medical practitioner is willing to demonstrate to the nurse practitioner abnormal findings as they present in patients, this will greatly assist you to recognize them independently. We will briefly mention some of the more common abnormal findings; those interested in this area may wish to consult a more advanced medical text for further information.

- Papilloedema: this is usually produced by increased intracranial pressure or cerebral oedema and results in swelling of the optic disc so that its normal cup shape is lost, veins are dilated and the margins become blurred. Venous haemorrhages may also be seen. Vision is not affected initially
- Glaucoma: the increased intraocular pressure disrupts the normal vascular supply to the optic nerve, resulting in blood vessels seemingly disappearing under the optic disc, which in turn shows cupping – it is depressed backwards. The disc also appears much paler than normal due to its diminished blood supply
- Haemorrhages: they can vary in size, shape and location depending upon their cause. Bleeding into the anterior chamber is known as a hyphaema and may initially appear as nothing more than a clouding of the chamber on ophthalmoscopy although later a distinct fluid level will be seen (Greaves *et al.* 1997). Glaucoma tends to lead to haemorrhages at the margin of the disc, while hypertension can lead to flame haemorrhages, which are superficial flame-shaped areas. A dark red blot indicates a deep haemorrhage although a microaneurysm usually cannot be distinguished from a deep haemorrhage. Both are seen in cases of diabetic retinopathy. In a vitreous haemorrhage the fundus view is usually lost altogether as blood has oozed throughout the vitreous humour
- Hypertensive retinopathy: hypertension is associated with disease of the arterial walls and this leads to the characteristic finding of arterioles causing venules to appear pinched where they cross. This is because the thickened arteriole wall is compressing the venule. Flame haemorrhages may be observed (see above) and papilloedema may also be present
- Diabetic retinopathy: haemorrhage has already been mentioned and is the early sign of diabetic retinopathy. Retinal ischaemia may become apparent later, as shown by venous dilation, creamy-coloured lesions known as hard exudates because of their well-defined borders (they consist of lipoproteins leaking from damaged blood vessels) and similar-looking but fuzzy-edged lesions, known as cotton wool spots, which represent infarcted nerve fibres. In advanced disease (proliferative diabetic retinopathy) new blood vessels may be seen developing; they are narrow and tortuous and may give rise to bleeds, causing loss of vision.

Visual function

Visual acuity should be tested first using the standard Snellen chart at a distance of 6 metres. It is useful to have a permanent mark, measured at 6 metres from a wall, ready to carry out this test if required. When asking the patient to read down the chart, the nurse practitioner is assessing which is the last line that can be read and noting the number of that line. The numbers (6, 9, 12, 18, 24, 36 and 60) represent the distance at which the normal eye can read each line of print. Visual acuity is then expressed as the distance in metres from the chart (usually 6) over the number of the last line read. A rating of 6/6 is therefore normal eyesight whereas a score of 6/9 means that at 6 metres the person can only read what a normal eye could read at 9 metres. The legal limit for driving is 6/12 and 3/60 is classified as legal blindness.

The test should be carried out on each eye in turn with the other eye obscured. In testing the second eye it helps to ask the person to read from right to left as this minimizes the memory effect. You should always check whether the person is wearing contact lenses before carrying out the test. If vision is less than 3/60, you should ask the person to count how many fingers they can see when you hold your hand up 1 metre away. It is also important to test whether they can detect movement or see light.

Visual fields

Peripheral vision can be tested simply with the confrontation test. Sit opposite the patient at a distance of 1 metre and ask him or her to cover the left eye. Cover your right eye, extend your left arm out wide horizontally and start to bring it inwards, asking the patient to tell you when he or she first sees your fingers. Compare your first perception of your fingers with the patient's to see if they are about the same or whether the patient is seeing your fingers significantly after you do, indicating a loss of peripheral vision. This should be repeated in the vertical plane, testing both above and below the patient's line of vision and also in the horizontal plane, but using the right hand to test peripheral vision from the midline (the nasal field will be less than the others because the nose limits this field of vision). The other eye may then be tested by reversing this procedure. It is important to be confident that you do not have any impairment of your own field of vision if the patient's responses are to be interpreted correctly.

Record any visual field defect and refer the patient on for more accurate determination of its extent (see

p. 74 for possible causes). In addition to defects in the periphery, the patient may report having an area of blindness surrounded by an area of vision – a scotoma. If attempting to fix the gaze on an object with one eye leads to the loss of vision of the object, this is a central scotoma and indicates disease of the macula, whereas if the scotoma occurs in the same area in each eye, this suggests an intracranial lesion affecting the visual pathway.

Summary

In carrying out a physical examination the following areas should be covered:

- External inspection of the area around the eye and the eyelids
- The vision in each eye – acuity and field of vision
- Peripheral vision by confrontation testing
- Ocular movements
- Pupil size and reaction
- Inspection of the cornea and testing the corneal reflex
- Ophthalmoscopy to examine the optic discs and retina

Laboratory studies and other investigations

A swab should be taken for culture and sensitivity if the patient presents with evidence of infection (inflammation and discharge leading to a 'sticky eye'). This is often the case with conjunctivitis although the infective organism may be viral rather than bacterial.

Other more specialist equipment includes the applanometer, slit-lamp and a perimeter. The applanometer is an electronic measuring instrument measuring intraocular pressure (normal 16–21 mmHg). This is an essential measurement in cases of suspected glaucoma and is now replacing the tonometer which was used to make the same observation. If you detect signs suggestive of glaucoma, intraocular pressure measurements are needed as a matter of urgency. The slit-lamp microscope permits detailed viewing of the eye and is particularly useful in dealing with foreign bodies, corneal abrasions and ulceration. A slit-lamp microscope is therefore extremely useful in A&E work. Fluorescein eye drops are used in conjunction with the slit-lamp to visualize corneal lesions. The perimeter is a semicircular instrument which permits accurate measurement in degrees of the patient's field of vision. If confrontation testing shows a defect, the patient should be referred for perimetry.

Detailed testing of visual acuity for a prescription for spectacles or contact lenses is of course the work of the optician. The nurse practitioner may be the first health professional who diagnoses the need for such specialist intervention.

Other highly specialized tests may be carried out in ophthalmology units, including gonioscopy to measure the angle of the anterior chamber, echo-ophthalmography using ultrasound to examine the interior of the eye when cataract prevents direct visualization or to check for retinal detachment, and fluorescein angiography, which assesses vascular structures within the eye and the condition of the retina.

Differential diagnosis

Sore red eye

When this is the presenting complaint, the nurse practitioner has to decide between the following possibilities:

- Foreign body: check history, examine for object; evert the upper lid in case it is a subtarsal body and use fluorescein eye drops
- Stye or chalazion: examine eye lids carefully
- Allergic reaction: check history, examine periorbital area for signs of oedema
- Conjunctivitis: characteristic pattern of inflammation, complaint of mild discomfort rather than severe pain
- Corneal abrasion or ulceration: painful; check history, including exposure to ultraviolet light; corneal damage is usually visible on examination with fluorescein eye drops; corneal discharge is present
- Acute glaucoma: painful, fixed dilated pupil; ophthalmoscopy shows raised intraocular pressure
- Iritis: small pupil, painful, redness restricted to immediate area of iris

Visual disturbance

It is important to obtain a clear history from the patient as the diagnosis is based upon essentially subjective information given by the patient. The main causes are likely to be:

- Refractive errors: history of eye strain; test visual acuity
- Double vision: check history, especially for any trauma. Observe movement of eyes; ascertain in which direction of gaze the diplopia is most pronounced to test whether this is an acquired paralytic condition caused by neuropathy affecting the oculomotor muscles
- Haloes, floaters and flashing lights: usually associated with a loss of vision (discussed below). Check whether migraine can be eliminated. Note that an occasional floater is not abnormal.

Loss of vision

A sudden loss of vision suggests a vascular cause rather than the progressive loss of vision associated with a space-occupying lesion, such as a pituitary tumour affecting the optic nerve or problems such as cataract formation. The following are the main causes of loss of vision:

- A lesion affecting the macula, or the optic nerve, anterior to the chiasma may produce total loss of vision in one eye only (assuming the lesion is on one side only)
- If the optic chiasma is affected by a lesion such as a pituitary tumour, visual loss will occur in both eyes but on opposite sides of the visual fields (bitemporal hemianopia)
- A lesion proximal to the optic chiasma produces loss of vision in both eyes but on the same side (homonymous hemianopia)
- Cataract leads to a history of gradual loss of visual acuity in one or both eyes and is readily visible on ophthalmoscopy as the lens appears opaque when viewed through the pupil
- Chronic glaucoma is associated with a history of progressively reduced peripheral vision, persistent haloes around bright lights and pain as a late symptom. Ophthalmoscopy and intraocular pressure measurement will confirm the diagnosis. Acute glaucoma is an ocular emergency caused by blockage of the drainage of aqueous humour. The dramatic rise in intraocular pressure leads to compression of the retinal blood vessels and destruction of the optic nerve cells. The patient will complain of rapid onset of severe pain, nausea and vomiting, blurred vision and haloes around bright lights. Characteristic changes include cupping of the optic disc and a much paler appearance than normal and these are visible on ophthalmoscopy
- Retinal detachment leads to sudden onset of floaters and loss of vision in the affected eye. Vitreous haemorrhage may be visible on ophthalmoscopy
- Diabetic retinopathy may lead to sudden loss of vision associated with sudden vitreous haemorrhage. There will normally be a significant history of diabetes and diabetic retinopathy

Treatment and management

This section will focus on those conditions that the nurse practitioner can manage alone. Other conditions that need referral to an optician or a medical practitioner who is possibly a specialist in ophthalmology will be briefly mentioned. You must appreciate that some disorders need urgent referral and be aware of any immediate first-aid steps. It is greatly to the patient's advantage if there are agreed referral pathways for the nurse practitioner, whether working in primary health care, a community hospital minor injuries unit or a general hospital A&E department, as this is no time for inter-professional political wrangles.

It is important in caring for patients presenting with an eye injury always to remember that the patient may be very anxious about possible blindness. You must consider the patient's psychological welfare and adopt a calm reassuring manner throughout. Social factors also need to be considered, such as how the patient will get home afterwards, whether s/he is safe to drive and how s/he will cope at home; this is particularly important in elderly individuals. As a general principle you should also be thinking about health education advice to prevent future problems.

Trauma

Simple lacerations around the eye may be closed in the normal way, preferably with steristrips or tissue adhesive to minimize scarring. If the laceration involves the eyelid or margin it is best to refer to a medical specialist. A history suggesting that a wound to the orbit may be penetrating should also alert the nurse practitioner to the need for medical referral as foreign material may be retained deep within the wound and intraocular structures may have been damaged. Radiography will reveal any metallic or stone fragments.

Blunt trauma involving an object the size of a squash ball can have serious consequences as the object fits within the orbit and may impact fully against the eye. The result may be haemorrhage into either the anterior chamber which will be visible as a collection of blood with a clear fluid level (a hyphaema) or into the vitreous, with the added risk of retinal detachment. Immediate referral to a medical specialist is indicated.

Foreign body

A subtarsal foreign body can be removed after everting of the lid. Local anaesthetic will usually be required (amethocaine 0.5% eye drops), after which a cotton wool bud moistened with normal saline can be used to remove the object gently. A good light source and a confident but gentle manner are essential.

If the object is located on the cornea it may be removed by irrigation using saline and either an eye undine or intravenous giving set. Jones (1998) recommends trickling the saline into the inner part of the eye and letting it run outwards, do not let it drop directly on to the cornea as this is painful. Alternatively a moist cotton wool bud may be used. Amethocaine 0.5% eyedrops should be instilled first.

They are rapid-acting (within a minute) but wear off after 20–30 minutes (Jones 1998). Local anaesthetic eye drops should never be used in the management of symptoms (*British National Formulary* 1999). If the eye remains sore after removal of the foreign body, local anaesthetic drops should *not* be given to the patient to take home as an anaesthetized eye is prone to further injury and may also have its healing impeded.

A foreign body may cause abrasion to the cornea and the traditional treatment has been to rest the eye with homatropine eye drops, instil an antibiotic ointment and pad the eye for 24 hours. There has been some debate as to how necessary a pad really is and a study by Hart *et al.* (1997) showed that there was no difference in pain relief for patients with corneal abrasions whether an eye pad was worn or not. A different approach has been described by Brahma *et al.* (1996); these authors showed that instillation of flurbiprofen 0.03% drops four times daily (a topical non-steroidal anti-inflammatory drug) combined with chloramphenicol ointment and an eye pad worn for only 6 hours produced better pain relief for patients than the traditional treatment.

If the object is not readily removed from the cornea, the patient should be referred to a medical specialist because of the risk of corneal damage and infection. In the meantime, an eye pad should be fixed over the eye as protection and the patient advised not to rub it.

Penetrating foreign bodies may leave little or no trace of their passing and therefore may be easily missed. The history is vital: if the patient was engaged in the kind of activity that may have produced high-velocity particles such as using a hammer and chisel, a drill or garden machinery, the nurse practitioner should suspect the possibility of a penetrating foreign body and seek a medical opinion. In some cases signs such as a distorted pupil or a vitreous haemorrhage may be apparent, but such is the potential damage from an untreated intraocular foreign body, even if there are no obvious signs, that you should act on the history and refer.

If chemical damage has occurred, copious irrigation with water should take place and any obvious solid particles should be removed from the conjunctival sac (e.g. cement or mortar, both of which contain lime). Local anaesthetic drops should be used to facilitate this process and an immediate medical referral is essential.

Do not miss a potential health education opportunity in the case of eye injury. The use of protective eye equipment should be emphasized, whether for work or for playing squash.

Disorders involving the eyelids

- Chalazion: some may be persistent, become infected and even lead to disturbance of vision by causing astigmatism. In these cases medical referral for surgical treatment is necessary. The large majority can be dealt with conservatively by advising warm compresses such as a face cloth soaked in warm water and the application of chloramphenicol ointment to deal with any infection. The patient should be asked to return if this regime fails to clear up the problem
- Stye: this should be treated in the same way as a chalazion. The warm compresses will help draw the stye and lead to its eventual discharge while the chloramphenicol ointment will deal with the infective organism
- Blepharitis: chloramphenicol ointment should be prescribed for application to the edge of the lid after it has been cleaned with a cotton wool bud dipped in warm water. This cleansing should take place at least twice a day. Artificial tears may also have to be prescribed. If little improvement occurs after follow-up, medical referral is necessary to treat the sebaceous gland dysfunction that probably lies at the root of the problem
- Acute inflammation of the eyelid: the cause of the inflammation may be a stye or chalazion, in which case the treatment described above will be sufficient. However, in the presence of a vesicular rash, herpes simplex or herpes-zoster ophthalmicus is likely to be present, either of which could lead to serious herpetic ocular disease. This indicates the need for a rapid medical referral. If orbital cellulitis is suspected, urgent specialist referral is needed as this can lead to blindness in a matter of hours (Elkington and Khaw 1988)
- Entropion: a first-aid solution involves taping down the lid and applying chloramphenicol ointment. Surgical correction is necessary for a long-term solution
- Ectropion: this too requires surgical correction; chloramphenicol ointment will assist in the short term
- Ptosis: as this may be a sign of serious systemic disease such as an aneurysm causing third cranial nerve palsy, prompt medical referral is necessary whatever the patient's age

Corneal damage

Whether the problem is caused by ulceration, abrasion or exposure to ultraviolet light, the approach to treatment is the same, although such are the potentially serious consequences of corneal damage (loss of vision) that rapid referral to a medical specialist is recommended. Fluorescein eye drops should be used for examination of the cornea as ulceration or abrasions will be readily apparent. Treatment aims to protect the eye in the interim (whilst waiting to see a specialist) with a pad and prevent infection with the use of chloramphenicol 1% eye ointment. The discussion on treatment of corneal abrasions on p. 82 should be borne in mind if any significant delay is expected in seeing an ophthalmology specialist or in transfer to an A&E department. Systemic analgesia (such as paracetamol) should also be recommended to relieve the pain. Before any chloramphenicol is used, swabs should be taken to help identify any organisms present.

Chloramphenicol ointment lasts longer than eye drops as it is less likely to be diluted by tears. It should be administered three to four times daily and you should carefully explain that it is only administered to the affected eye and that a thin smear along the lower lid is all that is required. If both eyes are affected, as in ultraviolet light exposure, one tube should be used for the left and another for the right eye, both clearly labelled. This is to prevent the risk of cross-infection. The patient should be made aware of the dangers of exposure to ultraviolet light when using an artificial sunlamp or when skiing (reflected sunlight off the snow surface). If welding has been the cause of the problem the opportunity should be taken to check the individual's understanding of health and safety regulations at work as protective wear must be provided for those working with welding equipment. It is essential to check how the patient intends to get home after treatment for corneal damage as driving is not advised.

Conjunctivitis

The infective organism may be bacterial or viral and in the latter case it is often associated with an upper respiratory tract infection. Viral conjunctivitis may produce a clear discharge as opposed to the mucopurulent discharge seen in bacterial cases. The treatment is the same in either case – chloramphenicol eye ointment (1%) in two tubes clearly labelled left and right. If it is a bacterial infection, the chloramphenicol will deal with it and if it is a viral problem, it will stop the secondary bacterial infection which often occurs, making the situation worse. Viral conjunctivitis is fortunately a self-limiting condition. Conjunctivitis is contagious so great care must be taken with measures to avoid cross-infection of other patients, staff or the nurse practitioner. Patients should be informed about the risk of infecting other family members and advised to use only their own face cloth and towel. It is wise to ask the patient to return if the problem does not resolve within a few days.

If the conjunctivitis is allergic in nature, antihistamine eye drops such as antazoline (2–3 times daily) or levocabastine (twice daily) may be prescribed together with oral antihistamines. It is important to ascertain the likely cause of the reaction and what steps can be taken to remove the patient from exposure to the causative agent.

Iriitis and uveitis

If either of these conditions is suspected you should refer the patient to a medical practitioner as there may be serious underlying pathology, either local (intraocular tumour, detached retina) or systemic, such as one of the arthropathies (ankylosing spondylitis, juvenile arthritis), sarcoidosis or infections such as syphilis, tuberculosis or herpeszoster ophthalmicus. Sometimes the cause remains obscure, but as the possible effects on the eye are serious, a medical practitioner should be involved at an early stage.

Other ophthalmic emergencies

Sudden visual disturbances, such as the appearance of:

- floaters due to possible detached retina or vitreous haemorrhage
- haloes due to the onset of acute open-angle glaucoma
- loss of vision in an eye due to arterial occlusion or disciform macular degeneration

Require prompt referral to an ophthalmic specialist, as would any case of penetrating eye trauma, chemical injury or severe pain in and around the eye which you are confident is not a migraine.

Other ophthalmic conditions

There are many other conditions which may present to the nurse practitioner as the first point of contact with the health care system. These vary from disorders such as squints and diplopia through to conditions such as cataracts or chronic open-angle glaucoma. Medical referral is necessary as these are serious disorders which may lead to loss of vision or even, in the case of diplopia, be signs of underlying pathology affecting the cranial nerves which innervate the extraocular muscles. Refractive errors of vision are best referred to an optician together with individuals seeking advice about contact lenses. A contact lens lost in the eye may be difficult to find but will usually be in the lower fornix or under the subtarsal plate (Jones 1998).

References

Bates B. (1995) *A Guide to Physical Examination and History Taking*, 6th edn. Philadelphia, JB Lippincott.

Brahma A., Shah S., Hiller V. *et al.* (1996) Topical analgesia for superficial corneal injuries, *Journal of Accident and Emergency Medicine*, **13**, pp. 186–188.

British National Formulary (1999) London, British Medical

Association, Royal Pharmaceutical Society of Great Britain.

Elkington A., Khaw P. (1988) *ABC of Eyes*, London, *British Medical Journal*.

Greaves I., Porter K., Burke D. (1997) *Key Topics in Trauma*, Oxford, Bios Scientific.

Hart A., White S., Conboy P., Quinton D. (1997) The management of corneal abrasions in A&E, *Injury*, **28**(8), pp. 527–529.

Jones G. (1998) Foreign bodies in the eye, *Accident and Emergency Nursing*, **6**, pp. 66–69.

Munro I., Edwards C. (1995) *Macleod's Clinical Examination*, 9th edn., Edinburgh, Churchill Livingstone.

Rees P., Williams D. (1995) *Principles of Clinical Medicine*, London, Edward Arnold.

Seidel H., Ball J., Dains I., Benedict G. (1995) *Mosby's Guide to Physical Examination*, 3rd edn., St Louis, CV Mosby.

Walsh M. (1996) *A&E Nursing: A New Approach*, Oxford, Butterworth-Heinemann.

CHAPTER 7
The cardiovascular system

Mike Walsh

Introduction

The importance of this system for survival needs no emphasis and, whilst nurses have traditionally undertaken basic measures such as blood pressure and pulse monitoring and, more recently, ECG recording, there is much more to learn that will enhance nursing practice. Enhanced knowledge and skills will assist the nurse whether s/he is working in a specialized field such as coronary care or in a more general nurse practitioner role in A&E or primary health care. This chapter will concentrate on the more commonly encountered conditions and, by acquainting the nurse with some history-taking and physical examination skills that have traditionally belonged in the medical sphere, we aim to show how nursing practice can be expanded to the patient's benefit. In each section of this chapter, the cardiovascular system will be considered in terms of the heart itself, the arterial system and the venous system.

Pathophysiology

The heart

Although mortality rates for coronary heart disease (CHD) are showing a decline, in 1995 it still accounted for one-quarter of all deaths in the UK (Department of Health 1997). The importance of this disorder therefore needs no emphasis, and in most cases the cause of CHD is atherosclerosis, although other less frequent causes include thrombus, embolism and coronary artery spasm. Atherosclerosis affects blood vessels elsewhere in the body, leading to peripheral vascular disease (p. 87). The main risk factors are well-known: hypertension, smoking, obesity, lack of exercise and diabetes, although controversy still surrounds the role of cholesterol in CHD.

Blood lipids are divided into high-density lipoproteins (HDL) and low-density lipoproteins (LDL). High levels of LDL associated with low levels of HDL are associated with increased risk of CHD. Cholesterol levels are poor predictors of the risk of a person having a CHD 'event' (such as a myocardial infarction) as studies have shown that 58% of UK males with an elevated cholesterol level (over 6.5 mmol/l) did not have a CHD event in the following 15-year period (York Centre for Review and Dissemination 1998).

Atherosclerosis causes narrowing of the artery lumen. When this exceeds 75% of the lumen and starts to compromise blood flow, symptoms of angina pectoris usually start to appear, especially when there is increased demand for oxygen by the myocardium. An abrupt reduction or complete loss of blood flow in the coronary artery may occur when an atheromatous plaque suddenly fissures and develops an associated thrombosis. This manifests itself as a myocardial infarction (Thompson and Webster 1992). Tissue beyond the obstruction loses its blood supply and rapidly dies before any collateral circulation can be established. One or more layers of the heart may be involved and the infarcted zone may be a volume of 1–2 cm across. Fibrous scar tissue eventually replaces the dead area of myocardium.

Heart failure is a common condition in the older population and is said to occur when cardiac output fails to meet the metabolic demands of the body. This usually occurs secondary to any disease which impairs cardiac function. Examples include myocardial ischaemia, myocardial infarction, established hypertension, cardiac arrhythmias and valvular disease (see below). Although reference is commonly made to left- or right-sided heart failure, the close relationship between the two sides of the heart means that, in practice, whichever side starts to fail, first the other will soon follow. The pattern of presenting signs and symptoms reflects this close association.

In left-sided failure, the problem is the heart's inability to pump blood efficiently into the systemic circulation, leading to congestion of the pulmonary vessels (backward heart failure) and accumulation of fluid in the alveoli (pulmonary oedema). This in turn causes symptoms of acute respiratory distress such as dyspnoea and coughing. The reduced cardiac output that follows from left-sided failure (forward failure) results in reduced renal perfusion. The body consequently retains sodium and water due to activation of the renin–angiotensin system and aldesterone production. Failure of the right side, which may be secondary to left failure, causes congestion of the venous system with congestion and oedema of peripheral tissues and organs.

Cardiac arrhythmias may produce no discernible effect and may only be discovered when a routine ECG is performed. Some arrhythmias are persistent but others are short-lived, consequently their effects may be transient and patients may present with a normal ECG even though they have a history of 'funny turns' or 'palpitations'. More persistent arrhythmias may have significant haemodynamic effects, reducing cardiac output and leading to heart failure (e.g. atrial fibrillation or bradycardia associated with heart block) or may predispose to thrombus formation. Most serious of all, some ventricular arrhythmias can be life-threatening (ventricular tachycardia) or result in complete collapse with cessation of cardiac output (ventricular fibrillation). Arrhythmias and ECG interpretation will be dealt with in more detail later in this chapter (p. 95).

Hypertension is associated with a substantial rise in mortality rates. It is either due to increased peripheral resistance in the arterioles (essential hypertension) or secondary to some other disorder such as renal disease, which usually involves the renin–angiotensin mechanism. Severe hypertension is defined as blood pressure (BP) in excess of 180/120 mmHg, whilst moderate hypertension is defined as a BP in the range 160/100 to 180/120 mmHg: in mild hypertension the BP lies in the range 140/90 to 160/90 mmHg (Rees and Williams 1995). There is evidence that Afro-Caribbean people are twice as susceptible to hypertension as Caucasians and in the USA are four times more likely to die as a result of the disease (Springhouse 1997). In many cases the patient is asymptomatic and hypertension is diagnosed as a result of a routine BP reading. In severe fulminating hypertension, the patient presents as an acute medical emergency with severe head-aches, vomiting, visual disturbances, papilloedema and retinal haemorrhages.

Disease of the valves within the heart may be either congenital or acquired, usually after rheumatic fever. Congenital problems usually cause stenosis of the pulmonary or aortic valves (a whole range of other congenital cardiac malformations are possible) whilst the mitral and aortic valves are most susceptible to the inflammatory response associated with rheumatic fever which leads to scarring and thickening of the valve tissue.

Congenital pulmonary stenosis leads to a build-up of back-pressure within the venous system and reduction in pulmonary blood flow and hence oxygenation. This leads in turn to chronic fatigue, shortness of breath and sometimes cyanosis. Although this is a congenital problem, the child may be several years old before symptoms become serious enough for the parent to bring him or her for attention. Aortic stenosis leads to reduced cardiac output and hence reduced arterial blood pressure.

Inflammatory disease of the valves can also produce stenosis which in turn increases the work of the heart chamber behind the damaged valve as it strives to force blood through the narrowed opening. In some cases loss of tissue occurs; this prevents the valvular cusps from coming together and consequently regurgitation or back-flow occurs – this is known as valvular incompetence. It is not uncommon for both conditions to exist together, seriously impairing the heart's ability to function normally and leading to serious damage (dilatation and hypertrophy) to the chamber behind the incompetent valve.

Other presenting conditions include pericarditis and infective endocarditis. The former is an inflammation of the pericardium, usually associated with a viral or bacterial infection, trauma or an autoimmune reaction. The inflammatory process leads to the accumulation of fluid in the pericardium which inhibits normal cardiac expansion (cardiac tamponade). Infective endocarditis may be associated with rheumatic fever, routine dental procedures, minor infections, parenteral drug use or valvular abnormalities. It may be acute and be caused by virulent organisms such as *Streptococcus pneumoniae* or *Neisseria meningitidis* or have a slower subacute presentation, which is usually associated with *Streptococcus viridans* or *Staphylococcus epidermidis* (Walsh 1997). Cardiac tamponade may occur in cases of trauma where an object penetrating the chest strikes the heart a glancing blow, leading to the accumulation of blood in the pericardium.

Arterial disorders

The same pathological processes that cause damage to the coronary arteries can affect arteries elsewhere in the body. Weakening of the wall of the aorta in the abdomen leads to the development of an aortic aneurysm which may present as an acute emergency or as a chronic problem. Symptoms are often not what might be expected (e.g. back pain) and this can cause a delay in diagnosis. As a leaking aortic aneurysm is potentially fatal, a high level of suspicion is necessary if seeing a male over the age of 65 with abdominal pain as, according to Munro and Edwards (1995), a leaking aneurysm is one of the commonest causes of abdominal pain in such patients.

Arterial disease may affect the main arteries of the legs in such a way as to produce a sudden blockage and loss of circulation (arterial embolism) or chronic deterioration in blood supply leading to intermittent claudication (pain on walking caused by a similar mechanism to anginal pain) and peripheral gangrenous ulcers (Table 7.1). Eventually the limb may be lost as a result of gangrene and the patient's life may be endangered through toxaemia and other metabolic disturbances secondary to gangrene if medical assistance has not been sought soon enough.

A less severe arterial condition is Raynaud's disease. The cause is unknown but it most commonly affects young adults (females more than males). The patient experiences severe episodes of vasospasm affecting the hands and sometimes the feet, which go white before turning red as the circulation returns, often causing significant pain and discomfort. These features may occur as a consequence of some other disorder (secondary Raynaud's), such as working with vibrating machinery, but then they are more localized.

Venous disorders

Deep venous thrombosis (DVT) is familiar to all nurses as a complication of prolonged immobility, usually affecting the iliac, femoral or calf veins. The associated risk of a pulmonary embolism due to a fragment of the clot dislodging is least if the thrombosis is only found within the calf veins. Other risk factors for DVT include heart disease, diabetes, use of the contraceptive pill and malignant disease.

Incompetence of the vein wall and/or valves is a common cause of varicose veins. Obstruction of venous return is also a contributory factor. The result is the development of distended and tortuous veins in the lower leg which, apart from being unsightly,

cause the patient considerable pain. Consistently raised venous pressure around the ankles is associated with peripheral oedema and venous insufficiency. It leads to the breakdown of the skin on the medial and lateral aspects of the lower leg and the formation of chronic ulcers which are notoriously difficult to heal, due to poor circulation, risk of infection and advancing age of the patient.

Taking a focused history

Cardiac disorder

Pain

The PQRST framework (p. 16) is valuable in evaluating the symptom of pain associated with the cardiovascular system. Chest pain which is provoked (P) by exertion but palliated (P) by rest is characteristic of angina, whereas the pain of myocardial infarction (MI) is usually unrelieved by rest or taking GTN. Emotional upset, cold weather and exertion after a large meal may also provoke an anginal attack. However, the patient frequently cannot point to anything which brings on the pain associated with MI. This is the key difference that will appear in the history between the two conditions. Other symptoms are similar, for example the patient usually describes the quality (Q) of the pain, whether due to angina or myocardial infarction, in terms of tightness, such as a crushing weight on the chest, although it may be described in terms of wind. The region (R) in both cases is retrosternal, located towards the base of the sternum, with radiation (R) occurring to the arm, hand, jaw (possibly leading to the patient presenting with toothache) or even the

Table 7.1   Differential diagnosis: causes of chest pain

	Angina	Gastrointestinal	Musculoskeletal	Respiratory
Provocation	Exercise Emotional upset	Related to food consumption	Related to trauma, physical effort	Increases with inspiration or trunk movement
Palliation	Rest GTN	Antacids	Mild analgesics, heat, rest	Little relief
Quality	Tightness	Burning, discomfort, wind	Ache	Sharp, grabbing (pleurisy, pneumothorax or pulmonary embolism) or dull, aching in pneumonia
	Stops patient activity	Patient carries on activity	Patient carries on activity	Lower chest, sometimes bilateral
Region	Retrosternal	Epigastric/retrosternal	Intercostal	Pneumothorax on entire side of chest
Radiation	Arm, wrist, hand, jaw	Unlikely, though possibly through to back	Backache	Pneumothorax radiates to back
Severity	Moderate	Variable	Moderate, though variable	Moderate to severe
Timing	Recent specific onset	Vague onset, though may waken patient from sleep	Shortly after physical effort	Sudden onset and then continual pain

ear. The pain may be severe (S), although some elderly patients may have an MI with little apparent pain. There is little association between the severity of chest pain and the seriousness of the illness (Hill and Geraci 1998). It is clearly important to know how long ago the pain began (time: T).

Chest pain is not uniquely caused by cardiac disorder. It is frequently musculoskeletal or associated with gastrointestinal problems. It may also be due to a respiratory disorder such as pneumothorax, pulmonary embolism, pneumonia or pleurisy. Table 7.1 is based on work by Hill and Geraci (1998) and should allow the nurse practitioner taking a focused history to distinguish between the most likely causes of the patient's chest pain.

Dyspnoea

Difficulty in breathing or shortness of breath brought on by lower than normal levels of exertion is a second major group of symptoms. The nurse practitioner needs to enquire into this area and try to ascertain exactly what the patient means by a phrase such as 'short of breath'. The PQRST framework guides the nurse practitioner into checking what brings on the symptom. If it is exertion, it is important to find out how much, such as climbing the stairs at home or walking up hills. The cause may be nothing to do with exertion as the patient may wake up suddenly short of breath with signs of pulmonary oedema and a frothy cough in left-sided heart failure (paroxysmal nocturnal dyspnoea). If the symptom is persistent even when resting during the day, this suggests severe heart failure, assuming a respiratory cause can be eliminated. Pulmonary oedema will be associated with dyspnoea in acute left-sided heart failure.

Other symptoms

Impaired cardiac output leads to fatigue and difficulty in keeping up a normal level of exertion. Cardiac arrhythmias may be perceived by the patient as palpitations or a sensation of feeling light-headed. Momentary loss of consciousness or syncope attacks may occur with some arrhythmias such as heart block (p. 95). The patient may complain of swollen ankles; oedema has been referred to above and is frequently found in heart failure or venous stasis. Alternative causes of oedema such as hepatic disorder or nephrotic syndrome should be eliminated before a cardiac origin is ascribed to this symptom.

Past medical history

Check whether the patient has a previous history of cardiac disorder such as hypertension, angina or a previous MI. Also enquire about associated diseases such as diabetes or rheumatic fever.

Family history

There is a genetic element associated with many cardiac diseases. Check whether there is any family history of diabetes, hypertension, hyperlipidaemia, congenital heart defects or other heart disease. Any unexplained sudden deaths in the family may also be significant evidence of cardiovascular disease.

Social history

Check known risk factors such as whether the person smokes (and if so, how much), diet, exercise, occupation, how s/he deals with stress and alcohol consumption.

Taking a focused history from the patient with peripheral vascular disease

Arterial disease

The previous medical, family and social histories should be explored as above because the underlying disease process is likely to be the same as that causing cardiac pain, i.e. atherosclerosis. The main difference is that the site of pain is in the leg. It is usually brought on by exercise such as walking and is due to diminished blood flow being unable to meet the tissues' metabolic demands. This type of pain is known as claudication; in more advanced cases the pain may be severe and present at rest. It is important to ascertain how far the patient can walk before the pain (P) comes on and how long s/he has to rest before it is relieved and the nature of the pain as it is typically a cramping pain (Q). Ask where the pain occurs (R) as this type of pain is usually in the calf; and enquire how severe it is (S). The effect on the person's lifestyle should also be noted as increasing difficulty in walking may be causing major problems. Time (T) since the patient first noted the problem is important: claudication usually has an insidious onset but an arterial embolus is a sudden event which the patient can pinpoint.

Venous disease

Pain is again the most common symptom and should be explored carefully in a focused history. Pain and swelling in the calf are suggestive of DVT; however, as Munro and Edwards (1995) point out, a potentially life-threatening DVT may produce no pain at all. The patient's previous medical history is important as an indicator of risk factors for DVT formation.

The pain of varicose veins typically gets worse during the day as the patient is standing: lying down and elevating the legs relieve the pain. The association between peripheral oedema and heart failure means that, although the patient may present with a complaint of swollen ankles, discoloured skin and possibly a venous leg ulcer, you must take a full cardiac history.

Physical assessment

General appearance

An initial decision must be made as to whether the patient is haemodynamically stable. If s/he is in a collapsed state with low blood pressure or absent pulse, then emergency resuscitation is necessary, However, if the patient has walked into the room then s/he may be assumed to be reasonably stable and a methodical assessment can be carried out, after obtaining the history.

The patient's general appearance holds several important clues. Dyspnoea on walking across the room clearly indicates a problem of cardiac or respiratory origin. Central cyanosis affecting the lips and mucous membranes of the mouth suggests impaired gas exchange in the lungs, raising the possibility of pulmonary oedema or respiratory disease. Congenital cardiac disorders may also cause central cyanosis. Peripheral cyanosis affecting the hands and feet, which look pale and feel cold with possibly weak or absent pulses suggests impaired cardiac output, peripheral vascular disease reducing blood flow to the extremities or vasoconstriction as found in Raynaud's disease. Inspection of the eye may reveal two significant signs of hypercholesterolaemia. Corneal arcus is the deposition of cholesterol at the edge of the cornea while xanthelasma is a yellowish deposit at the inner side of the eyelid of similar origin.

Pulse and BP

Check pulse and BP. The BP reading should be done carefully, ensuring that the right-sized cuff is used, the sphygmomanometer is at the same level as the patient's arm, there is no tight clothing around the arm, the patient is suitably relaxed and the arm is extended horizontally but well-supported. Modern electronic BP-measuring equipment requires the basic precautions described above to give accurate readings. If BP cannot be obtained at first, the end of the patient's finger should be compressed and the time taken for the colour to return to normal noted. If this is 2 seconds or greater, this indicates a profoundly shocked patient with a systolic BP of 60 mmHg or less.

Jugular venous pressure

Before moving on to examine the chest, the jugular venous pressure should also be recorded. This is a measure of pressure in the right atrium: raised pressure indicates either right-sided heart failure or an increase in the pressure in the pericardial sac which is restricting the return of blood to the right atrium (e.g. cardiac tamponade). Jugular venous pressure measurement is made relative to the sternal notch, which is always located 5 cm above the right atrium in the average adult, and is expressed as the vertical height above the sternal notch at which oscillations within the internal jugular vein can be seen. These oscillations are caused by pressure changes within the right atrium during the cardiac cycle.

In order to visualize these oscillations the patient should be reclining at 45° above the horizontal. If s/he is in a more upright position the oscillations become hidden by the clavicle and associated structures. If the jugular venous pressure is visible more than 4 cm vertically above the sternal angle, this is considered to be abnormally elevated (Figure 7.1). The exact angle that the patient is reclining at will not affect the measurement.

Chest examination

Useful information can be obtained by simply examining the chest visually. Privacy and a warm consulting room are essential. Evidence of old scars should be noted and their cause established (surgery or trauma). The general shape of the chest should be observed for any abnormalities. A simple but important observation is the location and extent of the apical beat, which should be visible in the mid clavicular line in either the fifth or fourth intercostal space. It is best seen with a tangential light source and may also be felt by gentle palpation. It is unlikely to be visible in muscular or obese individuals. If the apical beat is visible in two intercostal spaces, this suggests an enlarged heart – obviously a key observation.

Heart sounds and auscultation

We are all familiar with the basic 'lub dub' sound of a beating heart. In order to carry out a full physical exam, you must be able to use a stethoscope to check whether heart sounds are normal or abnormal. You must therefore understand the physiology behind what you are listening to in order to make a correct decision about referral.

The main heart sounds are caused by the closure of valves, their opening should be a silent event. It is the closure of the tricuspid and bicuspid valves at the beginning of systole that causes the first heart sound (S1). The opening of the aortic and pulmonic valves should be silent. Their closure at the end of systole, as the ventricles begin to fill with blood, produces the second heart sound (S2). This sound may be split as the two valves often do not close at exactly the same time. A deep inhalation may also produce a splitting of S2. Neither situation is abnormal. The tricuspid and bicuspid valves open to allow ventricular filling at this time, but these are silent events. The sound of blood filling the ventricles under the effect of gravity is faint but may just be heard as a third sound (S3). The contraction of the atria which expels the last fraction of blood into the

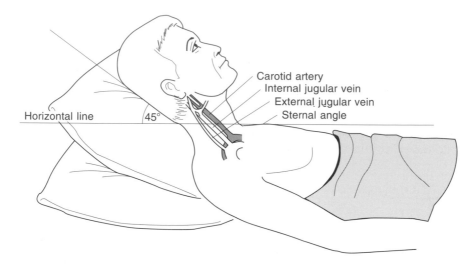

Figure 7.1 Measurement of jugular venous pressure (JVP). The JVP reading is the maximum height in centimetres above the sternal angle at which venous pulsations are visible

ventricles at the end of diastole may also produce a faint sound (S4). The soft, faint third and fourth heart sounds are best heard using the bell of the stethoscope placed over the apex, with the patient tilted on the left side at an angle of 45°.

Figure 7.2 shows the correct positions to place the stethoscope to carry out standard auscultation of the heart sounds. Positions 1 and 2 in the second intercostal space either side of the sternum will produce the clearest S2 sounds, while position 5 at the apex gives the best S1 sound (using the diaphragm). Work systematically through the five positions, slowly moving the stethoscope over the

chest wall, following each sound as you proceed. Continual practice will produce a smooth and competent technique allowing you to confidently recognize normal heart sounds.

Abnormal heart sounds may be due to many causes and may not even indicate pathology. The golden rule should be to refer to a doctor if abnormalities are detected. Diseased valves produce murmurs, clicking or snapping sounds; yet the presence of abnormal sounds may be benign. The S3 and S4 sounds are normally very faint; if they become pronounced the result is a gallop rhythm, rather than the normal 'lub dub'. Likely causes

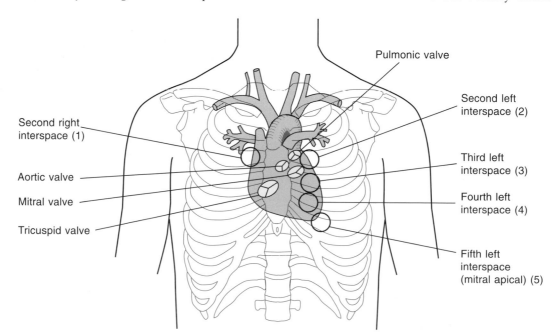

Figure 7.2 Sites for auscultation of heart sounds

include resistance to ventricular filling due to loss of compliance in the ventricular walls associated with hypertension and coronary artery disease or abnormally high stroke volumes associated with thyrotoxicosis, severe anaemia or pregnancy. Whenever an abnormal sound is detected, place it in the context of the patient's history and appearance, asking whether it can be linked to any obvious signs and symptoms, in order to assess its possible clinical significance. A medical opinion should always be obtained.

Peripheral examination

The patient's history and general appearance may indicate peripheral vascular disease. Cold, pale feet indicate a poor blood supply but the absence of *both* the dorsalis pedis and posterior tibial pulses (Figure 7.3) indicates significantly reduced arterial blood flow. The popliteal and femoral pulses should be assessed in such cases (Figure 7.4) and the results

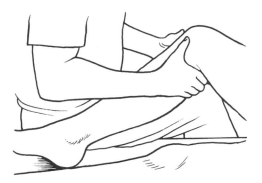

Figure 7.4 Examining the popliteal artery

recorded as suggested in Figure 7.5. A popliteal or femoral aneurysm may be discovered in this way. It will feel too obvious to be a normal pulse and is often described as expansile in that it pushes the examiner's fingers apart when gentle pressure is applied to both sides of the pulse.

If a Doppler probe is available, this can be used to assess the extent of peripheral ischaemia. A correctly sized BP cuff should be applied to the mid-calf region with the patient lying flat, and systolic BP estimated using the Doppler probe to detect arterial blood flow into the foot. This can then be divided by the systolic BP recorded in the arm to produce a ratio of ankle to brachial systolic BP. According to Munro and Edwards (1995), a ratio of between 0.7 and 1.0 is consistent with claudication, whilst severe ischaemia is present with a ratio < 0.4.

In severe ischaemia the foot may appear red but if it is elevated above the level of the heart it rapidly becomes pale, slowly turning red again if lowered below heart level due to capillary pooling. This is known as Buerger's test. Arterial ulcers may be seen on the toes or the sole of the foot and heel (dorsum). Gangrene and cellulitis may also be present.

Assess for peripheral venous disorder if the history is indicative of such problems. Both calves should

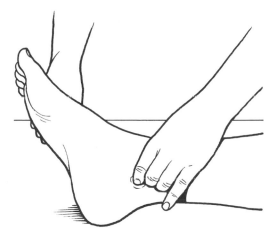

(a) Posterior tibial artery

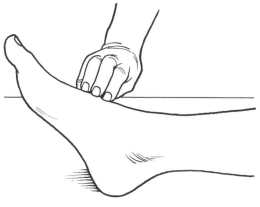

(b) Dorsalis pedis artery

Figure 7.3 Examining peripheral pulses in the foot. (a) The posterior tibial artery and (b) the dorsalis pedis artery

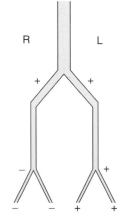

Figure 7.5 Recording peripheral pulses

be checked for size and tenderness (use a tape measure and ensure that circumference is measured at the same point on both legs with equal tension on the tape). The appearance, colour and warmth of the skin should be assessed for ulceration, oedema, varicose veins and engorgement.

Oedema in the lower limbs is associated with oedematous changes elsewhere if the cause is heart failure. Localized oedema indicates restriction of blood flow in the veins of the leg; the most probable cause is DVT. A red painful area close to a superficial vein is likely to be thrombophlebitis (superficial venous thrombosis), which does not carry the same serious potential threat as DVT. Prolonged immobility will produce localized oedema as the patient has lost the pumping action of the calf muscles.

Chronic venous insufficiency produces swelling and discoloration and may be associated with venous ulcers around the shins. This picture is usually seen in elderly patients and there are often other pathological processes at work, including arterial disease (giving a mix of arterial/venous signs and symptoms), diabetes and primary skin conditions.

Investigations

Electrocardiography

The electrocardiograph (ECG) is a useful adjunct to the physical examination and focused history. However it is just that, an adjunct, and you should always be mindful of caring for the patient rather than the ECG!

The 12-lead ECG is a three-dimensional picture of the electrical activity of the heart, as opposed to cardiac monitoring, which is concerned with arrhythmia detection, normally using chest leads only, in a coronary care or ambulatory setting. A correctly carried out 12-lead ECG can reveal evidence of myocardial ischaemia, myocardial infarction or ventricular hypertrophy. A short rhythm strip is routinely recorded as part of a 12-lead ECG which will help clarify any arrhythmia present, although continual monitoring is necessary if the arrhythmia is serious.

The ECG machine has electrodes attached to both wrists and ankles (only the left ankle is a recording lead as the right ankle serves as an earth) and has six separate chest (precordial) leads. The first six readings are designated I, II, III, aVR, aVL and aVF. The term bipolar or standard leads is used to describe I, II and III, while aVR, aVL and aVF are called unipolar leads. Each is the result of the machine making different combinations of the limb leads giving a three-dimensional picture of the heart's electrical activity: e.g. lead I is the voltage recorded in the left arm minus that recorded in the right. Figure 7.6 shows the views obtained.

The chest leads must be attached in the correct positions (Figure 7.7) which are as follows:

- V1: fourth intercostal space, immediately to the right of the sternum
- V2: fourth intercostal space, immediately to the left of the sternum
- V3: midway between V2 and V4
- V4: left fifth intercostal space, mid-clavicular line
- V5: left fifth intercostal space end of clavicle
- V6: left fifth intercostal space mid-axillary line

This ability to build up a three-dimensional picture of cardiac activity is of diagnostic significance, as will be seen. The interpretation of the ECG assumes that all the leads have been placed in the correct positions.

In order to take an ECG successfully it is important to explain carefully what is to happen to the patient in order to obtain complete cooperation. A simple explanation, such as: 'This machine will give us an accurate tracing of how your heart is beating' is more meaningful than a cryptic statement such as: 'I am just doing an ECG'. (At least one patient has confused ECG with ECT and become distressed as a result!) It is important to expose the chest fully, therefore privacy is required, especially for a female patient. Body hair seriously interferes with the trace so it must be shaved off as appropriate. Tremor will interfere with the recording so the patient must be still and relaxed. Calibration of the machine must

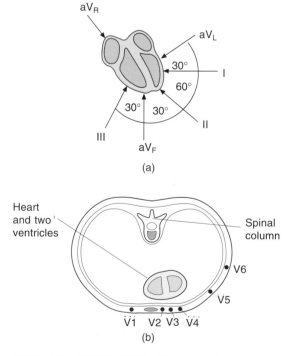

Figure 7.6 A 12 lead ECG showing (a) the views of heart obtained in the vertical plane by the limb leads and (b) views obtained by chest leads

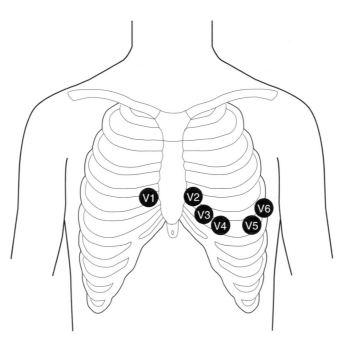

Figure 7.7   The correct positions of chest leads for a 12 lead ECG

be checked whenever it is used, along with paper speed. Interpretation assumes a vertical deflection of 1 cm corresponding to an electrical potential of 1 mV and that the paper speed is 25 mm/second. The most important piece of information on the ECG is the patient's name and date and time of the recording. Remember to write these on at the end.

Key findings

There are many advanced texts on ECG interpretation. This section will concentrate on the more common significant findings. A normal ECG is shown in Figure 7.8 and the key stages are as follows:

- P wave: sinoatrial node (pacemaker of the heart) discharges an electrical impulse through the atria
- PQ interval: time taken for impulse to travel from the atrioventricular node down the bundle of His and left and right bundle branches into the ventricles. Normally less than 0.2 second
- Q wave: beginning of electrical discharge in ventricles; occurs in the right lower section of the intraventricular septum and spreads into the right ventricle. As this electrical activity is normally moving away from the electrode it produces a downwards deflection as the machine is set to record in that way
- RST complex: electrical discharge throughout the rest of the ventricles; normally obscures the Q wave almost completely as it follows so quickly
- T wave: electrical activity associated with repolarization of cardiac muscle cells before next contraction.

One other key idea is the concept of the cardiac vector. A vector is any entity that has both magnitude and direction. An everyday example is the wind. The cardiac vector is the sum of all the electrical activity in the heart over one cycle. It has a magnitude which can be measured in normal electrical units and a direction which is normally aligned in the general direction of lead II. This explains why leads such as II normally produce the largest complexes whereas a lead such as aVL, which is at right angles to the normal cardiac vector, produces the smallest.

Armed with these basic facts about electro-

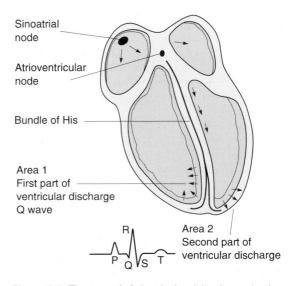

Figure 7.8 The spread of electrical activity via conducting mechanism

cardiography, it is possible to make some significant deductions from a 12-lead ECG. However, the patient's clinical condition remains of overriding importance.

Myocardial infarction

Ischaemic heart disease produces three characteristic changes on the ECG, any or all of which may be visible, depending on the individual patient's condition (Figure 7.9).

The Q wave may become more prominent than normal if the area of myocardium which normally obscures the Q wave is infarcted. As this myocardium now consists of dead tissue, there is no electrical activity taking place and therefore the full Q wave is now visible as if through an 'electrical window'. A pathological Q wave of this nature is more than 4 mm in depth and will be found in those ECG leads which are looking at the infarcted tissue, enabling the MI to be localized within the heart. As this is a record of dead tissue it tends to be a permanent characteristic of an ECG and therefore this limits its value as a diagnostic observation. The presence of an abnormally deep Q wave indicates that the patient has had an MI, but not when – it could have been last week or last year.

Of more use in diagnosing an acute infarct is the

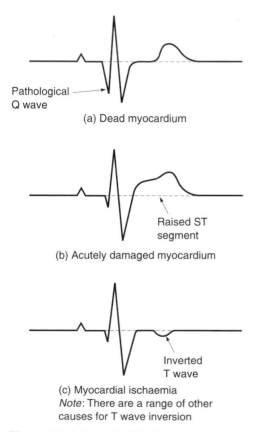

Pathological Q wave

(a) Dead myocardium

Raised ST segment

(b) Acutely damaged myocardium

Inverted T wave

(c) Myocardial ischaemia
Note: There are a range of other causes for T wave inversion

Figure 7.9   Ischaemic ECG changes

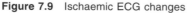

presence of an elevated ST section on the ECG. This section should normally be at the same baseline level as the rest of the trace. However, acutely damaged myocardial cells will leak potassium ions, each carrying a positive charge, with the result that after each myocardial contraction (QRS complex) there will be a surplus of positive charges with the result that the electrical baseline will be elevated above normal. This shows as an elevated ST segment of the ECG. This is therefore an acute change appearing within a short time of an MI and persisting for up to 2 weeks. It is possible that if the ECG is performed quickly after the patient complains of chest pain, the ST elevation will not have fully developed. This underlines the importance of treating the patient's clinical condition, not the ECG.

Myocardial ischaemia

Inverted T waves may be found associated with ischaemic tissue. There are also other causes for this phenomenon (see below). If a patient is experiencing anginal pain, s/he may show a depression of the ST segment. A patient with a history of angina who is experiencing no pain at present will probably have a normal ECG.

Ventricular hypertrophy

If one ventricle is abnormally enlarged (for example, in left- or right-sided heart failure), there will be an excess of electrical activity in that side of the heart compared with normal. This will pull the cardiac vector away from its normal alignment (towards the left in left ventricular hypertrophy and the right in right hypertrophy) and as a result produce changes in the size of various components of the ECG complex and in the whole complex. Recognizing these changes and knowing which leads they occur in can give useful information about the presence of ventricular hypertrophy.

Knowing the normal is the key to recognizing the abnormal. In a normal ECG the largest upright complex should be in lead II and leads I and II should both show an R wave which exceeds the S wave. Count how many squares the R wave stands above the baseline and how many the S wave lies below the baseline. R should exceed S – R > S, to use mathematical shorthand.

The following changes may be expected, though not all may be visible:

Right ventricular hypertrophy
- In lead I, S wave > R
- In V1, R wave > S
- In V6 there is an obvious S wave
- V1 and V2 show T-wave inversion

Left ventricular hypertrophy
- In lead II, S wave > R

- T-wave inversion in I, aVL, V5 and V6
- QRS complex is generally increased in height

This last point shows the importance of ensuring the machine is correctly calibrated: unusually tall QRS complexes should not be an artefact of an incorrectly calibrated machine but a real observation.

Arrhythmias

This section will briefly review the most significant and frequently encountered arrhythmias. This is a large field and you should study more detailed texts if ECG interpretation is an important part of your work. The key to rhythm interpretation is lead II: a lead II rhythm strip is automatically produced by most modern machines to allow arrhythmia detection. If your machine does not do this, then a 15-second lead II strip should be recorded after completing the 12-lead ECG.

Atrial fibrillation (Figure 7.10)

In this condition the normal regular firing of the sinoatrial node is replaced by disorganized atrial activity. As a result the regular P waves disappear and the normally flat baseline becomes irregular. It is important to distinguish this from movement or electrical interference, both of which also produce irregularities in the tracing of QRS complex. As the atrioventricular node is not receiving strong, regular electrical impulses, the bundle of His conducts electrical impulses of varying strengths at rapid but irregular intervals to stimulate ventricular contrac-

tion. This causes QRS complexes to occur at irregular intervals, and this is reflected in an irregular pulse rate which when palpated is also of unequal strength. This situation will eventually lead to heart failure as the heart's pumping mechanism becomes increasingly inefficient. Occasionally the chaotic atrial activity may become organized producing a sawtooth effect along the baseline with a regular pattern of two or four small atrial waves to each QRS complex. This is known as atrial flutter (Figure 7.11).

Paroxysmal supraventricular tachycardia (Figure 7.12)

Despite this daunting name, PST is simply an arrhythmia caused by an atrial impulse being recycled between the atria and ventricles. The result is sudden bursts of tachycardia which the patient experiences as palpitations or fluttering in the chest. Alarming though this may be, it is not a life-threatening arrhythmia.

Heart block (Figure 7.13)

This is a progressive condition which occurs as a result of ageing and degeneration of the conducting mechanism or as a result of acute damage to the bundle of His after an MI. First-degree block is shown on the ECG by lengthening of the PQ interval to 0.2 seconds or more as the electrical impulse is delayed in the conducting fibres. This in itself does not produce any clinical signs or symptoms. As the disease process advances some electrical impulses

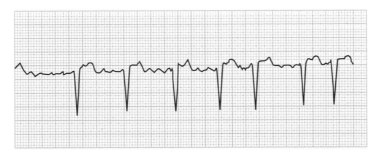

Figure 7.10 Atrial fibrillation. Note the irregular rhythm and absence of normal P waves

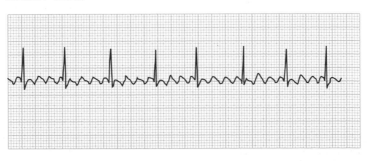

Figure 7.11 Atrial flutter. Note regular rhythm (P waves) but ventricular rhythm depends on conduction pattern

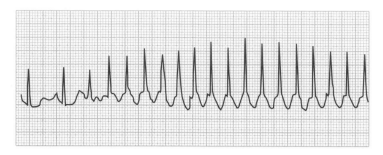

Figure 7.12   Paroxysmal supraventricular tachycardia. Note development from normal sinus rhythm.

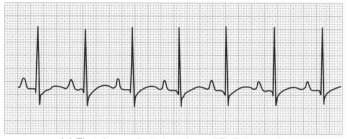

(a) First degree (note lengthened P–R interval)

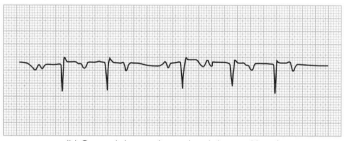

(b) Second degree (occasional dropped beat)

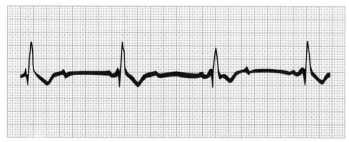

(c) Second degree (2:1 conduction)

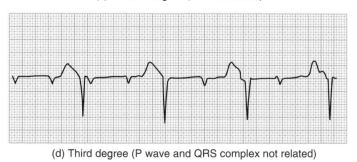

(d) Third degree (P wave and QRS complex not related)

Figure 7.13   Heart block

fail to make it through the conducting mechanism and therefore do not produce a ventricular contraction. A P wave is present but no associated QRS complex occurs. This may occur at random (Mobitz type 2 block) or in an organized way where the PQ interval progressively lengthens over 3 or 4 beats and then there is a completely missed QRS complex (Mobitz type 1 or Wenckebach's phenomenon). A more progressive form of the disorder sees a consistent pattern of alternate electrical impulses failing to make it through the bundle of His. This is known as 2:1 block as only alternate P waves produce a QRS complex and may start to produce symptoms of heart failure if the effective ventricular rate is slow enough.

Complete or third-degree heart block is present when there is a complete breakdown of the conducting mechanism and, despite regular P waves appearing on the ECG, there are no associated QRS complexes. An alternative ventricular pacemaker takes over. This may be located within the bundle of His below the blockage or elsewhere within the Purkinje fibres in the ventricles. The former produces narrow QRS complexes as conduction is quicker but the latter situation leads to slower conduction and a much broader QRS shape. The patient is likely to be in heart failure as with a slow heart rate (bradycardia) any exertion leads to dyspnoea. Syncope attacks are possible if there is any delay in the alternative pacemaker's action as the pulse may be only 20–30 beats/minute.

Ventricular extrasystole (Figure 7.14)
Extraventricular contractions as a result of stimulation by a group of cells outside the main conducting system are possible. The occasional ventricular extrasystole does not produce any clinical effect; however, if they become more frequent or organized this is a matter of concern for two reasons. If an extrasystole were to occur coincidentally with the normal T wave (R on T), this could trigger ventricular fibrillation which is effectively cardiac arrest, as cardiac output falls to zero. Ventricular extrasystoles may increasingly occur in short consecutive runs which unchecked may become ventricular

tachycardia – a serious life-threatening arrhythmia (Figure 7.15). In this situation an ectopic focus in the ventricle has taken over the pacing of the heart and is firing rapidly (150–200 beats/min). The oxygen demand of the myocardium increases dramatically whilst the filling time between beats is reduced by a half or two-thirds of normal and consequently cardiac output falls. This state of affairs will rapidly lead to ventricular fibrillation (Figure 7.16) and effective cardiac arrest unless it reverts to a normal sinus rhythm quickly. In ventricular fibrillation there is uncoordinated chaotic twitching of the ventricular muscle with no output; this quickly decays into asystole. Resuscitation with a defibrillator is possible if the patient is in ventricular fibrillation, but the outlook for resuscitation is poor in asystole.

Investigations

Bloods may be taken for enzymes as an aid to diagnosis of MI. An infarction damages cardiac muscle and it is this damaged muscle which releases certain marker enzymes into the circulation. Creatine phosphokinase (CPK) is the enzyme normally tested for as its levels start to rise within 4 hours of an infarction, peak within 24 hours and rapidly fall back to low levels thereafter. CPK may also be released from damaged skeletal muscle and an intramuscular injection may be sufficient to cause a rise in CPK levels so results must be interpreted with caution. Fortunately, enzymes have molecularly distinct subtypes, known as isoenzymes, which are specific to different body tissues. The isoenzyme of CPK specific to the myocardium is called CPK-MB: elevated levels indicate myocardial damage (this could also be caused by cardiac contusion, trauma or congestive cardiac failure). A blood sample taken too soon (e.g. within 2 hours of the infarct) may show a normal reading as the levels have not started to rise yet and a sample taken too late (e.g. 48 hours after the event) will miss the peak values as levels are now declining.

Other enzyme levels rise more slowly in response to muscle damage. Lactic dehydrogenase (LDH) is

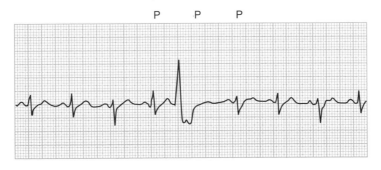

Figure 7.14   Ventricular ectopic with refractory period afterwards

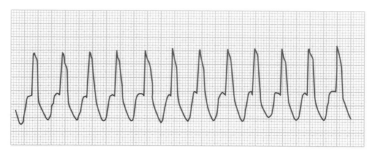

Rate: 100–170 beats/min, no P waves, broad QRS complexes

Figure 7.15   Ventricular tachycardia

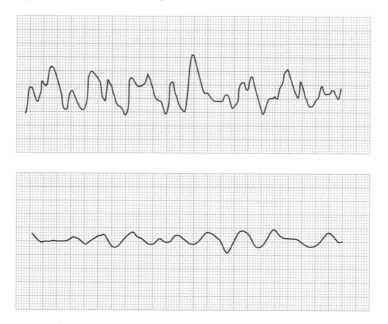

Figure 7.16   Ventricular fibrillation

an example: this peaks 3–6 days after the onset of symptoms. Again the problem of a non-specific response is resolved by the five isoenzymes of LDH. Normally LDH1 levels are less than LDH2, but after damage to the myocardium this ratio is reversed and stays reversed for up to 14 days (Owen 1995). LDH estimates are therefore useful to confirm a diagnosis in a patient who presents several days after an MI; this does happen, especially with in older patients.

Bloods may also be taken for serum cholesterol levels as hypercholesterolaemia is recognized as a risk factor in heart disease, although its usefulness as a predictor for any individual is limited (p. 85). The ratio of plasma total (or LDL) cholesterol to HDL cholesterol may be used as an aid to risk calculations as the greater the ratio, the greater the risk. In looking at any individual's cholesterol level it should be remembered that there is no threshold limit above which the person is suddenly at risk. The risk increases gradually as the cholesterol level

increases. The reliability of measurements of cholesterol levels is also open to question, as a combination of measurement error and natural variation in cholesterol levels over time can introduce significant inaccuracies (York Centre for Review and Dissemination 1998).

Differential diagnosis

The approach to history-taking, the physical examination and investigations discussed above should present sufficient information to enable you to make a differential diagnosis. The most likely scenario is the patient who presents with a history of chest pain: the nurse practitioner must decide whether this is a pain of cardiac origin rather than a gastrointestinal, respiratory or musculoskeletal problem. The history is usually sufficient to make this diagnosis (p. 87). Having decided that the problem is cardiac, next you need to decide between the two most likely causes, angina or MI. Again the history is likely to point one way or the other; an ECG and a physical exam should quickly confirm the diagnosis in most cases.

An alternative presentation is the breathless patient who is generally unwell. It is important to be able to distinguish between a cardiac problem such as heart failure and other possible causes such as respiratory disease. Again the history will give a strong pointer but a careful physical exam and ECG are essential to differentiate between heart failure (possibly secondary to an MI, especially in an elderly person) and respiratory disorders such as pneumonia or a pulmonary embolism.

Peripheral circulatory problems need careful consideration to distinguish between venous and arterial disorders; in some cases there may be a mixed presentation. As the approaches to treatment are different – and if the wrong diagnosis is made could be positively harmful – it is essential to combine careful physical examination with a good focused history to differentiate between peripheral venous and arterial disease.

If a patient is found to have above normal BP, it is necessary to consider whether this is a temporary effect due to stress and/or exertion, or a sign of hypertensive disease. In the former case it may be apparent that the patient is breathless after hurrying to keep an appointment or has just had a stressful experience. The diastolic pressure is relatively unaffected, even though the systolic may be above normal. When checked 15 minutes or so later, BP will have returned to normal. It is the sustained elevation of both diastolic and systolic BP with no apparent short-term cause that indicates hypertensive disorder.

Treatment

Cardiac disease

Acute disorders

MI has a mortality rate of 35–40% and about half these deaths occur within the first 2 hours (Rees and Williams 1995). The patient therefore needs to be admitted to a coronary care unit as soon as possible. Immediate treatment involves intravenous opioid analgesia and an antiemetic, oxygen therapy and psychologically supportive care in a quiet restful environment before transfer to coronary care. An intravenous line should first be secured. Diamorphine 2.5–5.0 mg should be given as it combines analgesia with a strong sedative effect. The dose may be repeated if it is not effective in controlling pain. Prochlorperazine is the standard antiemetic given as a 12.5 mg intramuscular injection.

Frequent observations of vital signs are necessary (15–30 minutes depending on the patient's condition) and, if an ECG monitor is available, the patient should be attached for rhythm monitoring. Ventricular fibrillation is the major danger in this initial period. A defibrillator should be readily available and the nurse practitioner should be trained to use it: the sooner the patient is defibrillated, the better the prognosis.

In recent years the introduction of fibrinolytic drugs which break up thrombi by degrading fibrin has significantly improved the outlook for patients who have had an acute MI. The benefits of treatment decrease rapidly as time elapses since the MI; however, administration within the first 12 hours can produce substantial benefits. It is important to consider the risk of bleeding caused by fibrinolytic therapy in patients with a history of cerebrovascular disease, recent surgery, trauma or known clotting disorders, before deciding whether the benefits of their use outweigh the risks. Streptokinase, alteplase and anistreplase have all been shown to reduce mortality when administered intravenously (*British National Formulary* 1999). Aspirin has an additive effect with streptokinase, and heparin should be given with alteplase to produce the best results. Local protocols will determine which drugs should be given and the nurse practitioner should be fully involved in this key therapeutic intervention.

The other acute presentation commonly encountered is the patient in acute heart failure. This is most likely to be due to left ventricular failure secondary to an MI or some other cardiac event such as failure of the aortic or mitral valves leading to aortic or mitral regurgitation. The patient has marked pulmonary oedema and is underperfused due to the failing pumping action of the left ventricle. This results in hypotension, cold extremities, possible confusion and a reduced urine output. Immediate hospital treatment is required, but in the interim the patient should be cared for sitting upright to help lung expansion and oxygen administered to help correct the hypoxic state that has arisen due to hypoperfusion. The immediate medical management should consist of intravenous morphine which will cause venodilation, respiratory suppression and relieve anxiety, all of which will relieve dyspnoea (Rees and Williams 1995). Intravenous frusemide will also assist by producing a prompt diuresis. If there is likely to be a delay in admission to hospital, these measures should be instituted at once.

The nurse practitioner may receive a phone call from a member of the public about someone experiencing chest pain. Briggs (1997) suggests that the following indications should dictate whether caller rings for an emergency ambulance: pain, tightness, pressure or discomfort in the chest, accompanied by any of the following:

- shortness of breath
- dizziness, weakness, nausea or vomiting
- cool moist skin
- pain affecting the neck, shoulders, jaw, back or arms
- heart palpitations
- pallor or blueness

Other factors which should alert you to advise immediate medical care are:

- if the chest pain is unrelieved by rest, antacids or nitroglycerine or if it has awoken the person
- it is accompanied by pain, swelling, warmth or redness in a leg
- sudden onset of swollen ankles
- recent history of childbirth, surgery, immobilization or blood-clotting disorder
- fever, cough, shortness of breath
- age over 60
- medical or family history of heart disease, diabetes or blood-clotting disorder
- heavy smoker

Chronic disease management

The nurse practitioner has a major role to play in the long-term management of patients with conditions such as heart failure, hypertension and ischaemic heart disease. A great deal of information is available about lifestyle modification such as smoking cessation, increasing exercise and losing excess weight. Such health education initiatives must be targeted to produce beneficial effects.

There is ample international evidence that screening the general population for cholesterol levels and giving advice about diet to those with elevated levels has little effect (York Centre for Review and Dissemination 1998). Low-fat diets perform poorly in cholesterol reduction due to non-compliance; they also often leave the LDL/HDL ratio unaffected as they merely substitute carbohydrates for total fat in the diet. The key goal should be to reduce CHD *risk* rather than cholesterol levels, as this is of little benefit in itself. The York Centre for Review and Dissemination also points out that there is no evidence to support the view that diets involving garlic, oats or soya protein have any effect on reducing CHD risk.

The nurse practitioner has the task of working with the individual patient to try and achieve cooperation in lifestyle modification. Leaflets and video material can be helpful, although there is no substitute for continual follow-up and encouragement. McDonnell *et al.* (1997) point out that the evidence which indicates the benefits of such changes is strong, but the evidence concerning which interventions are most likely to produce these changes is more debatable. The picture is confused by the changing nature of advice in the light of new research findings. Table 7.2 summarizes the current

best evidence-based practice for nurses working to achieve reduction in cardiovascular disease. It is in the nature of things that this table will soon become out-of-date as new research findings emerge.

The nurse practitioner plays a key role in securing adherence to drug therapy. An essential component of this work is fully explaining the benefits of drug therapy and the expected side-effects so that patients are fully informed about and involved in their

Table 7.2 Research-based indicators for nursing practice in relation to cerebrovascular disease (CVD) and stroke prevention

Smoking
Clear, repeated advice to stop smoking supported by a range of techniques:

- provision of leaflets
- negotiating dates for stopping
- giving patients feedback on exhaled carbon monoxide levels
- patient follow-up
- nicotine replacement therapy (particularly in those motivated to stop)

Hypertension
Referral of hypertensive patients to GP according to the following criteria:

- under 60 years: diastolic BP > 100 mmHg (or between 90 and 99 mmHg with target organ damage)
- aged 60–80 years: systolic BP > 160 mmHg
- above 80 years: systolic BP > 160 mmHg and/or diastolic > 90 mmHg

Non-pharmacological measures should be encouraged in all hypertensive patients, including limiting dietary salt and patient follow up

Raised blood cholesterol
Screening patients with existing CVD and family history of hyperlipidaemia. Population screening is contraindicated

Measurement should only be undertaken using regularly calibrated machinery, preferably within an accredited laboratory

Treatment with drugs or diet considered in those with a blood cholesterol level of more than 5.2 mm/l. Encouraging dietary modification (step 2 diet) with use of techniques such as:

- demonstrating hidden fat content
- assessing nutritional value of weekly shop
- written materials, e.g. diet sheets
- regular follow-up

Physical inactivity
Recommending 30 minutes of moderate exercises; e.g. brisk walking, at least 5 days per week

Diet and obesity
Advise to achieve and maintain weight within 'normal' range of BMI. Recommendation of a 'general lipid-lowering regime' supplemented with an increase in fresh fruit and vegetables

BP = Blood pressure; BMI = body mass index.
Source: Adapted from McDonnell *et al.* (1997).

treatment. This is consistent with the approach needed to secure lifestyle changes.

When enlisting the patient as a partner in care it is useful to follow the health belief model (Rosenstock 1974) which suggests that people make decisions about their health based upon judgements about several variables. These may be summarized as the perceived susceptibility to an illness, the effect upon the individual of that illness and the costs and benefits of seeking treatment.

To illustrate the model, consider a patient with hypertension being managed by the nurse practitioner in primary health care. Stress that the person already has high BP and point out the probabilities of a subsequent stroke or MI. This needs to be done in such a way as to make the patient perceive that s/he is highly susceptible but without causing undue anxiety and fear. The consequences of a stroke or MI to the patient and family should then be explored. Whilst there may be a fatal outcome, it is more likely that the person will be disabled. Who will look after the rest of the family? Who will look after the patient? These are the issues that need to be talked through sensitively without causing too much alarm, but in such a way as to motivate the patient to make a serious attempt to avert these possible future events. This brings the discussion on to drug therapy and lifestyle modification. The perceived costs or disadvantages should be carefully explored. Some may be removed from the equation as they may be mistaken beliefs or folk tales. Those that remain, such as the side-effects of drugs, have to be acknowledged so that at least there are no unexpected unpleasant surprises for the patient who, in the process, is becoming a real partner in care. It then remains to show the potential benefits of adhering to drug therapy, weight reduction, exercise and smoking cessation. It may take several consultations to work through these issues but at the end, you may well find a motivated patient who fully grasps the risks concerned and who is able to make an informed decision about antihypertensive therapy. The outcome is more likely to be positive adherence to the therapeutic regime than if you simply lecture the patient on the evils of smoking, supply a prescription and send him or her away with a leaflet on blood pressure.

The health belief model approach can be used to manage a wide range of chronic diseases other than hypertension. It is important to be fully aware of the main medications used and the possible side-effects to be explored with patients. The patient's understanding of the medication must be assessed as some patients may be vague and have little idea about each type of drug, how much to take and when, let alone know the side-effects to look out for. Detailed information can be found in the *British National Formulary*: the following list summarizes the most likely types of drugs used in treating cardiovascular disorders:

- calcium channel blockers: these drugs interfere with the displacement of calcium through active cell membranes, affecting cells in the myocardium, conducting mechanism and vascular smooth muscle. Myocardial contractility is reduced leading to arteriolar dilation, thereby reducing blood pressure. Different calcium channel blockers have slightly different effects. Thus nifedipine acts mostly on blood vessels, whereas verapamil has a stronger effect on the myocardium and should not be given to patients in heart failure. Constipation is a side-effect and verapamil may produce nausea, vomiting or dizziness
- beta-blockers: by blocking the beta-adrenoreceptors in the sympathetic nervous system, these drugs reduce cardiac contractility and heart rate. They also reduce renin release from the kidney and hence angiotensin II synthesis. The net effect is to reduce blood pressure and beta-blockers are often combined with thiazide diuretics to enhance this effect. Side-effects include bradycardia, conduction disorders, bronchospasm and peripheral vasoconstriction
- nitrates: both the above groups of drugs are used prophylactically to treat patients with angina. If an angina attack occurs, nitrates provide immediate short-term relief. Glyceryl trinitrate has been the standard drug for many years although its effects are short-lasting (20–30 minutes). It is usually administered sublingually or via an aerosol spray. It is also available as a transdermal patch for prophylaxis; each patch usually lasts 24 hours. Another commonly used nitrate is isosorbide mononitrate which is used prophylactically in tablet form. Nitrates may produce severe headaches, postural hypotension, dizziness and flushing as side-effects
- angiotensin-converting enzyme inhibitors (e.g. captopril): drugs which prevent the conversion of angiotensin I to angiotensin II have proved very effective as an alternative to beta-blockade and thiazide diuretic therapy in managing hypertension and also in treating heart failure, especially when combined with digoxin and diuretics. This group of drugs is best avoided in patients known or suspected to have renovascular disease and should only be commenced under medical supervision in hospital, as they may stop glomerular filtration and lead to renal failure (*British National Formulary* 1999)
- cardiac glycosides (e.g. digoxin): by increasing the force of myocardial contraction and reducing conductivity within the heart this group of drugs has proven effective in the treatment of atrial fibrillation and heart failure. Side-effects depend

not only on plasma concentrations but also on the sensitivity of the myocardium or conducting mechanism to the drug which varies considerably between patients. Bradycardias and other arrhythmias may occur in one patient but not in another, even though both are on the same dose. Simply monitoring plasma concentration is therefore not sufficient if toxicity is to be avoided. The nurse practitioner should follow up each patient on an individual basis, checking that the pulse remains in sinus rhythm with a rate above 60 beats/min, and that the patient has none of the other side-effects of toxicity, such as nausea, vomiting and loss of appetite

- diuretics: the thiazides such as bendrofluazide act by inhibiting reabsorption of sodium in the distal convoluted tubule. Loop diuretics such as frusemide inhibit reabsorption in the ascending loop of Henle in the renal tubule. Both types of diuretic produce an effect within 1–2 hours. This should be remembered in patient teaching as the individual should be advised to take the diuretic in the morning not the evening for this reason. Although useful in the management of heart failure and hypertension, these drugs have an extensive range of possible side-effects, including nausea, gastrointestinal disturbance and hypokalaemia. This latter problem has led to the development of drugs which are potassium sparing as an alternative to giving the patient potassium supplements; examples include spironolactone and amiloride

- statins: this class of drugs is effective in lowering LDL cholesterol levels by inhibiting a key enzyme involved in cholesterol synthesis, especially in the liver. The Standing Medical Advisory Committee (1997) based on evidence from a large randomized controlled trial, has recommended that patients with angina who have a total cholesterol level 5.5 mmol/l or more (or LDL 3.7 mmol/l) should be considered for statin treatment. However, the York Centre for Review and Dissemination (1998) in a systematic review point out that some antihypertensives, aspirin and beta-blockers are more cost-effective than statins in reducing the risk of *cardiovascular disease*.

- Warfarin: the prophylactic anticoagulation effects of warfarin are well-known. The number of patients for whom it is prescribed has increased substantially as it is now used to prevent embolization in patients with atrial fibrillation. Careful follow-up and monitoring of patients on long-term anticoagulation are essential and the nurse practitioner is ideally placed to provide that service

An earlier systematic review of the management of stable angina by the York Centre for Review and

Dissemination concluded that there was no long-term difference in effectiveness between the major types of drugs such as beta-blockers, nitrates and calcium channel blockers (CRD1 1997). This review also found powerful evidence for the effectiveness of aspirin therapy in reducing the incidence of MI amongst those with stable angina. Discussions with patients concerning surgical options for the treatment of their angina will usually be carried out by the GP. Patients may wish to discuss the options with the nurse practitioner, so it is useful to know that the CRD1 review showed that, while in the short-term angioplasty is more effective than drug therapy in relieving symptoms, after 2–3 years the beneficial effect had disappeared while overall angioplasty had no beneficial effect on survival rates. Coronary artery bypass improved quality of life and relieved angina more effectively than drug therapy over a much longer period (up to 10 years) but was associated with a significantly higher mortality rate in the initial period of treatment. There are therefore advantages and disadvantages and what might be best for one patient might not be the most appropriate option for another. The nurse practitioner can serve a useful function by allowing patients to rehearse the arguments and carefully consider which is the best option for them as individuals. Surgery is not a quick fix which allows the patient to forget about drug therapy and lifestyle modification – a key point to be reinforced.

Peripheral vascular disorders

Arterial problems

It is possible that the nurse practitioner may encounter a patient with an acute arterial embolism or leaking aneurysm. Both are major surgical emergencies and immediate transfer to a general hospital is essential after appropriate pain-relieving measures and once intravenous resuscitation has been started locally.

The nurse practitioner may see a patient with a history of intermittent claudication who may also have signs of peripheral arterial disease affecting the foot, such as small gangrenous ulcers. If these ulcers become infected they may worsen rapidly as the poor blood supply means that the body's natural defence mechanisms are ineffective in dealing with the infective organisms. Cellulitis may also develop. The patient requires urgent referral to a vascular surgeon. Meanwhile, an honest dialogue using the health belief model approach is necessary. The aim should be to persuade the patient to stop smoking immediately and to take great care of the affected foot. If s/he is also diabetic, compliance with the dietary and drug regime should also be explored. Dressings are necessary to any ulcers and a referral should be made to a chiropodist to deal with toenails and any other foot lesions such as corns and bunions. Patients should be dissuaded from home remedies or attempts to cut their own toenails as this may cause further skin damage which could rapidly lead to an infected ulcer.

Venous problems

If a DVT is suspected a medical opinion should be sought immediately in view of the potentially fatal outcome of a pulmonary embolism. Intravenous heparin should be commenced with oral warfarin for medium-term management.

Varicose veins are best managed by compression stockings and discussing the patient's daily routine. Periods of extensive standing should be identified and strategies explored to reduce these periods, especially at work. The importance of calf movements when standing to pump blood out of the affected veins should be emphasized together with the value of leg elevation when resting. It should be explained that to be effective this means elevating the legs above the level of the heart, not just sitting with the feet on a footstool. Referral to a doctor to consider the surgical option should always be offered.

Venous leg ulcers respond best to compression bandages which provide a pressure gradient within the lower part of the leg to reduce venous congestion. A systematic review carried out by the York Centre for Review and Dissemination indicates that best results come from the use of a high compression bandage involving a three- or four-layer system, while there is no place for drug treatment with medication such as stanozolol (CRD2 1997). A significant number of patients may have arterial as well as venous disease and high compression bandaging would be contraindicated for such persons. The York review emphasizes the importance of measuring ankle/brachial pressure index (ABPI, p. 91), as part of the assessment, noting that this is a more reliable indicator of peripheral arterial circulation than measuring whether peripheral pulses are present. However, nurses must be well-trained in the use of the equipment to obtain reliable results.

The patient should be encouraged to avoid sitting with the feet on the ground for long periods as this exacerbates venous congestion. A good dressing technique using one of the modern occlusive products, combined with the correct form of compression bandaging, has a major role to play in promoting healing of leg ulcers. Established ulcers can also be painful, therefore analgesia should be discussed with the patient and various analgesics may be tried until one is found that is effective for that patient. The elderly are increasingly susceptible to the side-effects of non-steroidal anti-inflammatory drugs (e.g. gastrointestinal disorders and hypersensitivity reactions), therefore other drugs such as paracetamol should be tried before these are used for pain control (*British National Formulary* 1999).

Summary

The nurse practitioner has a major role to play in the long-term management of patients with cardiovascular disorder, in primary health care or hospital outpatient settings. Other nurse practitioners working in community hospital minor injury units will encounter patients who have had an acute episode such as an MI or a bad angina attack, whilst those working in an A&E department will frequently encounter the full range of acute scenarios, though usually with the full range of medical services available. Whatever the situation, the nurse practitioner is likely to be the first point of contact with the health care system and, in many cases, the only point of contact for some considerable time. The principles of patient assessment and management outlined in this chapter, together with locally devised protocols and agreements, are therefore essential for the successful care of a large number of patients by nurse practitioners.

References

Briggs J. (1997) *Telephone Triage Protocols for Nurses*, Philadelphia, Lippincott.

British National Formulary (1999) London, British Medical Association/Royal Pharmaceutical Society of Great Britain.

CRD1 (1997) Management of stable angina, *Effective Health Care*, **3**(5) (York NHS Centre for Review and Dissemination).

CRD2 (1997) Compression therapy for leg ulcers. *Effective Health Care*, **3**(4) (York NHS Centre for Review and, Dissemination).

Department of Health (1997) *Mortality Statistics Cause 1995*, Series DH2: 22, London, Stationery Office.

Hill B., Geraci S. (1998) A diagnostic approach to chest pain based on history and ancillary evaluation. *Nurse Practitioner*, **23**(4), pp. 20–45.

McDonnell A., Crookes P., Davies S., Shewan J. (1997) Practice nurses and the prevention of cardiovascular disease and stroke: a literature review to promote evidence-based practice. Part 2. Hypertension, raised blood cholesterol, lack of exercise and obesity, *Clinical Effectiveness in Nursing*, **1**(4), pp. 198–205.

Munro J. Edwards C. (1995) *Macleod's Clinical Examination*, Edinburgh, Churchill Livingstone.

Owen A. (1995) The rise and fall of cardiac enzymes. *Nursing 95*, May, pp. 35–38.

Rees P., Williams D. (1995) *Principles of Clinical Medicine*, London, Edward Arnold.

Rosenstock I. (1974) Historical origins of the health belief model, *Health Education Monographs*, **2**, pp. 328–335.

Seidal H., Ball J., Dains J., Benedict W. (1995) *Mosby's Guide to Physical Examination*, St Louis, CV Mosby.

Springhouse (1997) *Handbook of Medical Surgical Nursing*, Pennsylvania, Springhouse.

Standing Medical Advisory Committee (1997) *The Use of Statins*, London, Department of Health.

Thompson D., Webster R. (1992) *Caring for the Coronary Patient*, Oxford, Butterworth-Heinemann.

Walsh M. (1997) *Watson's Medical Surgical Nursing*, 5th edn., London Baillière Tindall.

York Centre for Review and Dissemination (1998) Cholesterol and coronary heart disease: screening and treatment, *Effective Health Care Bulletin*, **4**(1).

CHAPTER 8
The respiratory system

Christina Clark

Introduction

Respiratory problems are among the commonest causes of illness and can range from a minor cold to a life-threatening asthmatic attack or pneumonia. The challenge is to be able to differentiate between minor, largely self-limiting conditions and more serious pathology requiring urgent intervention and/or specialist consultation. The health promotion role of the nurse practitioner is to the fore in areas such as asthma management and smoking cessation. The holistic nurse practitioner approach can therefore make a major contribution to respiratory health.

Pathophysiology

Some of the commoner or more serious conditions will be reviewed here before looking at the major symptoms of respiratory disease and how they relate to their underlying pathology.

The common cold

The cold is caused by viral infection from numerous different groups, e.g. rhinoviruses, respiratory syncytial virus, adenoviruses, influenza viruses and parainfluenza viruses (Chow *et al.* 1984; Simon 1995a). Incubation is from 1 to 5 days with viral shedding up to 2 weeks. Rhinoviruses are the commonest but there are over 100 types with no immunity after infection and it is not uncommon to be immediately reinfected with another type. The viruses are transmitted through inhaled droplet infection and direct contact from hands to mucous membranes. Recent studies suggest that host response to the virus is an important factor in developing a cold. Inflammatory mediators, particularly proinflammatory cytokines, appear to be significant instigators of symptoms and research is targeted towards interfering with their production. Being cold or damp does not contribute towards the risk of infection but increased stress may increase the risk of catching a cold (Simon 1995a).

Acute bronchitis and pneumonia

Infections involving the lower respiratory tract can vary between those easily managed at home and life-threatening conditions. Goroll *et al.* (1995) suggest that three basic issues need to be considered:

- Is the condition confined to the bronchi or does it affect lung tissue, as in pneumonia?
- Is the patient at risk for cardiopulmonary problems (such as an elderly person)?
- Is the infection bacterial or viral?

The same organisms may be implicated in acute bronchitis and pneumonia (Table 8.1). The patient may present with the same symptoms, such as productive cough, fever and feeling unwell. Usually the person with pneumonia appears ill and has higher fevers, chills and hypoxia. S/he is more likely to complain of breathlessness, pleuritic pain and, with bacterial infection, to have copious amounts of sputum. The diagnosis is made on clinical examination and confirmed by chest X-ray.

It is beyond the scope of this book to review all

Table 8.1 Comparison of physical findings in acute bronchitis and pneumonia

Bronchitis	Pneumonia
Hacking cough with thick sputum	Increased respiratory rate
	May have guarding of affected side
	Expansion may be asymmetrical
	Decreased on affected side
Resonant to percussion over area	Dull to percussion
Normal breath sounds	
Voice sounds normal	Increased clarity of voice with egophony whispered pectoriloquy
May have occasional wheeze	Bronchophony
	Crackles over area and sometimes low-pitched wheezes (rhonchi)

Source: Adapted from Jarvis (1992).

the possible causes of acute lower respiratory tract infections but, according to Rees and Williams (1995), the commonest cause of pneumonia (acquired outside hospital) is the bacteria *Streptococcus pneumoniae*, which accounts for 50% of cases. The other major causes are *Mycoplasma pneumoniae* (15%), viruses (14%) and *Haemophilus influenzae* (10%). Rarer causes include *Legionella pneumophila*, *Staphylococcus aureus* and *Chlamydia*. Nosocomial pneumonia in hospitalized patients is usually caused by different organisms, especially Gram-negative bacteria such as the *Klebsiella* species, *Pseudomonas aeruginosa* or *Escherichia coli*. *S. aureus* is the most likely Gram-positive bacteria involved.

Tuberculosis

There has been a significant increase in cases in the UK during the last few years. For example 1988 saw 5778 new cases but that number has risen to 6541 cases in 1993 (CSO 1995). This together with the finding of drug-resistant TB has alerted health professionals to be more vigilant. Poverty, malnutrition, overcrowding and poor living conditions reduce the effectiveness of the person's immune system, making him or her more likely to contract TB if exposed to the organism. Alcoholics and those with HIV are also at risk for TB. As has already been stated, there has been a recent increase in numbers in this country, which may partly reflect poor living conditions amongst the homeless and reactivation of the disease amongst immigrants from areas where the disease is common.

TB is caused by *Mycobacterium tuberculosis*. It most commonly affects the lungs but can migrate to other places such as lymph nodes, kidneys, bones and skin or wounds. It is spread by droplet infection from someone who has active respiratory disease. Systemic symptoms are fever, night sweats, weight loss, fatigue and loss of appetite. Respiratory symptoms include dry cough, dyspnoea, haemoptysis and chest pain.

Asthma

Asthma may be defined as: 'a disease characterised by wide variations over short periods of time in resistance to airflow in interpulmonary airways' (Rees and Price 1995).

It is a complex and not fully understood disease which, if not properly managed, can be fatal. It is estimated that in the UK there are 3 million people with asthma with a mean prevalence of 4% in adults and 4–6% in children. The figures rise to 15% in school-age children (Department of Health 1995).

There are two distinct patterns of presentation of asthma: the first has onset of symptoms during childhood accompanied by signs of atopic disease. There seems to be seasonal occurrence or a response to environmental stimuli such as dust mite or animal dander. Attacks are usually self-limiting but may at times be severe. Symptoms may have resolved by adulthood. The second pattern has onset of symptoms in adulthood with no identifiable allergen. There is often sputum production but no wheeze, which may confuse the picture with bronchitis. Coughing, dyspnoea and decreased expiratory flow rate are also present. Respiratory infections often trigger attacks. Bronchospasm from an asthma attack can linger for days to weeks, probably because the inflammatory response takes longer to resolve in more remote tissue. Further acute attacks are probably not a new attack but incomplete resolution of the first symptoms.

The main symptoms are wheezing, dyspnoea, cough (particularly at night when sleep may be disturbed) and a feeling of tightness in the chest. On physical examination there is usually prolonged expiration with diffuse wheezing and a decrease in expected values in peak flow. The reversible nature of the condition can be used to diagnose the disease. If the history is suggestive of asthma, the best of three successive peak flow readings should be noted. The patient can then be given two inhaled doses of a beta$_2$-agonist such as salbutamol and 15 minutes later the peak flow measurements repeated. An increase of 15% in peak flow after the salbutamol demonstrates the presence of reversible airway narrowing – asthma.

Pathological findings include inflammation, hypertrophy of smooth bronchial muscle, mucosal oedema, hypertrophy of mucous glands and thick mucus plugs which all lead to obstruction of the airways.

An asthmatic attack is severe if the peak flow is 50% of the person's normal or expected value. Other severe signs are a respiratory rate over 24 breaths/minute, pulse exceeding 110 beats/minute or if the person cannot complete a sentence in one breath. Life-threatening features include a peak flow of 33% (or less) of normal, cyanosis, feeble respiratory effort, a silent chest on auscultation, bradycardia, hypotension, confusion or coma. If pulse oximetry shows saturation levels dropping below 92% or there is any evidence of a general deterioration in the patient's condition, arterial blood gases should be taken if possible as severe hypoxia ($O_2 < 8$ kPa, $CO_2 > 5$ kPa and a low pH) is likely (Cross 1997a).

Many people with asthma are atopic and have allergic components to their disease but some sufferers cannot identify any allergen. The house dust mite seems to increase the risk of sensitization and other common triggers have been identified, such as:

• Animal dander
• Mould

- Pollens
- Aspirin and other non-steroidal anti-inflammatory drugs
- Emotional stress
- Exercise
- Respiratory infections
- Respiratory irritants, e.g. smoke and dust
- Occupational exposure to various agents

IgE antibodies are produced on first exposure to the allergen and attach to mast cells which stay at the tissue level and basophils which circulate in the blood. On subsequent exposure the allergen binds to IgE antibodies on mast cells. The cell releases potent chemicals or mediators of the allergic response – histamine, prostaglandin D, leukotrienes and eosinophilic chemotactic factor have all been implicated. They constrict the bronchial airways, stimulate secretion of mucus in the airways and increase the permeability of small blood vessels, causing wheezing, swelling of tissue and congestion of airways. A second or late-stage reaction can occur 6–12 hours later. It is believed to be a continuation of the inflammatory response at this stage and does not respond well to bronchodilator drugs.

There seems to be evidence for a neurological component to asthma. Stimulation of the vagus nerve causes the bronchioles to constrict. Emotional stress can bring about bronchial spasm by triggering vagal reflexes. The relationship between exposure and asthma symptoms is complex but asthma is usually more severe in sensitized patients exposed to a higher allergen level. Avoiding exposure to the allergen can be effective if the allergen is known.

Many people are unaware of having an allergy to the house dust mite or to animal dander. There is a particular risk of exposure to the dust mite allergen in the bedroom. This can be greatly reduced by opening the bedroom window. Dog and cat allergens are readily detectable in the homes of pet owners. It can take several months to remove allergens from a room after the last exposure to the animal, as shown by the fact that 25% of homes without a resident cat or dog have detectable levels of allergen (Custovic et al. 1998).

Chronic obstructive pulmonary disease (COPD)

This typically affects older people, men more than women, and unfortunately there is no known treatment that can halt the progression of the disease. Patients may receive combinations of drugs used in the treatment of asthma which may not be appropriate. The condition is defined as follows: COPD is a disorder characterised by reduced maximum expiratory flow and slow forced emptying of the lungs; features which do not change markedly over several months (Siafakas et al. 1995).

COPD is a mixture of two diseases – emphysema and chronic bronchitis. Sometimes one condition predominates but often symptoms coexist as part of a continuum that leads to progressive airway obstruction. In the past little treatment was offered as the outcome was thought to be inevitable disability. Recently evidence shows that with early identification and treatment some symptoms may be partially reversible. The goal for most symptoms is to preserve function and prevent complications.

Emphysema is defined by microscopic changes at the cellular level and characterized by abnormal permanent enlargement of air spaces distal to terminal bronchioles with destruction of their walls and without obvious fibrosis (Snider et al. 1985). Jeffery (1998) refers to a recent study that demonstrates that alveolar fibrosis remains in the lungs. The alveoli and capillary bed in the alveoli wall are slowly destroyed. This interferes with the lungs' elastic recoil, which may lead to hyperinflation and the collapse of poorly supported airways during expiration. In centrilobular or centriacinar emphysema, destruction affects the respiratory bronchioles. This type is associated with smoking and chronic bronchitis. Panlobular or panacinar emphysema destroys and distends the alveoli furthest away from the respiratory bronchioles and is more common in non-smokers. Clinically, dyspnoea is the main symptom, with minor cough and scant sputum. In advanced stages the patient is thin with pursed lip breathing without cyanosis. The anterior–posterior diameter of the chest is increased, the chest is hyperresonant to percussion and breath sounds are faint.

Chronic bronchitis may be recognized as the presence of bronchial secretions causing expectoration on most days for a minimum of 3 months of the year for 2 consecutive years. It is unclear how it develops, but repeated infection and hyper-reactivity are the hallmarks, along with, usually, a long history of tobacco smoking. Inflammatory cells are attracted into the lungs by smoking, releasing a proteolytic enzyme, elastase. Usually the lungs are protected by alpha-1 antitrypsin (AAT) but an imbalance ensues, causing destruction of tissue. Not all people who smoke develop COPD and not all those with COPD smoke, so other factors must be involved. Air pollution may cause respiratory problems such as chronic bronchitis. This was particularly evident before the dramatic reduction in open coal fires in the UK during the 1960s. Another less common cause (Mak 1997) is a genetic deficiency of the protective protease inhibitor, AAT. Low levels of AAT allow elastase to act on lung tissue, resulting in the destruction of alveoli. Exposure to passive smoking is also linked to increased respiratory infections and symptoms. Early childhood infections are often associated with respiratory symptoms and reduced lung function in adulthood. The viruses implicated are adenovirus and respiratory syncytial virus. Chronic bronchitis is four times more common than emphysema as the predominant condition. The typical patient is male, in his 50s and often with tobacco stains on fingers and teeth. There may be signs of cor pulmonale with distended neck veins and peripheral oedema. As COPD progresses increased effort must be expended in breathing to overcome the airway resistance and damage to the alveoli; gas exchange becomes more difficult and hypoxia may develop.

Bronchial carcinoma

The strong association with tobacco smoking is well-known, although factors such as exposure to asbestos dust, radiation and passive smoking are other important causes. The patient may present with a history of generally feeling tired, unwell and loss of weight and appetite. More localized chest symptoms include chronic cough, shortness of breath and possibly haemoptysis. Complaints of chest pain indicate probable involvement of the pleura. The prognosis is poor.

Other conditions

Sudden onset of chest pain and respiratory distress may be due to a spontaneous pneumothorax or pulmonary embolism. Chest trauma should always be taken seriously as a pneumothorax (or haemo-pneumothorax if bleeding into the pleura has occurred) is potentially fatal, particularly if it is a tension pneumothorax. Fractured ribs are always painful and will interfere with good chest expansion and coughing, leading to the risk of broncho-pneumonia. If ribs are fractured in two places, this segment of chest wall is known as a flail segment and, as it has become detached from the rest of the ribcage, will expand and contract out of step with the chest wall, giving rise to paradoxical respirations – the flail segment goes inwards on breathing in and vice versa.

Review of common respiratory symptoms

Dyspnoea can be caused by disease of the lung tissue, pleura or chest wall or may be due to extrapulmonary conditions such as heart disease, particularly heart failure, shock, anaemia, hypermetabolic states, abdominal distension, anxiety and a low level of physical fitness. It is a sensation of breathlessness, often described by the patient as feeling short of breath. The current severity of the symptom can be gauged by asking the patient to rate the breathlessness on a scale of 1–10 during your examination, where 10 represents the worst it has been and 1 the easiest since the problem started. Asking someone to estimate how far they can walk before feeling breathless is helpful. This establishes a baseline from which progress in treating the illness can be measured.

Paroxysmal nocturnal dyspnoea is a periodic attack of breathlessness that occurs at night or when lying down. This can occur in asthma and is usually triggered by a cough or wheezing episode.

Orthopnoea is discomfort in breathing, except when sitting or standing. It is often reported by people with left-sided heart failure and may also occur with asthma or COPD.

Coughing involves a forceful expulsion of air from lungs. The person may experience a single cough or episodes of repeated coughing. Everyone coughs from time to time during health to clear mucus from the pharynx or airways, but it is often a presenting symptom. It can be a voluntary or involuntary action, usually stimulated by secretions, irritation from a foreign body or inflammation.

Sensory nerve endings for the cough reflex are branches of the vagus in the larynx, trachea and bronchi. A cough may also be induced by stimulation in the external acoustic meatus which is supplied by the auricular nerve (Arnold's nerve), a branch of the vagus. A foreign body or wax in the ear, hair touching the tympanic membrane or a subphrenic abscess (pus beneath the diaphragm) can stimulate a cough. A cough lasting more than 3 weeks is considered abnormal.

Chronic cough is often associated with smoking, asthma and chronic bronchitis.
Other common causes are:

- COPD
- Postnasal drip due to chronic sinusitis, in which secretions flow from the postnasal area into the pharynx causing irritation and desire to cough
- Bronchiectasis; productive cough with copious amounts of purulent sputum
- Bronchial carcinoma
- Pulmonary tuberculosis
- Gastro-oesophageal reflux leading to aspiration at night
- Medication-related – angiotensin-converting enzyme inhibitors and beta-blockers produce a dry cough

Sometimes a cough from an upper respiratory infection can persist for 6–8 weeks due to induced airway inflammation and increased sensitivity, often referred to as hyper-responsiveness. Less common causes of chronic cough are congestive heart failure, occupational inhalation of bronchial irritants and psychogenic factors.

Croup is a barking cough common in infants and children. It usually begins at night after several days of an upper respiratory infection.

Haemoptysis is the term used for coughing up blood or blood-tinged sputum. Vigorous coughing may bring up a minimal amount of blood. Bright red, frothy blood is usually from the bronchial area and this may indicate bronchiectasis, carcinoma or TB. Frothy, pink sputum indicates pulmonary oedema whereas coughing up mostly blood with little mucus is usually associated with a pulmonary embolism. Haemoptysis is a serious symptom that should be investigated. The amount of blood, colour and whether mixed with sputum should be ascertained. It is important to find out if the blood is truly coming from the lung and not from the nose or pharynx.

Other abnormalities

A *wheeze* is a musical sound. Air is forced through narrowed airways which vibrate, producing a high-pitched sound as in asthma, or low-pitched sound as in bronchitis. A wheeze is most pronounced on expiration.

Stridor is a harsh, crowing sound caused by the turbulent flow of air through a narrowed upper airway. It is a musical sound of constant pitch which is most prominent on inspiration and can be heard at some distance from the patient. Stridor is usually produced in central airways and may be due to an obstruction, laryngeal spasm or oedema.

Chest pain related to the respiratory system usually arises from the pleura, chest wall or from the bronchial tree. Inflammation of the pleura (pleurisy) produces sharp, stabbing pain made worse by coughing, breathing or laughing. It usually makes the person try to stop and hold the breathing movement to avoid the pain. The parietal pleura has many sensory nerve fibres joining the intercostal nerve branches that also innervate the overlying skin. Pleural pain is caused by stretching the inflamed pleura or by separation of fibrous adhesions between the two pleural surfaces. The visceral pleura has no sensation. Rib fractures produce localized bony tenderness over the fracture site and pain is also produced by pressing on the same rib but away from the fracture. Costochondritis of the rib is common, starting with a dull pain which increases with respiratory motion. It is diagnosed by palpation and finding tenderness at the junction of the rib and cartilage.

Burning pain along the path of a dermatone on one side that does not cross the midline might suggest the beginning of herpes-zoster. Erythema on the skin is followed by clusters of tiny blisters which burst and scab over. The discomfort can vary from minimal to disabling pain and sometimes subside in a week, or may persist long after the skin has cleared, as in postherpetic neuralgia.

Diaphragmatic pain is sharp and may be localized along the costal margins, epigastric area and lumbar regions or radiate to the shoulder. The peripheral area of the diaphragm is supplied by the intercostal nerves but the central portion is served by the phrenic nerve that also supplies the neck. Mediastinal pain from organs behind the sternum is usually deep, poorly localized pain. Oesophagitis usually has a burning sensation and tumours or lymphadenopathy are associated with dull central pain.

When a patient complains of chest pain it is important to rule out angina. The diagnosis is made from the history (p. 87).

Review of common signs of respiratory disease

Tachypnoea is rapid shallow breathing, usually greater than 18 breaths/minute in an adult. Hyperventilation or overbreathing leads to an increase in air entering the alveoli, causing hypocapnia (arterial $PCO_2 < 5$–6 kPa).

Asymmetrical chest movement can be caused by scoliosis, chest wall injury or loss of lung volume on one side. Symmetrically reduced lung expansion can be a sign of emphysema or neuromuscular disease. Asymmetrical chest movement during inspiration can be a sign of airway obstruction on one side, pleural or pulmonary fibrosis or splinting due to chest pain.

Cyanosis a bluish discoloration of skin and mucous membranes, is caused by increased amounts of unsaturated haemoglobin in the blood. Central cyanosis occurs in respiratory failure, pulmonary oedema and congenital cardiac defects can best be seen in the tongue and mouth and are a late sign of serious respiratory failure with oxygen saturation levels of around 80–85%. Peripheral cyanosis is more likely to be due to a circulatory problem.

Clubbing – bulbous swelling seen in the nail beds and fingertips – can indicate serious respiratory disease such as bronchial carcinoma, bronchiectasis, fibrosing alveolitis and empyema. It is also found with congenital heart defects, hepatic cirrhosis and imflammatory bowel diseases such as ulcerative colitis and Crohn's disease. It is said to exist when the anteroposterior thickness of the index finger at the base of the fingernail exceeds the thickness of the distal interphalangeal joint. There is also flattening of the angle between the nail plate and proximal skin fold. When healthy nails of the left and right hands are held together a diamond-shaped space appears between them, but in fingers with clubbing this disappears (Figure 8.1). Patients rarely complain of clubbing so it is up to the nurse

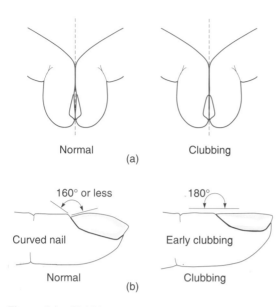

Figure 8.1 Clubbing

practitioner to observe this important sign and find out if this is a recent change in appearance.

Taking a focused history

The main symptoms of concern in respiratory illness are cough, sputum production and changes in breathing pattern or sensations of feeling short of breath. Any report of chest pain must also be carefully checked to rule out a cardiac origin.

The PQRST approach to symptom analysis can be useful when exploring a patient's cough. Enquire what brings the cough on and what relieves it (P). To help the patient describe the quality (Q) of the cough, ask if it is dry or whether it produces phlegm. The nature of the cough should also be checked (hacking, barking or bubbling) and whether it feels like it comes from a tickle in the back of the throat or deeper in the chest (R). Encourage the patient to rate the severity of the cough on a scale of 1–10 (S) and link this to the timing of the cough to check whether the severity varies with time of day (cough causing sleep disturbance is common in asthma but less so in COPD; Munro and Edwards 1995). You also need to check how long the symptom has been present (T).

If sputum is produced, a description should be obtained, including the quantity, consistency, colour (clear, white, creamy, yellow, green, brown) and presence of blood.

Breathlessness can also be checked using a PQRST approach. The key finding is how far the patient can walk without feeling out of breath, such as 10 paces on level ground or a flight of stairs. Ask whether the patient has noticed any hoarseness which might indicate laryngeal problems.

Previous medical history should check whether there has been any past respiratory disease, chest trauma or cardiac disease. Immunization status should be checked, specifically immunizations related to the respiratory system, e.g. BCG vaccination, pneumococcal and influenza vaccines. When asking about current health it is important to take a careful smoking history and also to note any allergies.

The current medication part of the history is particularly important as many drugs have pulmonary side effects. Angiotensin-converting enzyme (ACE) inhibitors can cause a dry cough. They are valuable in treating hypertension and heart failure; however, coughing occurs as a side-effect in 5–20% of patients but this usually resolves when the drug is withdrawn (Philip 1997). Beta-blockers can also stimulate a cough, which resolves when the medication is stopped. Aspirin, other non-steroidal anti-inflammatory drugs and beta-blockers can all trigger asthmatic episodes and should therefore only be used with great care by a person with asthma (Stauffer 1997). The respiratory-depressant effect of drugs such as alcohol and the opioids should always be borne in mind if called to deal with a collapsed, unresponsive individual where alcohol and drug abuse are suspected.

In the psychosocial history, occupation should be carefully checked. Ask about exposure to environmental hazards such as passive smoking, silica, asbestos or coal dust. Hobbies should be noted as pets such as pigeons, parrots and parakeets can spread disease to their owners, such as pigeon fancier's lung. Travel abroad to areas where there is a risk of exposure to specific respiratory pathogens should also be checked.

The family history should enquire whether there is any history of TB, allergic disorders or asthma. The review of systems should check overall health and for any general symptoms such as fevers, night sweats, fatigue or weight loss. You should ask about any nose and throat complaints, in particular sinus congestion, postnasal drip or allergic rhinitis, and any cardiac symptoms to rule out pulmonary problems linked to heart failure.

Table 8.2 summarizes how to take a focused history, incorporating the PQRST tool (Chapter 2) for a typical patient with a respiratory complaint.

Physical examination

The basic anatomical landmarks of the chest are shown in Figure 8.2. These will be useful in finding your way around and in documenting examination findings. You should familiarize yourself with the exact location of underlying structures such as the diaphragm and lungs in relation to the surface appearance of the chest.

Table 8.2 Summary of focused history for respiratory system

1 Identifying data	Patient's name, etc.
2 Chief complaint	Cough going to my chest

3 History of present illness
   Cough: symptom analysis using PQRST tool:
   - Provocation/palliation: what brings the cough on? What relieves it?
   - Quality: patient's description, e.g. rattling. Is it productive? If so, what of?
   - Region: is it in the chest or does it feel more in the throat?
   - Severity: is it keeping you awake at night? Does it cause pain?
   - Time: how long have you had it? Is it worse at different times of the day?
   Type of sputum: colour, smell, consistency, blood?
   Shortness of breath: how far can you walk without getting out of breath?
   Hoarseness
   Pain: any associated chest pain.

4 History of previous illness:
   Hospitalizations/specialist consultations
   TB/pneumonia/chest infections
   Chest injuries/deformities

5 Current health:
   Current Medications
   Allergies
   Immunizations

6 Psychosocial history:
   Smoking
   Recreational drugs
   Occupation
   Hobbies
   Travel

7 Family history:
   TB, asthma, allergic disorder

8 Review of systems:
   General
   ENT
   Cardiac

A common mistake in examining the respiratory system is to rush in to listening to the breath sounds before systematically examining the person. It is important to have a good view of the chest and to take a moment to stand back and observe how the person holds himself or herself, body shape and the movement of the chest wall on breathing.

Explain to the patient you are going to examine the chest and that it is necessary to remove clothing from the upper body. Offer a gown that can be slipped off easily at the appropriate time. The patient should sit comfortably on an examination table with the chest at your eye level so that you have a good view.

The order of examination for the chest is:

- Inspection
- Palpation
- Percussion
- Auscultation

Always compare one side with the other, looking for symmetry. Each step in the examination builds on the last to direct you towards any abnormality so that by the time you use the stethoscope you will have a good idea of the location of any problem.

Usually the posterior chest is examined while the patient is sitting. Ask the patient to fold his or her arms across the chest with hands touching opposite shoulders. This serves to separate the scapula so that you avoid trying to listen through bone. If the patient cannot sit, ask someone to hold him or her in a sitting position or roll the patient to one side and then the other. The anterior chest can be examined with the patient sitting but many recommend a lying position, especially for a female patient because it is easier to move the breast during the examination.

Inspection

Observe the general state, height and weight of the person. The speed at which the person undresses may help you gauge the degree of respiratory impairment. Note the rate, rhythm and effort of breathing. Normally the rate is around 14 breaths/minute. Rapid shallow breathing may be a sign of

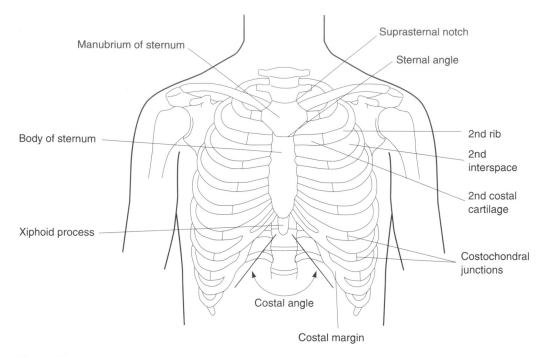

Figure 8.2   Anatomical landmarks of the chest

pleuritic pain and prolonged expiration may show airflow obstruction. In health the chest wall should move smoothly and symmetrically. Inspiration involves the external intercostal muscles and diaphragm while expiration is passive and dependent on the elastic recoil of the lungs. Women use more intercostal breathing than men and infants.

Look for use of accessory muscles such as the sternocleidomastoids, scaleni and trapezii. This indicates increased effort in breathing. If the person is breathing using mainly intercostal muscles there may be something interfering with the diaphragm, e.g. abdominal distension, ascites or pregnancy. If he or she is breathing using more abdominal muscles, consider pleural pain, ankylosing spondylitis or intercostal paralysis. Retraction of interspaces during respiration can indicate rib fracture.

Check for breathlessness, audible wheezing, cough or sputum. If the patient coughs, note the frequency during examination and if it is productive or dry. Observe the colour and amount of sputum. It is useful to have a specimen container available to collect an expectorated sample.

Observe skin colour for pallor or cyanosis as seen in chronic bronchitis or emphysema. Look for any skin rashes, nodules or scars. Check for neck vein distension. An increase in jugular venous pressure may indicate heart failure secondary to lung disease (p. 89). In COPD there may be distension of veins on expiration and collapse of veins on inspiration. The expiratory distension is caused by positive pressure in the chest from the effort of breathing. Look for clubbing and/or nicotine stains on the fingertips.

Check the extremities for peripheral oedema which may be linked with right ventricular failure. Facial puffiness is seen in supraventricular obstruction which often indicates bronchial carcinoma.

Identify anatomical reference points on the patient to help pinpoint the location of an abnormal finding and observe the shape of the chest, looking for any deformities such as pectus carcinatum (pigeon chest) or pectus excavatum (funnel chest). Assess the anterior–posterior diameter and compare to the lateral diameter. The normal ratio is 1:2. In emphysema this may increase to 1:1 and this is known as barrel chest.

Palpation

You should always feel any areas of reported tenderness. Palpate the lymph nodes, particularly cervical, supraclavicular and axillary. With the patient's chin in the midline position and neck slightly flexed, check that the trachea is midline. Chest expansion can be checked by asking the patient to sit upright, then from behind, placing your thumbs at the level of the 10th rib (posteriorly). The thumbs should be nearly touching with a loose fold of skin in between. Ask the patient to inhale deeply and observe the degree and symmetry of expansion. Tactile fremitus may also be assessed (Seidel *et al.*, 1999).

Percussion

Percussion is the technique of tapping the body to produce sounds which indicate if the underlying structures are air-filled, fluid-filled or solid. A resonant note is produced over normal air-filled tissue. A large air-filled space such as a pneumothorax may produce a hyper-resonant note. Increased resonance is also found in emphysema. When lung tissue is fluid-filled or thickened it may have a dull percussion note. Percussion is usually carried out on the intercostal spaces; the exception is the clavicle where percussion may detect lesions in the upper lobes.

The technique involves placing the left hand over the region to be percussed and pressing firmly downwards with the second phalanx of the middle finger. This part of the left middle finger is then struck by the end of the right middle finger, rather like a hammer and anvil. The movement should come from the right wrist and not involve the arm. The exam should be conducted in an orderly manner comparing left and right sides. In health there should be a symmetrical distribution of sounds. The areas to be compared are shown in Figures 8.3 and 8.4.

- Anterior chest wall:
  Clavicle
  Infraclavicular area
  Second to sixth intercostal spaces
- Lateral chest wall:
  Fourth to seventh intercostal spaces
- Posterior chest wall:
  Trapezius
  Above level of scapula
  Every 4–5 cm from scapula to 11th rib

Auscultation

Stethoscopes
The modern stethoscope contains a diaphragm, a bell-shaped funnel, tubing, headset and ear tips. The open bell conducts sound well and is used to hear low-pitched sounds such as extra heart sounds or murmurs. The diaphragm screens out lower-pitched sounds and allows higher-pitched sounds to be heard more easily. The ear tips should closely fit the ear canal and incline towards the nose, matching the angle of the ear canal to block out outside noise.

Assessment of lung sounds
Breath sounds have frequencies which are hard for the human ear to hear. It is therefore important to listen to respiratory sounds in a quiet room with little external stimulation. It is helpful to listen with eyes closed to focus attention on the sound.

Breath sounds originate with the turbulent flow of air through the larynx during breathing. This causes vibration of the vocal cords and these sounds are transmitted to the chest wall via the trachea, bronchi and then normal lung tissue. It is the normal

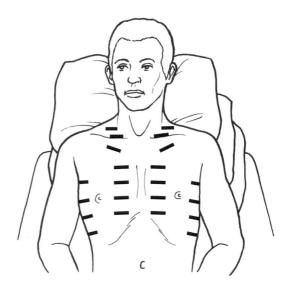

Figure 8.3 Anterior and lateral chest wall sites for percussion

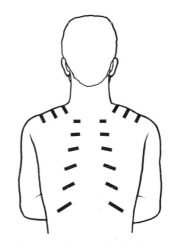

Figure 8.4 Posterior chest wall sites for percussion

spongy structure of the lungs, due to the alveoli, that modifies these sounds until they have a rustling sound. These are the sounds normally heard with a stethoscope at the chest wall and they are described as vesicular breath sounds. The sound on inspiration lasts longer than expiration. Usually breath sounds are soft in the lower lobes and at the lung bases and

Table 8.3 Percussion notes and their significance

Note	Abnormal finding
Resonant	(Normal lung)
Hyper-resonant	Pneumothorax
Tympanitic	Hollow, air-filled space
	Large pneumothorax
Dull	Pulmonary consolidation
	(e.g. pneumonia) or collapse
Flat	Pleural effusion

they appear of shorter duration than in the upper airways.

If, however, the area of lung has lost the small air sacs that are normally present (alveoli) due to consolidation or fibrosis, and the main bronchus is still patent, this alters sound conduction so that the sounds detected are much more like the original sounds produced in the larynx. These are known as bronchial breath sounds and, apart from having a different quality to vesicular sounds, the sound on breathing out is of equal volume and duration as inspiration. Bronchial breath sounds can be heard by the manubrium in the normal person. It is important therefore to be able to distinguish between vesicular and bronchial breath sounds as the latter indicates significant lung pathology such as an area of consolidation asociated with pneumonia.

Adventitious sounds

Two main categories of abnormal sounds can be heard in addition to the usual breath sounds: crackles (crepitations) and wheezes. Crackles are intermittent, non-musical sounds such as the sound produced by rubbing hair next to your ear. If they are clearly heard on inspiration it is thought that this is due to the sudden reopening of collapsed airways that have become occluded during expiration. They may also be produced by air bubbling through secretions, as in pulmonary oedema. Crackles that clear with coughing are usually benign. Early inspiratory crackles may be heard with bronchitis.

Wheezes (rhonchi) are continuous musical sounds caused when air is forced through narrowed airways and usually heard on expiration. Spasm of the airway and mucosal oedema are the usual causes of narrowing and wheezes. If the sound is constant and low pitched this may indicate a partial obstruction of a major bronchus by an inhaled foreign body or a tumour. Polyphonic wheezes (made up of several different notes) on expiration are heard in asthma, chronic obstructive airway disease and emphysema. There may be a relationship between the degree of bronchial obstruction and the presence of wheezes. There does not seem to be a relationship between the loudness or pitch of a wheeze and lung function (Messier *et al.* 1995).

A pleural rub is described as a leathery or creaking sound (Munro and Edwards 1995) and is caused by movement of the visceral pleura over the parietal pleura when both surfaces have become roughened with a fibrinous exudate and are in contact. It is best heard at the end of inspiration and beginning of expiration and indicates pleurisy.

Transmitted voice sounds

When speaking, the sound of the patient's voice undergoes significant alteration as it passes through the lungs. Consequently, voice sounds heard with a stethoscope placed on the chest wall can give useful information on lung pathology. The following terms are commonly used.

Egophony describes change in sound caused by consolidation in the lung. This may be tested for by asking the patient to say 'ee'. In normal tissue the sound is a muffled 'ee' but when the stethoscope is located above abnormal tissue, such as in pneumonia, it sounds like 'ay'.

Whispered pectoriloquy: whispered sounds are not usually heard through a normal chest, but through consolidated tissue the high-pitched sounds are transmitted and the whispering can be heard loud and clear.

Bronchophony: normal speech is usually muffled as high-frequency sounds are screened out by healthy lung tissue. In an area of consolidation the sound becomes louder and clearer than normal. This may be tested for by asking the patient to say '99'.

Using a stethoscope for auscultation

In examining the respiratory system the bell end will give the best results. Place the stethoscope on the chest wall in the same positions used in percussion (Figures 8.3 and 8.4). Each position is matched symmetrically with the same location on the opposite side so that the examiner can compare sounds in both lungs. The examiner listens at each position for a complete breath (both inspiration and expiration) and evaluates the sounds produced by breathing and any additional abnormal sounds. If there are abnormal sounds the additional technique of using the patient's voice to transmit sound through the tissues is used. You should compare areas of normal with abnormal sound transmission to allow you to localize the problem area.

It is usually necessary to demonstrate how you want the patient to breathe and coach him or her through the examination. If breath sounds are faint, ask the person to breathe more deeply. Listen to a full breath in each location and pace the auscultation according to patient comfort, watching for hyperventilation. Concentrate on listening to inspiration, its length and any abnormal sounds, and then when you are clear about the sounds that go with inspiration, focus on expiration. Note the pitch, intensity and duration of inspiratory and expiratory sounds. Sometimes chest hair can cause extra crackles. Wetting the hair may help reduce this sound. Also make sure that the stethoscope tubing does not touch anything else, such as clothing, or you may hear extra sounds. Never listen through clothing as breath sounds are difficult enough to hear without going through an extra layer.

Examination of the respiratory system may be summarized as shown in Table 8.4.

Table 8.4 Examination of the respiratory system

General	
Vital signs	Pulse; blood pressure; respiratory rate; temperature
Hands, fingers and nails	Clubbing
	Peripheral cyanosis
	Nicotine stains
Head and neck	Jugular venous pressure
	Horner's syndrome (carcinoma of the bronchus)
	Hoarseness
Lymph nodes	Cervical and axillary nodes
Chest	
Inspection	Scars; prominent veins
	Pattern of breathing
	Shape of chest
Palpation	Tracheal deviation
	Chest expansion
Percussion	Resonant, hyper-resonant
Auscultation	Breath sounds
	Adventitious sounds
	Vocal resonance

Diagnostic tests

Sputum

During physical examination of the chest the patient with a productive cough may produce a specimen of sputum. Always have a specimen pot available. Observe colour, consistency and odour. The ideal time to collect a sputum specimen is the first expectorated sputum on waking. Sputum can also be induced by inhalation of saline mist which induces coughing.

Sputum samples can be sent for examination under the microscope after Gram stain, culture and sensitivity to identify bacteria and appropriate sensitivity to antibiotics, staining for acid-fast bacilli (TB) or cytology (e.g. for *Pneumocycytis carinii*).

Pulmonary function tests

Most tests depend on the patient's best effort so if the patient is too ill or unable to make a good attempt, the test results may not be valid.

Peak expiratory flow

Peak flow meters are familar to most nurses and widespread, hence they will be considered separately from other instruments used in spirometry (see below). It simply measures the rate at which a patient can forcefully exhale and has the advantage of being simple and portable so patients can use it to monitor their symptoms at home. Serial peak flow measurements are useful in monitoring asthma and can guide titration of medication to prevent a flare-up of symptoms. The disadvantage is that accuracy depends on the user's effort and technique. The normal range is 400–650 l/min in healthy adults and varies with height, gender and age. It is reduced in asthma and COPD.

Spirometry

Spirometry (Mak and Vince 1997) is thought to provide a more objective measure of lung function. As well as normal function it can reveal three patterns of lung function: obstructive, restrictive and a combination of obstructive and restrictive.

A normal pattern shows lung volumes and flow rates within the expected range for a person of that age, sex and height. An obstructive pattern is produced by someone who has any disease that decreases the diameter of the airways by excessive mucus production, inflammation or constriction, e.g. asthma and chronic bronchitis. Restrictive patterns are produced by people with diseases of the lung tissue or a reduced capacity to expand the lungs and hold air, e.g. someone with pneumoconiosis, or a physical deformity. A combined pattern has obstructive and restrictive components, e.g. in cystic fibrosis which causes excess mucus production and damage to the lung tissue.

Tests may be either static, where time is not a factor, or dynamic, where performance is measured against time.

STATIC TESTS

- vital capacity (VC) measures the change in volume of gas in the lungs from complete inspiration to complete expiration. The normal is around 5 litres
- forced vital capacity (FVC) measures the maximum volume that can be forcefully exhaled after a maximum inspiration. The best of three readings is usually taken

DYNAMIC TESTS

- forced expiratory volume in first second (FEV_1) is the volume of air expelled in the first second of a forced expiration, starting from a full inspiration, and is normally around 4 litres, i.e. 80% of VC
- peak expiratory flow rate (PEFR) has already been discussed. It is the greatest flow that can be sustained for 10 ms on forced expiration starting from full inflation

The effort involved means that spirometry is contraindicated if the patient is in respiratory distress, is experiencing chest pain, may have a pneumothorax, has active TB or has suffered a haemoptysis.

Examples of obstructive pulmonary dysfunction include asthma, chronic bronchitis and emphysema. It is graded according to the reduction in the ratio of FEV_1 to FVC. In obstructive disease the FVC is low as the airways are partially closed, limiting expiration and there is high airway resistance.

Restrictive pulmonary dysfunction is associated with reduced lung volumes due to pulmonary infiltrates, pleural diseases, chest wall disorders, reduced diaphragm movement and neuromuscular disease. It is measured by the reduction in the FVC from the expected value. The FVC varies with gender, age and height. In restrictive disease, e.g. when pulmonary infiltrates are present, the FVC is low because of the limited expansion of the lung, but the airway resistance is normal.

Spirometry measurements are recommended for investigating COPD and spirometers are widely used in clinical practice. With improving technology they are now available at affordable prices and the hand-held models make them convenient for the primary care setting. Spirometry devices record air movement against time whereas peak flow records the greatest flow in a short burst. Serial peak flow measurements are useful in asthma care as patients can do repeated measurements at home. In asthma there is good correlation between peak flow and FEV_1. In COPD the amount of airway collapse varies between patients: the correlation between PEF and FEV_1 varies, therefore PEF is not an accurate guide in a patient who has COPD.

Pulse oximetry

A pulse oximeter measures oxygen saturation. It is a non-invasive technique that is quick and accurate at saturation levels above 70%. A plastic clip is attached to the patient's index finger (or earlobe). The top arm of the clip sends red and infrared light out to a photodetector in the other arm of the clip. The instrument measures the 'redness' of the transmitted light and is calibrated to convert this into a measure of oxygen saturation. It is important to remember that the relationship between saturation and partial pressure of oxygen is not linear. The clinical accuracy is reduced in conditions of anaemia, abnormal haemoglobin (e.g. carboxyhaemoglobin found in carbon monoxide poisoning), decreased flow in the vascular bed (in cases of hypovolaemic shock) or if the patient is wearing nail polish (Durren 1992).

Management of common conditions

The common cold

Most people treat colds by themselves at home but it is important to recognize the symptoms, be familiar with the common non-prescription remedies and know how to advise those who seek help with their condition (Simon 1995a).

The best advice to prevent colds is to avoid others with a cold and wash hands frequently. High-dose vitamin C and zinc, although popular, have not been proven in clinical trials to prevent colds (Simon 1995a). Millions of pounds are spent on cold remedies which are often combination analgesics and decongestant, some at subtherapeutic levels. Decongestants may be helpful in relieving symptoms and also in preventing sinusitis or eustachian tube obstruction. Sympathomimetic agents are often used as decongestants. They work quickly to relieve nasal congestion and improve sinus drainage. They stimulate the alpha-receptors, causing vaso-constriction which reduces the formation of mucus but have the side-effect of increasing blood pressure. They are often used in the form of nasal sprays which are effective but should only be used in the short term due to the hazard of rebound congestion leading to an increase in use and dependence. Expectorants are of little value, although they are widely used. It is better to increase hydration by warm fluids while steam inhalations are also useful (Simon 1995a). Antihistamines are often in combination cold remedies but may only benefit because of their sedating effect. They may act as an irritant as they tend to dry mucous membranes.

The most important patient education is to explain that colds are viral infections that will not respond to antibiotics. Relief from symptoms seems to be brought about by resting, increasing fluids, particularly water, with steam inhalations and treating the discomforts of temperature, headache and muscle aches with aspirin or paracetamol.

Acute bronchitis or pneumonia

Leiner (1997) suggests it is best to refrain from treating acute bronchitis with antibiotics as it is usually self-limiting. The patient should be told to increase fluids and report if symptoms do not resolve.

Antibiotic therapy is essential for pneumonia but often has to be started before the causative organism can be identified from sputum samples. Local protocols may determine the drugs used but, whatever the choice, the antibiotic must be effective against *Streptococcus pneumoniae* as this is by far the most likely cause of the infection. Amoxycillin or ampicillin is recommended in the *British National Formulary* (1999), with the addition of flucloxacillin if a *Staphylococcus* infection is suspected. Erythromycin should be used for atypical pneumonia and a broad-spectrum cephalosporin in case of nosocomial infection.

With early diagnosis and appropriate treatment, many patients can be managed at home. They should be encouraged to rest but not lie in bed and sit in an upright position which encourages maximal lung expansion. Deep breathing and coughing are important to clear secretions. Fluid intake should be increased. A humidifier in the room may help loosen secretions and soothe irritated airways. It is generally best not to suppress coughs but if the person is exhausted from coughing, codeine can be used to calm the cough. Aspirin or non-steroidal anti-inflammatory agents may be useful to ease chest pain; taken with great caution if the patient has asthma, any history of peptic ulceration or is a child.

Patient education plays a key role in treatment. Rest should be encouraged and the importance of deep breathing and coughing to clear airways discussed. Patients should be taught to monitor their temperature at home. The importance of increasing fluid intake and stopping smoking should also be discussed.

Vaccination will prevent infection and should be considered for high-risk groups. The pneumoccocal vaccine contains purified polysaccharide from 23 of the commonest strains of *Streptococcus pneumoniae*. Antibody production after immunization depends on the immune function. After injection there is local erythema in 50% of patients and some tenderness. It is only recommended once in a lifetime for most people. However, repeat vaccination is recommended after 5–10 years in people who have had a splenectomy or who have nephrotic syndrome as their antibody levels decline more rapidly than normal people.

Influenza vaccination may also be considered here. The influenza viruses A and B change every year, consequently the World Health Organization recommends each year which strains should be included in the vaccine. These are made ready to be given in the autumn, prior to the flu season from the end of November to mid-February. Only those at high risk are vaccinated, i.e. with chronic conditions or residents of residential homes (Department of Health 1996). It is not thought necessary to vaccinate staff unless they have a medical condition.

Tuberculosis

Diagnosis is usually made by sputum examination for evidence of acid-fast bacillus on smear and the culture is positive for *Mycobacterium tuberculosis*. Most cases also show a positive reaction to TB skin tests (Mantoux or Heaf) and chest X-ray shows pulmonary infiltrates. People with active pulmonary TB are contagious but relatively few organisms are airborne, so it is usually a household member or someone with close contact over a prolonged period who is at risk rather than a brief encounter.

Treatment is usually with a combination of three to four antibiotics for 6–9 months. The simplest regime is rifampicin, isoniazid and pyrazinamide for 2 months followed by rifampian and isoniazid for 4 months (Gleissberg 1997). After 2 weeks of treatment patients are not considered to be an infection risk to others.

Skin tests are used to identify people who have been exposed to TB but who do not have active disease. The Heaf and Mantoux tests are placed subdermally and read in 72 hours. A grade 3–4 Heaf test and greater than 10 mm diameter wheal (not erythema) indicates exposure to TB. To prevent activation of TB, isoniazid is given for 6 months or isoniazid and rifampicin for 3 months.

Vaccination with BCG (bacille Calmette-Guérin) is recommended for all children aged 10–14 years in the UK to prevent TB. Also it is offered to high-risk neonates.

Asthma

In treating asthma the focus is firmly on prevention of acute attacks and managing the condition so that it has the minimum possible impact upon normal everyday life. It is particularly important to work with patients as partners in care as successful treatment depends on effective self-care by the patient. Patient education is important to ensure s/he understands and complies with the medication regime. Self-administered peak flow readings allow the patient to recognize any deterioration in performance and adjust the medication to prevent an acute attack.

Using inhalers takes some mastery and inadequate technique is often implicated in flare-ups of the disease. Spacer devices have been developed for those patients who find it difficult to coordinate breathing with hand movement (to press and activate the inhaler). These are chambers which can be attached to the inhaler, allowing the patient to breathe from the chamber after spraying the inhaler inside. With the opportunity to demonstrate technique and frequent reinforcement at nurse consultation, patients are more likely to gain effective pharmacological control and comply with their drug regimen. The nurse practitioner must keep up-to-date in the rapidly changing field of spacer technology.

The importance of self-management is demonstrated by the fact that many people admitted to hospital with severe asthma have usually misjudged the severity of their asthma and made errors in their treatment. In a group of people admitted to hospital with severe asthma Kole *et al.* (1998) found that there was a high frequency of psychological influences, especially anxiety and major socioeconomic disadvantage. These factors have powerful effects on learning about asthma and understanding behaviours necessary to manage asthma successfully. This is consistent with the work of Harrison (1998), who found in a review of the literature that those most likely not to follow a treatment plan were younger, depressed and worried about the side-effects of steroids or addiction to medications. Deprivation, life crises, family conflict, social isolation, substance abuse, unemployment, bereavement and emotional disturbance all place people with asthma at increased risk of premature death. It highlights the need for a full psychosocial assessment and patient-centred treatment – themes central to the nurse practitioner approach.

The British Thoracic Society and National Asthma Campaign have published step guidelines for the treatment of asthma. Anti-inflammatory agents are the mainstay of therapy, bronchodilators should only be used if required (Cross 1997b). This approach involves titrating drug therapy against the severity of symptoms and the control achieved. The reader is referred to Cross (1997b) and the British National Formulary (1999) for a comprehensive description.

Leukotriene receptor antagonists are a recently introduced new group of drugs. Leukotrienes are important mediators in the inflammatory response produced by mast cells. Their inhibition prevents bronchospasm and inflammation hence drugs such as montelukast and zafirkulast can be used for prophylaxis but should not be used to treat an acute attack (BNF 1999).

Most authorities point to improper inhaler technique as the reason for failure of treatment. This is particularly important in reducing the systemic effects of inhaled steroids. The mouth should always be washed out after inhaling steroids for this reason. A common mistake is overdependence on the bronchodilator to relieve symptoms and underuse of anti-inflammatory agents such as sodium cromoglycate to prevent problems occurring in the first place. There are many types of inhalers available and this whole area underlines the importance of good patient teaching if effective technique is to be learnt.

The following measures are useful for reducing house dust mite allergen response (Custovic et al. 1998):

1   Encase mattress, pillow and quilt in impermeable covers
2   Wash all bedding in the hot cycle (55–60°C) weekly
3   Replace carpets with linoleum or wood flooring
4   If carpets cannot be removed, treat with acaricides and/or tannic acid
5   Minimize upholstered furniture or replace with leather furniture
6   Keep dust-accumulating objects in closed cupboards
7   Use a vacuum cleaner with integral HEPA filter and double thickness bags
8   Replace curtains with blinds or easily washable (hot cycle) curtains
9   Hot-wash/freeze soft toys

The patient with an acute attack of asthma presents as a potentially life-threatening emergency. Figure 8.5 summarizes the main steps to take depending on the patient's condition, and care should be based on this protocol at all times. Every effort must be made to transfer the patient to an A&E department by ambulance as quickly as possible if his or her condition indicates.

Chronic obstructive pulmonary disease

The classic patient with COPD has a history of smoking, probably for more than 20 years. The main symptoms are breathlessness and productive cough with grey, white or yellow sputum. Most patients generally feel unwell and have difficulty with strenuous activity. They have frequent respiratory infections. Anorexia with weight loss may occur or there may be weight gain due to oedema. The breathing pattern shows prolonged expiration with pursed-lip breathing and tachypnoea (rapid respiration). A barrel-shaped chest with increased resonance on percussion is common.

The most objective test for COPD is spirometry to measure forced expiratory volume. Hypoxaemia occurs in advanced disease and would be shown by a low oxygen saturation. Arterial blood gas may be helpful in severe bronchitis when there is low PaO_2 but may show no abnormality in the early stages of COPD.

Sputum culture may reveal secondary infection with organisms such as *Streptococcus pneumoniae*, *Haemophilus influenzae* or *H. pneumoniae*, or *Moraxella catarrhalis*. Chest X-ray may show hyperinflation, barrel chest or a flat diaphragm. Sometimes enlarged air spaces (bullae) are seen with emphysema and blunting of the costophrenic angle on posterior–anterior view. A chest X-ray is helpful in detecting complications such as heart failure, pneumonia or a pneumothorax.

Treatment of COPD involves:

• stopping smoking
• bronchodilators, which help to control the symptoms but do not alter the progression of COPD. Antimuscarinic drugs such as ipratropium seem to be more effective than beta$_2$-agonists (Barnes 1998)
• chest physiotherapy
• treat infections promptly as well as other complications such as heart failure
• oxygen therapy to improve function and quality of life
• patient education and involvement in care plan

Drugs commonly used include ipratropium, beta$_2$-agonists such as salbutamol and terbutaline, long-acting beta$_2$-agonists such as salmeterol, theophylline and corticosteroids. However Barnes (1998) argues that there is little evidence that inhaled steroids are beneficial in COPD. The small percentage (10%) of patients who do respond

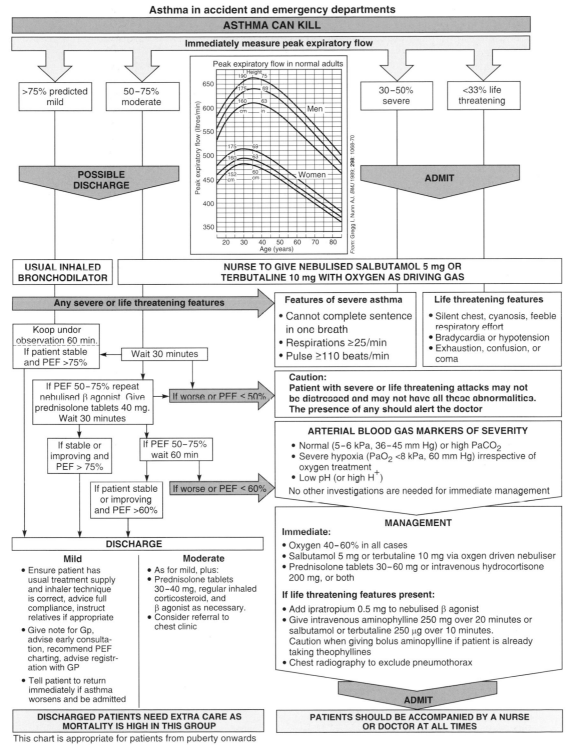

Asthma in accident and emergency departments

ASTHMA CAN KILL

Immediately measure peak expiratory flow

>75% predicted mild | 50–75% moderate | 30–50% severe | <33% life threatening

Peak expiratory flow in normal adults

From: Gregg I, Nunn AJ. *BMJ* 1989; **298**: 1068–70

POSSIBLE DISCHARGE

ADMIT

USUAL INHALED BRONCHODILATOR

NURSE TO GIVE NEBULISED SALBUTAMOL 5 mg OR TERBUTALINE 10 mg WITH OXYGEN AS DRIVING GAS

Any severe or life threatening features

Features of severe asthma
- Cannot complete sentence in one breath
- Respirations ≥25/min
- Pulse ≥110 beats/min

Life threatening features
- Silent chest, cyanosis, feeble respiratory effort
- Bradycardia or hypotension
- Exhaustion, confusion, or coma

Keep under observation 60 min. If patient stable and PEF >75%

Wait 30 minutes

If PEF 50–75% repeat nebulised β agonist. Give prednisolone tablets 40 mg. Wait 30 minutes

If worse or PEF < 50%

Caution:
Patient with severe or life threatening attacks may not be distressed and may not have all these abnormalities. The presence of any should alert the doctor

If stable or improving and PEF > 75%

If PEF 50–75% wait 60 min

ARTERIAL BLOOD GAS MARKERS OF SEVERITY
- Normal (5–6 kPa, 36–45 mm Hg) or high PaCO$_2$
- Severe hypoxia (PaO$_2$ <8 kPa, 60 mm Hg) irrespective of oxygen treatment
- Low pH (or high H$^+$)

No other investigations are needed for immediate management

If patient stable or improving and PEF >60%

If worse or PEF < 60%

DISCHARGE

Mild
- Ensure patient has usual treatment supply and inhaler technique is correct, advice full compliance, instruct relatives if appropriate
- Give note for Gp, advise early consulta-tion, recommend PEF charting, advise regist-ration with GP
- Tell patient to return immediately if asthma worsens and be admitted

Moderate
- As for mild, plus:
- Prednisolone tablets 30–40 mg, regular inhaled corticosteroid, and β agonist as necessary.
- Consider referral to chest clinic

MANAGEMENT

Immediate:
- Oxygen 40–60% in all cases
- Salbutamol 5 mg or terbutaline 10 mg via oxgen driven nebuliser
- Prednisolone tablets 30–60 mg or intravenous hydrocortisone 200 mg, or both

If life threatening features present:
- Add ipratropium 0.5 mg to nebulised β agonist
- Give intravenous aminophylline 250 mg over 20 minutes or salbutamol or terbutaline 250 µg over 10 minutes. Caution when giving bolus aminopylline if patient is already taking theophyllines
- Chest radiography to exclude pneumothorax

ADMIT

DISCHARGED PATIENTS NEED EXTRA CARE AS MORTALITY IS HIGH IN THIS GROUP	PATIENTS SHOULD BE ACCOMPANIED BY A NURSE OR DOCTOR AT ALL TIMES

This chart is appropriate for patients from puberty onwards

Figure 8.5   The main steps for treating asthma

Source: Thorax 1997: **52** (supplement 1). The British Guidelines on Asthma Management 1995 Review and Position Statement. Copyright BMJ Publishing Group. Reproduced with permission

probably have an asthma component to their disease. In acute flare-ups of COPD corticosteroids are probably effective because of the anti-inflammatory effect. Again the reader is referred to the *British National Formulary* (1999) and the British Thoracic Society guidelines (1997) for a comprehensive review of drug treatment.

The focus should be on prevention of respiratory infections and preserving lung function. Immunizations should be given to protect against influenza and pneumococcal pneumonia (p. 117). Exercise treatment is important to maintain lung function. Different regimens have been suggested but walking is accessible to most people. It is good aerobic activity which does not overtax the upper body and a programme can be tailored to most individuals' needs. Recommendations vary from 20–30 minutes 3–5 times per week to 5–15 minutes four times daily. Teaching breathing techniques may be helpful to slow breathing but increase the tidal volume.

Psychosocial support is an essential part of treatment. As with any chronic illness, patients need to be involved in decision-making concerning their care, developing a personalized plan that addresses their problems. Involving the rest of the family is usually helpful. Although COPD is a chronic and progressive disease, patients can still have some choice and control over their illness.

Oxygen therapy can be prescribed for continuous use, or at night or with exercise only. People most likely to benefit from therapy are hypoxaemic patients with pulmonary hypertension, chronic cor pulmonale, erythrocytosis, impaired cognitive function, exercise intolerance, nocturnal restlessness or morning headache (Stauffer 1997). In advanced COPD oxygen therapy improves survival, reduces the need for hospitalization and gives the patient better quality of life. Home oxygen may be supplied in compressed gas cylinders or oxygen concentrators. The concentrators use room air and are best for long-term continuous use. The large tanks are best for intermittent use. Most patients benefit from both a stationary and portable oxygen system. Oxygen is usually given by nasal cannula rather than a mask, at a flow rate of 1–2 l/min.

Cigarette smoking is a major cause of disease in the UK and there is strong evidence to suggest that stopping smoking, even for elderly long-term smokers, is beneficial (Rigotti 1995). In treating any respiratory complaint it is important to inform smokers of the hazards of smoking and suggest that they stop. Smoking is a complex habit which often starts in adolescence and is linked to peer pressure and parental influence. Once smoking becomes a habit it is difficult to change.

To promote health the nurse practitioner needs to develop expertise in strategies to help patients stop smoking. There are many techniques available and

knowing how and when to use them is important. Often nurses become frustrated because they invest a lot of time in counselling, only to find that patients continue without any change in their habit. It is always important to ask patients if they would like to stop smoking as it is a waste of time attempting a smoking cessation programme with someone who has no intention of giving up the habit. There is evidence to suggest that a simple recommendation to stop smoking by a health professional can have a positive effect (Sanders 1992; Rigotti 1995). The Agency for Health Care Policy and Research offers the following smoking cessation guidelines. It suggests:

- Everyone who smokes should be offered smoking cessation at every visit
- Clinicians should ask and record the tobacco use status of every patient
- Cessation treatments – even as brief as 3 minutes – are effective
- More intense treatment is effective in producing long-term abstinence from tobacco
- Nicotine replacement therapy (patches or gum), clinician-delivered social support and skills training are particularly effective components of smoking cessation

Change is complex and it may be years later that the person is ready and the message remembered. It is also important that relapse is an important phenomenon in any change of habit. Relapse should be viewed as part of learning to change and not as total failure for either patient or nurse. It is often 6–9 months after stopping that patients relapse because of life events or a stressful period, when old habits are associated with comfort and the familiar. It is helpful to warn patients of the possibility of relapse and develop strategies to avoid it. Also keep an open door so that if someone starts smoking again they can return quickly for guidance if desired. Most people who stop smoking are able to do so by themselves without outside help.

Summary

The broader approach used by nurse practitioners, taking into account psychosocial influences and patient preferences, contributes greatly to the successful management of many respiratory conditions. Health education plays a major part in the management of respiratory illnesses. Recent improvements in the management of asthma demonstrate what can be achieved when nurses and doctors work together with patients as equal partners. There remains a great deal to do in the promotion of respiratory health, especially given the worrying rise in the numbers of youngsters taking up smoking and the possible harmful effects of air pollution.

References

Barnes P. (1998) New therapies for chronic obstructive pulmonary disease, *Thorax*, **53**, pp. 137–147.

British National Formulary (1999) London, British Medical Association/Royal Pharmaceutical Society of Great Britain.

British Thoracic Society (1997) Guidelines on the management of asthma, *Thorax*, **52**(1).

Butler C., Pill R., Stott N. (1998) Qualitative study of patients' perceptions of doctors' advice to quit smoking: implications for opportunistic health promotion, *British Medical Journal* **316**, June 1998.

Central Statistics Office (1995) *Annual Abstract of Statistics*, London, HMSO.

Chow M., Durand B., Feldman M., Mills M. (1984) *Handbook of Pediatric Primary Care*, 2nd edn., New York, John Wiley.

Cross S. (1997a) The management of acute asthma, *Professional Nurse*, **12**(7), pp. 495–497.

Cross S. (1997b) Revised guidelines on asthma management. *Professional Nurse*, **12**(6), pp. 408–410.

Custovic A., Simpson A., Chapman M., Woodcock A. (1998) Allergen avoidance in the treatment of asthma and atopic disorders, *Thorax*, **53**, pp. 63–72.

DeGowin E. (1987) *DeGowin & DeGowin's Bedside Diagnostic Examination*, 5th edn., New York, Macmillan.

Department of Health (1995) *Asthma: An Epidemiological Overview*, Central Health Monitoring Unit Epidemiological Overview series, London, HMSO.

Department of Health (1996) *Immunisation against Infectious Diseases*, London, HMSO.

Durren M. (1992) Getting the most from pulse oximetry, *Journal of Emergency Nursing*, **18**(4), pp. 340–342.

Gleissberg G. (1997) A shadow of the past: tuberculosis today, RCN nursing update 3 unit 067, *Nursing Standard*, **11**(1).

Goroll A., May L., Mulley A. (1995) *Primary Care Medicine, Office Evaluation and Management of the Adult Patient*, 3rd edn., Philadelphia, JB Lipincott.

Harrison B. (1998) Psychosocial aspects of asthma in adults, *Thorax*, **53**, pp. 519–525.

Jarvis C. (1992) *Physical Examination and Health Assessment*, Philadelphia, WB Saunders.

Jeffery P. (1998) Structural and inflammatory changes in COPD: a comparison with asthma, *Thorax*, **53**, pp. 129–136.

Kole J., Vamos M., Fergusson W., Eikind G. (1998) Determinants of management errors in acute severe asthma, *Thorax*, **53**, pp. 14–20.

Leiner S. (1997) Acute bronchitis in adults: commonly diagnosed but poorly defined. *Nurse Practitioner, 22,* January 1997.

Mak V. (1997) Chronic obstructive pulmonary disease; COPD: the UK perspective. *Chest Medicine On-line* http://www.u-net.com/priory/cmol/copd.htm.

Messier N., Charbonneau G., Racineux J.L. (1995) Wheezes. *European Respiratory Journal*, **8**(11), pp. 1942–1948.

Munro J., Edwards C. (1995) *Macleod's Clinical Examination Skills*, Edinburgh, Churchill Livingstone.

Omerod P. (1996) Tuberculosis in the UK, 1994: current issues and trends, *Thorax*, 49.

Philip E. (1997) Chronic cough. *American Family Physician*, **56**(5).

Rees J., Price J. (1995) *ABC of Asthma*, London, British Medical Journal Publications.

Rees P., Williams D. (1995) *Principles of Clinical Medicine* London, Edward Arnold.

Rigotti N. (1995) Smoking cessation. In: Goroll A.H., May L.A., Mulley A.G. (eds), *Primary Care Medicine*, Philadelphia, JB Lipincott.

Sanders D. (1992) *Smoking Cessation Interventions: Is Patient Education Effective?* London, Health Promotion Sciences Unit, London School of Hygiene and Tropical Medicine.

Seidel H., Ball J., Dains J., Benedict G. (1999). *Mosby's Guide to Physical Examination*, 4th edn., St Louis, Mosby.

Siafakas N. (1995) Optimal assessment and management of chronic obstructive pulmonary disease (COPD), *European Respiratory Journal*, **8**, pp. 1398–1420.

Simon H. (1995a) *Management of the Common Cold* in Primary Care Medicine. In: Goroll A.H., May L.A., Mulley A.G. (eds.) *Primary Care Medicine*, Philadelphia, JB Lipincott.

Simon H. (1995b) *Approach to the Patient with Acute Bronchitis or Pneumonia in the Ambulatory Care Setting*. In: Goroll A.H., May L.A., Mulley A.G. (eds.) *Primary Care Medicine*, Philadelphia, JB Lipincott.

Snider G.L., Kleinerman J., Thurlbeck W.M. (1985) The definition of emphysema, Report of the National Heart and Blood Institute, Division of Lung Diseases Workshop, *American Review of Respiratory Disease*, **132**, pp. 182–185.

Stauffer J. (1997). The lung. In: Tierney L., McPhee S., Papadakis M.A. (eds). *Current Medical Diagnosis and Treatment*.

CHAPTER 9

The abdomen

Alison Crumbie

Introduction

The abdomen extends from the diaphragm to the pelvis. The major system which concerns the nurse practitioner when examining the abdomen is the gastrointestinal system. The genitourinary, cardiovascular and neurological systems can also be examined in the abdominal area. The focus of this chapter is the gastrointestinal system, which includes the processes of digestion, secretion, absorption and metabolism and therefore includes the liver, pancreas and gallbladder and the urinary system, including the kidneys and the bladder. The nervous, cardiovascular and reproductive systems will be mentioned briefly; a more detailed review of these systems can be found in Chapters 5, 7, 10 and 11 respectively.

Pathophysiology and clinical presentations

Patients may present with a variety of signs and symptoms which may lead you to carry out an abdominal examination. You may consider an examination of the abdomen for example in a patient who presents feeling tired all the time and has signs of jaundice or a person who complains of abnormal weight loss. The following clinical presentations are common general complaints encountered in general practice or the hospital setting. The aim is to present these general complaints in a logical order from mouth to anus, followed by the structures that lie outside the gastrointestinal tract.

Dysphagia

Difficulty in swallowing may be a symptom of oesophageal disease or due to conditions which influence gut motility such as parkinsonism, multiple sclerosis and motor neurone disease. The most common causes of dysphagia include benign oesophageal stricture, carcinoma of the oesophagus, achalasia of the cardia and old age (presbyoesophagus).

Heartburn

Galloway (1993) states that 65% of the UK adult population have suffered with heartburn at some stage, 7% use indigestion aids every day and 3% have been doing so for more than 3 years. Heartburn is clearly a common condition that nurse practitioners can expect to encounter in any setting. The patient may complain of a variety of symptoms including a burning sensation or pain in the stomach which may move up to the mouth. The pain is usually intermittent, occurs after meals, gets worse on lying down and is relieved by antacids and some people complain of an unpleasant taste in the mouth (Ingram Tagg 1996). The patient's discomfort results from gastric acid, pepsin and bile refluxing from the stomach into the oesophagus; the mucosa becomes damaged and this produces muscle spasm and retrosternal pain. The damage to the oesophagus is caused by the intense acidity of the gastric juice irritating the oesophageal mucosa, which does not have the same acid tolerance as the stomach. A variety of medications can produce this result by stimulating acid secretion or increasing acidity in the stomach. Coffee, tea, cocoa, chocolate, tomato products, citrus fruits and milk are all potent stimulators of acid secretion or add to the acidity of the stomach contents (Ingram Tagg 1996). Other foods or medications produce the same symptoms through a different mechanism as they reduce tension in the lower oesophageal sphincter. Central nervous system depressants such as morphine or diazepam can reduce the normal input to the lower oesophageal sphincter and certain fatty foods, alcohol and smoking produce the same response (Norwak and Handford 1994). Increase in pressure in the abdominal cavity (e.g. from pregnancy or obesity) can also cause oesophageal reflux. Herniation of the stomach into the thoracic cavity is known as hiatus hernia and may be associated with reflux oesophagitis.

Dyspepsia and indigestion

The terms indigestion, heartburn and dyspepsia are

often used interchangeably by both clinicians and patients and there is clearly some confusion and overlap. The terms dyspepsia or indigestion refer to a sensation of fullness in the epigastrium which is frequently accompanied by belching, nausea or heartburn. Jones and Murfin (1993) state that dyspepsia can be classified as:

- ulcer-like dyspepsia
- reflux-like dyspepsia
- dysmotility-like dyspepsia
- idiopathic dyspepsia

Ulcer-like dyspepsia can be experienced in the area over the stomach. Reflux-like dyspepsia refers to symptoms which tend to be retrosternal and may be accompanied by regurgitation of acid. Dysmotility is accompanied by vague abdominal symptoms such as bloating and bowel dysfunction and idiopathic dyspepsia encompasses conditions which do not fit well into any of the other three categories.

One of the causes of dyspepsia is peptic ulceration. Peptic ulcers arise throughout the oesophagus, stomach and small intestine. It is thought that two factors are involved in the development of peptic ulceration – gastric hypersecretion and impaired defences in the mucosal lining of the intestine. There are several theories relating to the causative factors associated with hypersecretion: cigarette smoking is one suggestion. In folk wisdom, psychological stress has been linked to peptic ulceration; however, there is a lack of evidence to substantiate this link and it is therefore now generally discounted (Nowak and Handford 1994). Milk and products containing caffeine have been found to be potent stimulators of acid secretion (Ingram Tagg 1996). The mucosal defences can be interrupted by a variety of factors. The bacterium *Helicobacter pylori* is thought to predispose the gastric mucosa to ulceration by inducing gastritis, and non-steroidal anti-inflammatory medications such as aspirin, indomethacin and ibuprofen have been found to cause damage and bleeding in the gastric mucosae. Exposure of the deeper layers of the stomach lining results in further damage caused by the gastric enzyme pepsin, resulting in peptic ulceration. There is a familial tendency to peptic ulceration, which suggests that genetics probably play a part in this disease process (Nowak and Handford 1994). Smoking may also play a role in compromising the mucosal defence mechanisms.

Clearly there are many factors involved in the development of peptic ulceration and it appears that a combination of factors produce the ulceration. Of major concern are the complications of ulceration which include haemorrhage from the ulcer and perforation of the stomach wall. The most serious complication of infection with *H. pylori* is gastric cancer. *H. pylori* is not the carcinogen *per se* but it appears to set the scene for cancer development (Harris and Misiewicz 1996).

Nausea, vomiting and haematemesis

Nausea and vomiting result from a complex process involving the vomiting centre in the brain. The vomiting centre receives input from the gastrointestinal tract, the vestibular apparatus, the chemoreceptor trigger zone in the medulla oblongata and the cortex of the brain. The gastrointestinal tract responds to the ingestion of toxins and communicates with the vomiting centre via the vagus nerve; the vestibular apparatus responds to motion; the chemoreceptor trigger zone responds to toxins in the blood and inputs from the cortex result from disagreeable sights and sounds. The vomiting centre receives stimuli which eventually exceed a certain threshold and nausea, retching and vomiting follow (Williams 1994).

The characteristics of the vomit are important factors in assessment of the patient. Of particular importance is the presence of blood in the vomit (haematemesis). Vomiting blood indicates bleeding from the stomach, duodenum or oesophagus. The blood may be bright red or dark brown depending on the amount of time it has been in contact with gastric acid. Causes of gastrointestinal bleeding include gastric cancer, duodenal ulcer, gastritis, oesophagitis or oesophageal ulcer, duodenitis, varices, tumours or Mallory–Weiss tear (a tear which occurs at the gastro-oesophageal junction).

Abdominal pain

There are many causes of abdominal pain. The history-taking process and physical examination are essential in differentiating between a number of potentially life-threatening diagnoses. It is helpful to understand the difference between visceral, parietal and referred pain. The peritoneum is a serous membrane system in the abdominal cavity, the parietal layer lines the inner walls of the cavity and the visceral layer is adherent to the surfaces of the organs. Visceral pain refers pain caused by stretching or inflammation of a hollow organ and it is often associated with visceral symptoms such as anorexia, sweating, nausea and pallor. This pain is often described as a dull ache and tends to occur near the midline. Movement does not aggravate visceral pain so the patient may writhe or double up in response to it. The parietal layer of the peritoneum is innervated with pain-sensitive fibres and therefore the sensation is well-localized and movement or stretching aggravates the discomfort. Patients describe parietal pain as sharp or stabbing and find palpation extremely painful; the pain is exacerbated when the palpating hand is released (rebound tenderness). Figure 9.1 outlines the location of

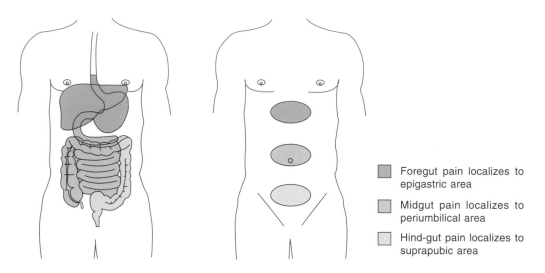

Figure 9.1 The location of visceral pain on the abdominal surface. *Source:* Adapted from Epstein *et al.* 1997

visceral pain on the abdominal surface related to the structure within the abdominal cavity.

Epstein *et al.* (1997) state that appendicitis is an excellent example of the difference between visceral and parietal pain. Acute appendicitis starts with a dull ache around the periumbilical area and the patient often complains of nausea. As the appendicitis develops, the inflammation advances through the visceral layer to the parietal peritoneum. The pain then shifts to the right lower quadrant, typically at a place which is named McBurney's point (the mid-point between the symphysis pubis and the right iliac crest) and the character of the pain changes from dull to sharp. Palpation becomes extremely painful and the patient displays reflex guarding with contracted abdominal muscles and rebound tenderness.

Inflammation in the abdominal organs can result in referred pain to other parts of the body. For example, inflammation in the gallbladder may be experienced as pain over the scapula and diaphragmatic pain may be felt as pain in the shoulder. Table 9.1 is adapted from Seller (1993) and Seidel *et al.* (1995) and outlines the potential differential diagnoses of abdominal pain according to location on the abdomen.

It is worthwhile entertaining a number of potential differential diagnoses for patients who present with abdominal pain. The locations shown in Table 9.1 provide a general guide for your problem-solving process; however, unusual presentations occur and are particularly common in the elderly. As the incidence of cancer increases with age, it is worth remembering that, in a study of patients presenting with non-specific abdominal pain over the age of 50, 10% had a malignant tumour (Seller 1993).

Mesenteric angina

Blood supply to the bowel may be interrupted by atherosclerotic arteries. There is a good collateral blood supply to the bowel and therefore ischaemia associated with stenosed arteries usually becomes apparent as pain on eating. The pain is experienced as severe periumbilical pain which causes anorexia and weight loss. It is visceral in nature and therefore has several of the characteristics described above in the definition of visceral pain.

Wind

Flatulence (excessive belching) and flatus (the passage of wind through the anus) can cause considerable distress and patients often feel helpless and unsure about managing their symptoms. It is always worth exploring dietary causes for flatus, such as the excessive consumption of legumes or recent changes in dietary habits as fermentation of certain foods can cause excessive gas throughout the intestine. Flatulence is usually caused by swallowing air during eating (aerophagy) and often occurs in patients who have a hiatus hernia, peptic ulcer or chronic gallbladder disease.

Changes in bowel habit

Changes in bowel habits can take several forms: the patient may experience constipation, diarrhoea or a change in the type of stool being produced. A change in bowel habit can be a subtle first sign of serious disease and therefore it is essential to explore this area in detail with the patient.

Constipation

Constipation can be caused by organic disease such as hypothyroidism, strictures in the colon or electrolyte imbalance. A motility disorder or physical immobility can cause constipation and a variety of drugs such as the opiates and antidepressants have the same effect in reducing the motility of the

Table 9.1   Location of abdominal pain

Diffuse pain
Peritonitis, pancreatitis, leukaemia, sickle cell crisis, early appendicitis, mesenteric adenitis, mesenteric thrombosis, gastroenteritis, aneurysm, colitis, intestinal obstruction, metabolic, toxic and bacterial causes

Right upper quadrant	**Left upper quadrant**
Cholecystitis	Gastritis, gastric ulcer
Hepatitis	Pancreatitis
Hepatic abscess	Splenic enlargement, rupture
Hepatomegaly	infarction, aneurysm
Peptic ulcer	Renal pain
Pancreatitis	Herpes-zoster
Renal pain	Myocardial ischaemia
Herpes-zoster	Pneumonia
Myocardial ischaemia	Aortic aneurysm
Pericarditis	
Pneumonia	

Periumbilical
Intestinal obstruction
Acute pancreatitis
Early appendicitis
Mesenteric thrombosis
Aortic aneurysm
Diverticulitis

Right lower quadrant	**Left lower quadrant**
Diverticulitis	Diverticulitis
Intestinal obstruction	Intestinal obstruction
Appendicitis	Appendicitis
Leaking aneurysm	Leaking aneurysm
Ectopic pregnancy	Ectopic pregnancy
Ovarian cyst or torsion	Ovarian cyst or torsion
Salpingitis	Salpingitis
Endometriosis	Endometriosis
Ureteral calculi	Ureteral calculi
Renal pain	Renal pain
Seminal vesiculitis	Seminal vesiculitis
Regional enteritis	Strangulated hernia
Cholecystitis	Ulcerative colitis
Perforated ulcer	
Strangulated hernia	

Source: Adapted from Seller (1993) and Seidel *et al.* (1995).

gastrointestinal tract. A low-residue diet will also slow peristalsis and depression or dementia can cause constipation. The fear of pain associated with passing stools when a patient has haemorrhoids is a further cause. The pathophysiology therefore depends upon the cause of the constipation.

Diarrhoea

Diarrhoea is defined as increased faecal fluidity (Nowak and Handford 1994). It is caused by increased fluid volume in the colon which produces distension and activates the defecation reflex. Three processes result in fluid gathering in the intestine – secretion, osmosis and impaired water absorption. Secretion of water into the lumen of the intestine is a response to irritation which may be caused by bacterial toxins. Intestinal secretion can also be caused by certain gastrointestinal tumours, laxatives or unabsorbed fatty acids. Problems with digestion can result in an increase in the osmotic pressure in the intestinal lumen. This is caused by several mechanisms, including lack of bile or enzymes necessary to break the food macromolecules into smaller subunits, a diet that has a high indigestible content such as legumes or carbohydrates, or bacterial growth within the lumen. The osmotic pressure rises and water is drawn into the lumen from the intestinal wall, resulting in an increase in the fluidity of the stool. The small intestine and colon absorb approximately 8600 ml/day and therefore any condition that impairs the absorption of this fluid will result in diarrhoea. Coeliac disease and Crohn's disease are examples of malabsorption conditions that impair absorption of water in the intestine, resulting in increased frequency and fluidity of the stool.

Alcohol and certain medications such as anti-biotics can also produce diarrhoea by interfering with fluid absorption or promoting fluid secretion due to irritation of the intestine. Whatever the cause of the diarrhoea, the consequences can be severe, particularly in elderly or very young patients. Increased fluid loss may result in dehydration and acidosis as alkaline bicarbonate ions are expelled from the system and these are important considerations in your treatment and management of the condition.

Seller (1993) states that the acute onset of diarrhoea in a previously healthy individual with no signs of other organ involvement is likely to be caused by an infectious agent that is most commonly viral. Differential diagnoses for diarrhoea according to Seller (1993) can be divided into acute and chronic. In a patient who presents with acute diarrhoea, consider a viral or bacterial cause, toxin-mediated such as *Clostridium* or *Staphylococcus*, use of laxatives, antibiotics or other drugs or dysentery syndrome. Also consider rotavirus, *Salmonella* and *Shigella*, all of which occur more commonly in children than in adults. Chronic diarrhoea can be caused by irritable bowel syndrome, diabetes, giardiasis, inflammatory bowel disease (Crohn's or ulcerative colitis, for example) or lactase deficiency in infants or adults of African or Mediterranean descent.

Rectal bleeding

Polyps, diverticular disease, inflammatory bowel disease, carcinoma, haemorrhoids, anorectal lesions and ischaemia of the intestine can all produce rectal bleeding. The patient's description of the blood loss will help you gain some idea of the origin of the bleeding, although a diagnosis should be made with caution as bleeding from benign haemorrhoids can mask the signs of bleeding from a more serious disease which originates further up the intestinal tract. Sixty per cent of rectal bleeding is caused by haemorrhoids, however, as the patient's age increases your level of concern relating to the possibility of malignancy should also increase. The incidence of cancer in people who present with dark rectal bleeding in the 75–80-year-old age group is 1 in 40.

Rectal bleeding can present as bright red, plum or maroon, black and sticky or microscopic (occult) blood. Bright red blood loss tends to originate from the anus or rectum and plum or maroon coloured from the colon. Blood loss which presents as black and sticky originates from higher up the gastrointestinal tract, for example the stomach or oesophagus. Blood which has been denatured by gastric acid and enzymes develops a characteristic smell and the consistency of tar, this is known as melaena. In the instance of microscopic blood the patient may present to you with anaemia and it is therefore always worth considering gastro-intestinal blood loss as the cause of iron-deficiency anaemia.

Diverticular disease

Diverticula are pouch-like sacs which occur in the intestinal mucous membrane and bulge out through the wall of the large intestine. It is widely thought that low-residue diets have a part to play in the development of diverticular disease. The dry small stools that result from low-residue diets require a greater strength of colonic contraction to force them along the colon. This raises pressures in the wall of the colon and promotes formation of diverticula at areas of weakness in the walls. The presence of diverticula is described as diverticulosis. In many cases this condition is asymptomatic; however in a few people it can cause mild to severe bleeding into the lumen of the colon or may result in cramping pain and constipation. Irritation and bacterial damage may produce inflammation in the diverticula known as diverticulitis. This results in left lower abdominal pain, fever, diarrhoea or constipation and can cause a great deal of discomfort.

Liver disease and biliary obstruction

The liver can be damaged in two ways – damage to the liver cells (hepatocellular disease) or biliary tree obstruction (intrahepatic or extrahepatic cholestasis). When hepatocytes are damaged, enzymes leak into the blood where they can be detected in the plasma. In cirrhosis there is extensive damage to the liver which results in obstruction of the blood flow and one of the consequences is portal hypertension. The early symptoms of liver damage include malaise, fatigue, anorexia and nausea and the signs include darkening of the urine, lightening of stool colour and the gradual development of jaundice. Brain function is depressed in patients who have severe liver damage due to the reduced ability of the liver to detoxify potentially neurotoxic products from the gut. In the case of a person who has developed portal hypertension, the blood bypasses the liver and the brain becomes exposed to toxic substances, resulting in changes in sleep patterns and in some cases personality changes. As the damage to the liver progresses, the patient may develop hepatic encephalopathy. A further complication of liver disease is ascites. This is an accumulation of fluid in the abdominal cavity and resulting from high portal pressure and low serum albumin levels, causing noticeable weight gain and increasing girth.

When sufficient hepatocyte damage occurs, glycogen storage and glucose secretion become impaired and bilirubin excretion fails, resulting in jaundice as the bile pigment deposits in the tissues. Epstein *et al.* (1997) divide the causes of jaundice into prehepatic, hepatocellular, intrahepatic cholestasis and extrahepatic cholestasis. Prehepatic relates to haemolytic anaemias and Gilbert's syndrome (a disorder where the patient may show signs of jaundice intermittently but is otherwise essentially asymptomatic). Hepatocellular disease includes viral hepatitis (A–E), alcoholic hepatitis, autoimmune hepatitis, drug hepatitis and decompensated cirrhosis. Intrahepatic cholestasis disorders include drugs, primary biliary cirrhosis and primary sclerosing cholangitis and extrahepatic cholestasis includes bile duct stricture, common duct stone and cancer of the head of the pancreas.

Pancreatic disease

Pancreatitis is an inflammatory response to the damage of the exocrine tissue of the pancreas. This may take the form of acute pancreatitis or chronic pancreatitis. Acute pancreatitis commonly presents with severe epigastric or left upper quadrant pain which may radiate to the back. Intense attacks are associated with pancreatic necrosis, and vascular shock, renal failure and adult respiratory distress syndrome may threaten the patient's life. Factors linked to the cause of acute pancreatitis include gallstones, tumours and alcohol. Alcohol is known to have an irritant effect on the duodenal mucosa and the resultant inflammation at the sphincter of Oddi obstructs the passage of pancreatic juice into the lumen of the duodenum. The pancreatic juices back up and digestion of the pancreas by its own enzymes occurs. Chronic pancreatitis involves repeated moderate attacks of acute pancreatitis. Successive episodes result in the formation of scar tissue in the pancreas and diabetes mellitus can occur as the islets of Langerhans are destroyed. People most at risk of chronic pancreatitis are those who have severe persistent cholelithiasis and those who continue to indulge in alcohol after an initial alcohol-related attack (Nowak and Handford 1994).

Kidney and bladder disease

A variety of diseases occur in the kidneys, ureters and bladder. The result of any disease process in these organs is usually a change in the frequency and volume of urination and pain or discomfort for the patient. Epstein et al. (1997) list the variety of symptoms which can be found in the renal system and their possible causes (Table 9.2).

Disorders of the renal system can be divided into prerenal, postrenal and renal disease. Prerenal disease is caused by renal ischaemia resulting in inadequate glomerular filtration and postrenal disease is caused by urinary obstruction, creating back-pressure in the kidney and a destruction of kidney tissue. Renal disease results from changes

Table 9.2 Renal symptoms and signs and their causes

Symptoms and signs	Causes
Frequency	Irritable bladder (infection, inflammation, chemical irritation)
	Reduced compliance (fibrosis or tumour)
	Bladder outlet obstruction (prostatism, detrusor muscle failure)
Polyuria	Chronic renal failure
	Diabetes mellitus
	Diabetes insipidus
	Diuretic treatments
Dysuria	Bacterial infection of the bladder
	Inflammation of the urethra
	Infection or inflammation of the prostate
Incontinence	Sphincter damage or weakness after childbirth
	Sphincter weakness in old age
	Prostate cancer
	Benign prostatic hypertrophy
	Spinal cord disease, paraplegia
Oliguria or anuria	Hypovolaemia
	Acute renal failure (acute glomerulonephritis)
	Bilateral ureteric obstruction
	Detrusor muscle failure
Haematuria	*Painful*
	Kidney stones
	Urinary tract infection
	Papillary necrosis
	Painless
	Infection
	Cancer of the urinary tract
	Acute glomerulonephritis
	Contamination during menstruation

Source: Adapted from Seller (1993) and Epstein *et al.* (1997).

within the kidney itself and an example of this is glomerular nephritis. Damage to the kidney through whatever cause results in renal failure which may be acute or chronic. There are many disorders of the renal system. The more common disorders are mentioned here, and you are advised to consult a specialist text on the subject if you need greater detail.

Others

The male and female reproductive systems are found within the abdominal cavity. An assessment of the abdomen would not be complete without considering the prostate, the male genitalia, the uterus, fallopian tubes, ovaries and the female genitalia. Each of these systems is dealt with in Chapters 10 and 11.

History-taking

Abdominal problems commonly present as non-specific symptoms. When the patient first presents for consultation with the nurse practitioner, it is likely that you will have several differential diagnoses to consider. A thorough history-taking process will enhance the potential accuracy of your diagnosis and will help to narrow your differential diagnoses and guide your physical examination. The following is a guide to specific questions which might be useful when a patient presents to you with identifiable complaints. The history-taking process as outlined in Chapter 2 is useful as a general guide to your approach.

Dysphagia

Dysphagia caused by carcinoma usually progresses quickly over 6–10 weeks and is worse for solids than liquid. If the dysphagia is caused by a disease of the swallowing centre in the brain (e.g. pseudobulbar palsy) or damage to the vagus nerve (e.g. bulbar palsy caused by polio) the symptom is accompanied by coughing and spluttering as food spills into the larynx and trachea (Epstein *et al.* 1997). It is therefore worthwhile asking questions which focus on the duration, precipitating factors and associated factors such as pain, cough or weight loss in patients who present with dysphagia. Other questions might include:

- At what level does the food stick?
- Has the symptom been intermittent or progressive?
- Are both food and drink equally difficult to swallow?
- Is there a history of reflux symptoms?

Heartburn

The pain of heartburn is described as burning or scalding and may radiate to the throat. The patient's description may be accompanied by a gesture with the hand, showing the upward movement of the retrosternal pain. An acid or bitter taste may develop in the mouth, resulting in reflex salivation, known as water brash. It is important to carry out the usual assessment of pain including radiation, precipitating factors, palliating factors and timing. Fisher and Tyler (1997) state that in the case of heartburn it is also useful to ask the patient to describe his or her bowel pattern and whether it has changed recently. A description of black tarry stools might lead you to consider an upper gastrointestinal bleed or a malignancy of some kind.

A major concern of most nurse practitioners is the differentiation between heartburn and myocardial infarction. Epstein *et al.* (1997) provide an overview of the distinguishing features of reflux and myocardial ischaemic pain (Table 9.3).

Weight loss and anorexia

Weight loss and anorexia are both non-specific symptoms that may accompany acute or chronic conditions. Enquire about appetite, eating habits, average daily diet and any discomfort caused by eating or swallowing (odynophagia). Weight loss may be due to an inappropriate loss of calories in conditions such as thyrotoxicosis or diabetes mellitus. Marked weight loss and anorexia should alert the nurse practitioner to serious pathology such as malignancy and failure of the major organs. Some useful questions to ask when a patient presents with weight loss include the following (Epstein *et al.* 1997):

- Is your appetite increased or decreased?
- Over what time span has the weight been lost?
- Do you enjoy your meals?
- Describe your average daily intake
- Do you experience nausea, abdominal discomfort or pain?
- Describe your bowel motions
- Have you experienced a fever?
- Do you pass excessive volumes of urine?
- Have you noticed a change in how you tolerate the weather?

Dyspepsia and indigestion

Ask the patient if the discomfort is associated with

Table 9.3   Differentiating between the pain of reflux dyspepsia and myocardial ischaemia

	Position	Character	Associated features	Aggravating factors	Relieving factors
Reflux	Radiates towards the chest from the epigastrium	Burning, scalding	Water brash	Bending, lying down, eating	Antacids
Myocardial ischaemia	Radiates across the chest into the jaw and down to the left arm	Gripping, vice-like pressure	Nausea, shortness of breath	Exercise	Ceasing exercise, nitrates

Source: Adapted from Epstein *et al.* (1997).

belching, nausea, vomiting, haematemesis, change in bowel habits or interruption in sleep. The timing of the dyspepsia is particularly useful in determining its association with food and fluid intake. It is useful to enquire if the patient has been diagnosed with *Helicobacter pylori* in a previous episode of dyspepsia as the course of treatment will change if the patient has received eradication therapy.

Nausea, vomiting and haematemesis

There are a variety of causes of nausea, vomiting and haematemesis and the history-taking process will help you differentiate between those causes. Some key questions include:

- Is the vomiting worse in the morning?
- Does it occur in relation to meals?
- Is there associated abdominal pain?
- Is the vomit blood- or bile-stained?
- Is there recognizable food or coffee grounds in the vomit?
- What drugs are being taken?

The patient's responses to these questions will provide clues for diagnosis. For example, a woman complaining of nausea in the mornings could possibly be experiencing hyperemesis. If there is knowledge or evidence of liver disease, it is worth considering oesophageal varices in the case of a person who has complained of haematemesis. If there is a history of weight loss associated with haematemesis, it is worth considering gastric cancer. Digoxin, morphine and anticancer drugs are all known to stimulate the vomiting centre – in one rare case timolol eyedrops were found to cause severe nausea and vomiting in a 77-year-old woman (Wolfhagen *et al.* 1998). It is therefore always worth enquiring about all types of medication.

Abdominal pain

An assessment of abdominal pain should include the usual structured history-taking process associated with all forms of pain (PQRST), as described in Chapter 2. In particular it is worth exploring with the patient how long s/he has been experiencing pain, whether it is constant or intermittent and what relieves or aggravates the discomfort. If you consider the pathophysiology associated with visceral and parietal pain it is worth asking the patient to describe the type of pain and whether movement aggravates or relieves the pain. Associated symptoms such as vomiting, nausea, sweating and weight loss may provide a clue that the pain is visceral in nature. It is also worthwhile including in the history-taking process an exploration of the patient's bowel habits and if there have been any recent changes. The exact location of the pain will help you determine if the patient is experiencing the diffuse discomfort of visceral pain or the specific discomfort associated with parietal pain. Always ask whether there is any sensation of pain elsewhere in the body, as referred pain to the shoulders or scapula could indicate problems within the abdominal cavity.

As with all history-taking, it is important to ask about medication, not only what the patient is currently taking but also what s/he has taken in the past. A history of non-steroidal anti-inflammatories for example might provide a clue to potential damage to the stomach and duodenum.

Changes in bowel habits

Always begin by asking what the patient's normal bowel habit is.

Constipation

Drossman *et al.* (1990) state that the diagnostic criteria for constipation can be defined as the presence of two or more of the following symptoms for at least 3 months:

- Two or fewer bowel movements per week
- Stool weight of < 35 g/day
- Straining on more than 25% of occasions
- Hard, lumpy stool on more than 25% of occasions
- Sensation of incomplete evacuation on more than 25% of occasions

It is worth exploring all of the above factors with the patient in the history-taking process. Epstein *et al.* (1997) state that you should also ask the patient if there is any associated nausea, abdominal pain, distension, nausea or vomiting. Ask about use of medication and particularly whether the patient has used constipating drugs such as opiates or codeine.

Diarrhoea

Important points in the history of a person who complains of diarrhoea include the duration of the problem and the number of motions per day. Ask the patient to describe the stools, including signs such as the presence of blood or mucus, colour and consistency of the stools and any aroma. Ask whether the patient is taking any medication, if s/he is awoken from sleep with the diarrhoea and if there is any recent history of travel abroad. If the patient states that it has been necessary to get out of bed at night to empty the bowels, this is a significant finding. Functional diarrhoea almost never occurs at night (Seller 1993) and rarely wakens the patient. It is also worth considering other medical conditions such as diabetes mellitus. Diabetes is associated with neurological dysfunction, which can also result in diarrhoea.

It is always necessary to extend the history-taking process to include the patient's family in the case of diarrhoea. Complaints of family members with the same symptoms may provide a clue to the infectious nature of the disease. Ask if the patient has recently ingested seafood. Shellfish poisoning can present within 30 minutes of ingestion of the contaminated food, causing abdominal pain, nausea, vomiting and diarrhoea which may last for more than 8 hours (Scoging and Bahl 1998). If the patient describes symptoms which may be caused by a bacterium or virus, it is also extremely important to enquire about occupation and possible transmission to other people in the food trade (Johnson and Johnson 1997).

Rectal bleeding

The history-taking process is limited in providing you with a definitive diagnosis in the case of a patient with rectal bleeding. Always maintain a high level of suspicion in any patient who presents with a change in bowel habit, particularly rectal bleeding. Ask the patient to describe the blood loss in terms of colour, smell, frequency and duration. As a general guide, a complaint of a smear of blood on the toilet tissue may increase your suspicion of haemorrhoids, a squirt of blood may be due to an anorectal lesion, complaints of blood on the surface of the stools or clots originate from the rectum or descending colon, plum or maroon-coloured blood is due to colonic bleeding which may be linked to diverticula or a malignant tumour, tarry stools result from bleeding in the upper gastrointestinal tract and green or black stools are a side-effect of treatment with iron. If pain is associated with the bleeding this is significant, as haemorrhoids are often uncomfortable but rarely painful. A complaint of pain therefore should make you consider other causes for the patient's problems. Remember that there is sensory innervation in the anal canal and lesions in this area will cause the patient some degree of pain. Indeed, symptoms vary according to the origin of the tumour and subtle differences can be noted between tumours arising in the caecum, sigmoid colon and the rectum. Tumours which form in the caecum can present with chronic bleeding or anaemia, however, tumours in this area are commonly large before the patient experiences any symptoms at all. The sensory innervation to the sigmoid colon results in the patient experiencing pain, there is noticeable bleeding and often patients report a change in bowel habits. Tumours which arise in the rectum can cause the patient to report a sensation of incomplete evacuation (tenesmus) and, as in the case of the sigmoid colon, the sensory innervation to the rectum results in reports of pain from the patient.

Liver disease and biliary obstruction

In patients who present with liver disease it is certainly worth taking a history relating to alcohol consumption. Foreign travel, the use of intravenous drugs and past exposure to blood products are important factors in the patient's history as exposure to viral hepatitis should be considered. One of the key questions in the history-taking process is whether the patient has developed a painless jaundice or whether there is any associated abdominal discomfort. Painless jaundice suggests chronic obstruction of the common bile duct which may have been caused by cancer of the bile duct or the head of the pancreas. If the patient complains of severe epigastric and right hypochondrial pain accompanied by fever, this suggests a gallstone in the common bile duct.

Consider the physical consequences of hepatic disease and focus your questions on these possible symptoms. As the bile acids build up in the patient's system it is common for a pruritus to develop, followed by the signs of biliary obstruction such as dark urine, lightening stools, steatorrhoea and weight loss. The patient may have thought that these symptoms were of no consequence and may not offer the information unless you ask for it in a direct manner. The responses to your questions will help provide clues to the cause of the disease process.

Pancreatic disease

The pain of acute pancreatitis is often severe and accompanied by nausea and vomiting. It is useful to enquire about alcohol consumption and the use of drugs such as corticosteroids and frusemide. If a patient has recurrent bouts of pancreatitis, bear in mind the gradual destruction of the pancreatic tissue associated with chronic pancreatitis and ask about symptoms and signs of jaundice. In later disease ask the patient about the symptoms of diabetes mellitus such as excessive thirst and polyuria.

Kidney and bladder disease

If a person presents with a history suggestive of renal system disease it is important to enquire about past medical history and the medications which may be nephrotoxic. Cover the patient's normal fluid intake and ask him or her to describe normal pattern of urination. Areas to cover in the history-taking process include hesitancy, frequency, dribbling, urgency, sense of incomplete emptying of the bladder, flank pain or discomfort on passing urine.

Medications

It is essential in the history-taking process associated with problems in the abdominal cavity to enquire specifically about the use of medications. Many drugs are associated with side-effects in the gastrointestinal tract and the renal system and it is always worth checking the *British National Formulary* (1999) for side-effects of those medications being taken by the patient. Tricyclic antidepressants, anti-Parkinson drugs, morphine, anticholinergic drugs, ferrous sulphate and certain antacids can cause constipation and digoxin, thyroxine, laxatives, antibiotics and magnesium-containing antacids can cause diarrhoea (Jones and Murfin 1993).

Physical examination

As with all examinations, it is unlikely that you will be able to focus on one discrete area to provide you with the clues for diagnosis and management. Patients may present complaining of left-sided upper abdominal pain which is of cardiac origin; alternatively, a person may present with leg oedema caused by a problem in the abdomen such as a pelvic mass or renal disease. Barkauskas *et al.* (1998) provide an overview of signs and symptoms which occur in systems other than the abdominal area which may relate to the abdominal examination.

Table 9.4 Signs and symptoms which occur outside the abdominal systems and are relevant in the abdominal examination

Sign or symptom	Possible pathological condition
Shock or orthostatic hypotension	Acute pancreatitis, obstruction, ruptured tubal pregnancy, hypovolaemia due to fluid loss
Mental status deficit	Haemorrhage, duodenal ulcer
Hypertension	Aortic dissection, abdominal aortic aneurysm, renal infarction, glomerulonephritis
Pulse deficit	Aortic dissection, aortic aneurysm or thrombosis
Bruits	Aortic dissection, aortic aneurysm, dissection or aneurysm of splenic renal or iliac arteries
Atrial fibrillation	Ischaemia of the mesentery
Pleural effusion	Oesophageal rupture, pancreatitis, ovarian tumour
Flank tenderness	Renal inflammation, stone, infarct and thrombosis
Leg oedema	Iliac obstruction, pelvic mass, renal disease
Lymphadenopathy	Hepatitis, lymphoma, mononucleosis
Jaundice	Excessive haemolysis, liver, biliary disease
Dark yellow/ brown urine	Blood as a result of a stone, infarct, pyelonephritis or glomerulonephritis, liver, biliary disease
Fever and chills	Peritonitis, pelvic infection, cholangitis, pyelonephritis

Source: Adapted from Barkauskas *et al.* (1998).

Having considered the signs and symptoms occurring in systems beyond the abdominal cavity, we will now focus on physical examination of the abdomen. As with all physical examinations, you need to ensure that your patient is comfortable, warm and relaxed. The patient can feel extremely vulnerable when exposing his or her abdomen, particularly where the patient has abdominal pain, as he or she may be afraid that you will exacerbate the pain. Therefore a careful and thorough explanation should be offered before carrying out the exam. In some cases you may need to ask patients to help you by using their hands for palpation; this will be explained in more detail below.

A further consideration before performing the abdominal examination is that the patient should be allowed to empty the bladder as a full bladder will interfere with the exam. The patient should be placed in a supine position with arms resting on the couch and should be allowed to cover areas of the body which do not need to be exposed for the examination. Ensure you have a good source of light and approach the patient in a calm, gentle manner. If the patient has been experiencing pain, ask him or her to point to the area of tenderness and make a mental note of its location. You will find that it is beneficial to examine painful areas last as the discomfort caused by palpating over an area of tenderness will result in a patient who is anxious and no longer relaxed.

In order to report your findings and to provide you with a structure for the abdominal examination, it is helpful to divide the abdomen into sections. Different clinicians use different methods; the two commonest methods are quadrants and nine regions. The quadrants are left upper quadrant, right upper quadrant, left lower quadrant and right lower quadrant. The nine regions include the right hypochondriac, epigastric, left hypochondriac, right lumbar, umbilical, left lumbar, right inguinal, hypogastric (pubic) and left inguinal. It is worthwhile becoming familiar with both systems as you will find that with certain conditions one system enables you to describe the area more specifically than the other. Both systems allow you to consider which organs lie beneath each region and therefore help you to link areas of tenderness with specific organs in some situations. A description of the organs which lie beneath each region can be found in Tables 9.5 and 9.6.

Inspection

Inspect the abdomen from a variety of positions. Sitting beside the patient and then standing above him or her will allow you to review the contour of the abdomen and to notice any lack of symmetry. Ascites will result in a taut glistening appearance

Table 9.5 Anatomical correlates of the abdomen

Right upper quadrant	Left upper quadrant
Liver and gallbladder	Left lobe of liver
Pylorus	Spleen
Duodenum	Stomach
Head of pancreas	Body of pancreas
Right adrenal gland	Left adrenal gland
Portion of right kidney	Portion of left kidney
Hepatic flexure of colon	Splenic flexure of colon
Portions of ascending and transverse colon	Portions of transverse and descending colon

Right lower quadrant	Left lower quadrant
Lower pole of right kidney	Lower pole of left kidney
Caecum and appendix	Sigmoid colon
Portion of ascending colon	Portion of descending colon
Bladder (if distended)	Bladder (if distended)
Ovary and salpinx	Ovary and salpinx
Uterus (if enlarged)	Uterus (if enlarged)
Right spermatic cord	Left spermatic cord
Right ureter	Left ureter

over the abdomen. Seidel *et al.* (1995) have outlined an easy way to remember the causes of abdominal distension – the Fs of abdominal distension:

- Fat
- Fluid
- Flatus
- Fetus
- Faeces
- Fibroid
- Full bladder
- False pregnancy
- Fatal tumour

If you ask the patient gently to breathe in and out you should notice the abdomen move symmetrically and smoothly during the manoeuvre. If you ask the patient to lift his or her head off the table, you may find that a previously unnoticed mass appears as the diaphragm compresses the contents of the abdominal wall within the abdominal cavity. You may notice peristaltic movement during inspection, this is most often associated with an obstruction. You may also notice pulsations in the midline which are quite normal in thin adults; if they become marked they may be related to the increased pulse pressure of an abdominal aortic aneurysm. During inspection you are also looking for any discoloration and scars.

Auscultation

Auscultation is carried out before percussion and palpation in the examination of the abdomen as percussion and palpation may alter the bowel sounds. All four quadrants of the abdomen should be covered and it is not possible to state that there are no bowel sounds without 5 minutes of continuous listening. Use a warm stethoscope and place the diaphragm gently on the abdomen in the desired location. The frequency and character of the bowel sounds should be noted. Clicks and gurgles which occur in a range of 5–35 per minute are quite normal. Increased bowel sounds may occur with gastro-enteritis, hunger or intestinal obstruction and decreased sounds may occur with peritonitis or paralytic ileus. High-pitched tinkling sounds may suggest early obstruction.

It is also possible to listen for vascular sounds during the abdominal examination. Using the bell of the stethoscope placed over seven different locations (Figure 9.2), it is possible to listen for bruits. Friction rubs over the spleen and liver are rare but

Table 9.6 Anatomical correlates of the abdomen

Right hypochondriac	Epigastric	Left hypochondriac
Right lobe of liver	Pyloric end of stomach	Stomach
Gallbladder	Duodenum	Spleen
Portion of duodenum	Pancreas	Tail of pancreas
Hepatic flexure of colon	Portion of liver	Splenic flexure of colon
Portion of right kidney		Upper pole of left kidney
Suprarenal gland		Suprarenal gland
Right lumbar	**Umbilical**	**Left lumbar**
Ascending colon	Omentum	Descending colon
Lower half of right kidney	Mesentery	Lower half of left kidney
Portion of duodenum and jejunum	Lower part of duodenum Jejunum and ileum	Portions of jejunum and ileum
Right inguinal	**Hypogastric (pubic)**	**Left inguinal**
Caecum	Ileum	Sigmoid colon
Appendix	Bladder	Left ureter
Lower end of ileum	Uterus (in pregnancy)	Left spermatic cord
Right ureter		Left ovary
Right spermatic cord		
Right ovary		

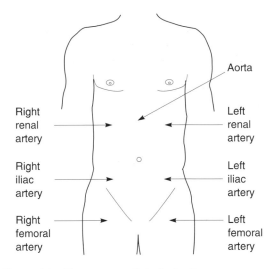

Right renal artery

Left renal artery

Aorta

Right iliac artery

Left iliac artery

Right femoral artery

Left femoral artery

Figure 9.2 Sites to auscultate for bruits

can be heard with respiration if there is a tumour or some other source of inflammation over the peritoneal surface of these specific organs.

Percussion

Percussion is used to detect the presence of air, fluid or solid masses. You need to develop a structured approach to percussion, ensuring that you cover all regions of the abdomen in a logical order. The main sound you should hear is tympany – a high-pitched musical note. Dullness is heard over organs and solid masses, this is a short, high-pitched note. Resonance is a sustained sound of moderate pitch which can be heard over lung tissue and sometimes over the abdomen. You may hear hyper-resonance, which is a pitch lying between tympany and resonance.

Percussion can be used to estimate the location and size of the liver. Locate the mid clavicular line on the patient's right side and percuss along this line from an area of resonance in the lung downwards to an area of dullness. Note this point and repeat the procedure from an area of tympany in the abdominal mid clavicular line to an area of dullness. It is always useful to percuss towards the area of dullness as it is easier to hear the change in the sound rather than from a dull area to an area of resonance or tympany. When you measure the distance between the two points located through percussion you should find that the liver measures approximately 6–12 cm. It should lie approximately 2–3 cm below the costal margin and should appear no higher than the fifth intercostal space. If the liver lies outside any of these dimensions it may be enlarged, atrophied or displaced by lung tissue in pulmonary disease or abdominal fluid or masses.

Palpation

You may need to enlist the patient's assistance in palpation. Patients who are ticklish or particularly frightened of you touching their abdomen may find the procedure more acceptable if you ask them to place their own hand on their abdomen and you place yours on top of theirs. You can palpate gently and slowly together and eventually the patient will allow you to palpate without his or her own hand being in place.

Begin with light palpation, using a systematic approach over the four quadrants, initially avoiding painful areas. Use the palmar surface of your hand to depress gently and smoothly over the abdominal surface at a depth of approximately 1 cm. A patient who is in pain will watch your every move and may guard certain areas; a more relaxed patient may lie on the couch with eyes closed. Continue palpating and gradually increase the depth of the pressure you apply. In thin adults you may be able to locate several of the abdominal organs; in some abdominal examinations you may find it difficult to feel anything at all.

Examining the groins

The abdominal examination is not complete without an examination of the groins for femoral or inguinal herniae. This has been covered in more detail in Chapters 10 and 11.

Liver

To feel for the liver, rest you hand against the bottom of the right ribcage. Ask the patient to breathe in and you may be able to feel the smooth edge of the liver move under your hand. You can carry out the same manoeuvre by standing towards the patient's head, grasping the lower edge of the right ribcage by hooking your fingers over the costal margin and again asking the patient to take a deep breath.

Spleen

A similar procedure can be used to palpate for the spleen. Place your left hand behind the patient's left ribs and your right hand at the lower edge of the left ribs. Ask the patient to take a deep breath and push slightly forward with the left hand and down with the right. This pushes the spleen slightly forward to enable you to palpate it; it is unusual to be able to feel the spleen as it has to be approximately three times its normal size before you can feel anything (Walker 1995).

Gallbladder

A healthy gallbladder is not palpable. One which is palpable and tender indicates cholecystitis, whereas non-tender enlargement indicates common bile duct obstruction. If you are considering cholecystitis as a potential diagnosis you can demonstrate the presence of an inflamed gallbladder by eliciting a response called Murphy's sign. To demonstrate Murphy's sign, place your hand over the lower right rib margin with your fingers facing towards the centre and during deep palpation ask the patient to take a deep breath. As the inflamed gallbladder moves against your examining fingers, the patient will experience pain and will momentarily halt breathing.

Kidneys

The kidneys are not usually palpable; however, it is important to practise the technique of palpation for the kidneys to ensure that you find an enlarged one when a patient presents to you with renal problems. The technique is similar to the assessment of the spleen. For the right kidney, place your left hand behind the patient just below the 12th rib and lift, trying to displace the kidney anteriorly. Place your right hand in the right upper quadrant and ask the patient to take a deep breath in. At the peak of inspiration, press your right hand into the right upper quadrant and try to capture the kidney. Ask the patient to exhale and feel for the kidney's return to its expiratory position. It is occasionally possible to palpate the right kidney, in thin women in particular. The same procedure is carried out on the left side to palpate for the left kidney.

The kidneys can also be assessed for tenderness by placing the ball of one hand in the costovertebral angle. You then strike your hand with the ulnar surface of the fist of your other hand. You need to use sufficient force to cause a thud (Bates 1995). This should be a painless exercise. If the pressure from this manoeuvre causes pain, this suggests the possibility of kidney infection or possibly a musculoskeletal problem.

Bladder

The bladder is not usually palpable unless it is distended with urine. If the bladder is distended it is possible to palpate a smooth rounded mass in the midline. It is possible to percuss a distended bladder and this will produce a lower percussion note than the surrounding air-filled intestines.

Reflexes

The abdominal reflexes can be tested by lightly but briskly stroking each side of the abdomen above and below the umbilicus. Above the umbilicus tests the superficial reflexes of T8, T9 and T10 and below the umbilicus tests the reflexes of T10, T11 and T12. You should note the contraction of the abdominal muscles and the deviation of the umbilicus toward the stimulus. If the abdominal reflexes are absent there may be a central or peripheral nervous system disorder or a patient's obesity may obscure the response. In this case, place your finger on the patient's umbilicus, pulling slightly away from the side to be stimulated and you should be able to feel the response as the muscles contract during the reflex action (Bates 1995).

The anus and rectum

It may be necessary to carry out an examination of the rectum and anus and patients should be reassured that it should not be a painful experience, although it is certainly uncomfortable and may stimulate a feeling of rectal fullness. Position the patient in the left lateral position with the hips and knees well flexed. It is important to make sure that the patient is as relaxed and comfortable as possible, as tension and anxiety will make the examination impossible. Gently separate the buttocks and inspect the anus and describe what you see by viewing the area as a clockface. Twelve o'clock is the anterior position and six o'clock the posterior position (Figure 9.3).

Lubricate your index finger, place it at the 6 o'clock position and slide it into the anal canal and then into the rectum, directing your finger posteriorly. Explore the posterior and posterolateral walls of the rectum by sweeping your finger around 180° in both directions. The normal rectum should feel smooth and pliable. A palpable mass in the anterior position is possibly the prostate in a man and may be the cervix in women who have a retroverted uterus. You may wish to ask the patient to contract the muscles of the anus around your finger. In doing this you can assess the tone of the anal muscles. When you withdraw your finger, check your gloved hand for stool. Blood, melaena or mucus may be present and all of these signs will help you in your problem-solving process.

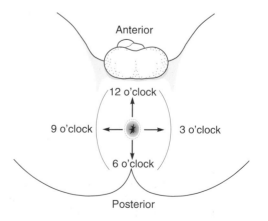

Figure 9.3 Clockface positions around the anus

Management and patient education and investigations

The management of patients who present with gastrointestinal disorders or problems with the renal or urinary system may vary according to the patient's general health status, age and the severity of the symptoms. The common conditions of heartburn and diarrhoea will be explored here, followed by a brief overview of irritable bowel syndrome, as patients who receive this diagnosis often have questions about the management of their condition.

Diarrhoea

Watson (1993) states that there is still an appreciable mortality from diarrhoeal disease in the UK due to dehydration in infants and the elderly. It is therefore important to take this condition seriously and to advise about fluid intake and monitoring for signs of deterioration. The symptoms of dehydration are reduced consciousness, dry mucous membranes, reduced tissue turgor, sunken and tearless eyes, tachypnoea, hypotension and peripheral vaso-constriction, sudden weight loss and oliguria; in infants, a sunken fontanelle is an important sign (Johnson and Johnson 1997). Sachets of oral rehydra tion salts are useful to maintain fluid during the severe stages of the disease process and patients should be advised that this is generally a self-limiting condition which should settle within 2–3 days. The fluid should be taken little and often; in young children sips of the fluid every 10 minutes are useful even in the presence of vomiting (Watson 1993). As viruses are the usual causative agents in diarrhoea the use of antibiotics is limited. Treatment with antibiotics should be considered, however, in severe cases of infection with *Shigella* spp. and *Campylobacter jejuni*, in immunosuppressed patients, the very young and the very old who are infected with *Salmonella*, in severe cases of infection with *Clostridium difficile* and in giardiasis (Watson 1993). The use of loperamide and diphenoxylate is contraindicated in severe infective diarrhoea as they slow the clearance of the infecting organism and their use should be limited to moments of social necessity. Stool samples are only indicated if the condition persists beyond 7 days, if there is blood or there is persistent fever.

Traveller's diarrhoea is caused in up to 75% of cases by *Escherichia coli* and is treated with trimethoprim or ciprofloxacin together with vigorous rehydration. Travellers should be educated about the possibility of suffering from diarrhoea whilst travelling abroad and advised to seek medical help if the diarrhoea is associated with abdominal pain or a fever exceeding 38.5° (Watson 1993).

Heartburn

Patients should be assessed for lifestyle factors, food consumption and medications which may be contributing to the causes of their heartburn and should then be advised accordingly. Some useful tips for patients include avoiding caffeine, fatty foods, tomato, milk and citrus products. Small regular meals are preferable to large ones and the patient should be encouraged to eat slowly and sit in an upright position when eating. The evening meal should be consumed at least 3 hours before going to bed and it may help to be slightly elevated in bed. The patient should be encouraged to stop smoking, reduce alcohol consumption, wear loose-fitting clothing and, if overweight, lose weight. Drink water after eating to clear the oesophagus. Many of these suggestions require major changes to the patient's lifestyle and this may only be achieved with consistent empathic advice over several consultations.

It may be useful to screen the patient for *Helicobacter pylori* and initiate eradication therapy according to local protocols if the result is positive. This action may depend on the practice's policy on *H. pylori* and on the patient's past medical history and current condition.

Heartburn may be managed with a variety of medications including antacids, alginates, H_2-receptor agonists, prokinetics and proton pump inhibitors. Antacids are constipating and care must be taken in the presence of renal disease and glaucoma; similarly, care must be taken in renal disease and hepatic disease with H_2-receptor agonists. The side-effects of proton pump inhibitors include rash, headache and diarrhoea.

It is important for the nurse practitioner to be aware of the need to refer on to a colleague if the patient presents with anything other than straightforward heartburn. Indications for referral are:

- If the symptoms are not relieved or have worsened even after initiation of medication
- If there is associated weight loss, anaemia, melaena, vomiting, anorexia or dysphagia
- If the patient is over 45 years of age and this is the first presentation with heartburn

A high level of suspicion for other causes of the discomfort must be maintained with all patients but particularly in older people as the incidence of malignancy increases with age.

Irritable bowel syndrome

Irritable bowel syndrome occurs in approximately 20% of the general population (Fisher 1997; Carlson 1998). It is characterized by pain, irregular bowel habits (constipation or diarrhoea) and abdominal bloating with flatulence. The patient may complain of pain as the intestines go into spasm; symptoms are usually intermittent and may last for days or weeks at a time. Of the people who are diagnosed with irritable bowel syndrome, 25% will have a complete remission. The remaining 75% have to learn to live with a chronic condition and the nurse practitioner can assist in offering advice and support for this group of patients.

Drossman *et al.* (1990) state that the diagnostic criteria for irritable bowel syndrome are:

- Persistence or recurrence of the following for a period of at least 3 months abdominal pain or discomfort, relieved by defecation or associated with a change in the frequency or consistency of the stool
- An irregular (varying) pattern of defecation at least 25% of the time with two or more of the following:

  - Altered stool frequency
  - Altered stool form (hard or loose, watery stool)
  - Altered stool passage (straining or sensation of urgency, or a feeling of incomplete evacuation)
  - Passage of mucus
  - Bloating or a feeling of abdominal distension

Moriarty (1993) states that the characteristic features of irritable bowel syndrome are abdominal distension, relief of pain with the bowel movement, loose and frequent movements with the onset of pain, the passage of mucus and incomplete evacuation. The motions tend to be small-volume, pencil-like and accompanied by urgency. The symptoms rarely disturb sleep and often occur before breakfast. The symptom criteria are wide and it is therefore essential to rule out any other organic cause of the patient's problems before confirming the diagnosis. Once the diagnosis has been confirmed, the nurse practitioner can reassure the patient that irritable bowel syndrome is simply the abnormal movements of essentially healthy normal bowels. The condition is not fatal and can be managed with lifestyle adjustments and a change in diet (Fisher 1997).

It is useful to explain to the patient that antibiotics, gastroenteritis, food intolerance, stress, anxiety, menstruation and smoking are all aggravating factors for irritable bowel syndrome and in some cases this may explain the timing of the patient's presentation. Eating too quickly can exacerbate symptoms by causing bloating and belching. Drinking water and fizzy drinks with meals can also increase the bloating and excessive bran or natural fibre can exacerbate pain during periods of constipation. Patients often ask if there are certain foods which should be excluded from the diet in trying to manage the symptoms of irritable bowel syndrome; any exclusion diet should be carried out with the advice of a dietician to ensure that the patient is able to consume all the necessary nutrients even in the absence of the food which has been excluded. Carlson (1998) lists the foods which have most commonly been linked to the symptoms of irritable bowel syndrome:

Milk	Cheese	Butter	Alcohol
Citrus	Barley	Yoghurt	Corn
Chocolate	Rye	Yeast	Nuts
Onions	Coffee	Oats	Fruit
Potatoes	Tea	Eggs	Wheat

It can take considerable time for a patient to find the foods which cause the symptoms of irritable bowel syndrome and therefore a food diary may help. The patient should be encouraged to drink approximately 1.5 litres of fluid daily and to engage in exercise. It may be helpful for patients to increase their fibre intake to approximately 25–35 grams daily (Carlson 1998); however, Moriarty (1993) states that a high-fibre diet may lead to an improvement or deterioration or have no effect at all. When the patient is constipated it seems that an increase in fibre may exacerbate the flatulence and therefore increase the patient's discomfort. The advice relating to diet should therefore be flexible according to the patient's needs.

Pharmacological management of irritable bowel syndrome may be necessary in a few individuals. Some patients require a combination of therapies to control the symptoms, whilst others may require a single medication on an 'as required' basis. Examples of the medications used include antispasmodics, bulk laxatives, antimotility drugs and antidepressant therapies. The treatment regime will vary according to the patient's symptoms. Education and support will be necessary to ensure that the patient understands when and how to use treatments in conjunction with dietary therapy.

It is important to refer patients on if they present with the symptoms of irritable bowel syndrome, are over 40 years of age, have experienced a recent change in bowel habit, have noticed weight loss or rectal bleeding or have been woken from sleep with the pain.

References

Barkauskas V.H., (ed.) (1998) *Health and Physical Assessment*, 2nd edn., St Louis, Mosby. Cited in: Seidel H.M., Ball J.W., Dains J.E., Benedict G.W. (1999) *Mosby's Guide to Physical Examination*, 4th edn., St Louis, Mosby.

Bates B. (1995) *A Guide to Physical Examination and History Taking*, 6th edn., Philadelphia, JB Lippincott.

British National Formulary (1999) London, British Medical Association/Royal Pharmaceutical Society of Great Britain.

Carlson E. (1998) Irritable bowel syndrome, *Nurse Practitioner*, **23**, pp. 82–91.

Drossman D.A., Funch-Jensen P., Janssens J. *et al.* (1990) Identification of subgroups of functional bowel disorders, *Gastroenterology International*, **3**, pp. 159–172.

Epstein O., Perkin G.D., deBono D.P., Cookson J. (1997) *Clinical Examination,* 2nd edn., London, Mosby.

Fisher P. (1997) Irritable bowel syndrome, *Practice Nursing*, **8**(9), pp. 41–44.

Fisher P., Tyler M. (1997) Heartburn, *Practice Nursing*, **8**(12), 41–44.

Galloway J. (1993) Oesophageal disorders. In: Jones R. (ed.) *Gastrointestinal Problems in General Practice*, Oxford, Oxford University Press.

Harris A.W., Misiewicz J.J. (1996) *Helicobacter pylori*, London, Blackwell Healthcare.

Ingram Tagg P. (1996) Heartburn, *Nurse Practitioner*, **21**, (suppl): pp. 9.

Johnson S., Johnson W. (1997) Diarrhoea, *Practice Nursing*, **8**(5), pp. 41–44.

Jones R., Murfin D. (1993) Gastrointestinal problems in the community and in general practice. In: Jones R. (ed.) *Gastrointestinal Problems in General Practice*, Oxford, Oxford University Press.

Moriarty K.J. (1993) The irritable bowel syndrome In: Jones D.J., Irving M.H. *ABC of Colorectal Diseases*, London, British Medical Journal Publishing Group.

Nowak T.J. Handford A.G. (1994) *Essentials of Pathophysiology. Concepts and Applications for Health Care Professionals,* Dubuque, Iowa, Wm C Brown.

Scoging A., Bahl M. (1998) Diarrhetic shellfish poisoning in the UK, *Lancet*, **352**, July 1998, pp. 117.

Seidel H.M., Ball J.W., Dains J.E., Benedict G.W. (1999) *Mosby's Guide to Physical Examination*, 4th edn., St Louis, Mosby.

Seller R. (1993) *Differential Diagnosis of Common Complaints*, 2nd edn., WB Saunders. Philadelphia.

Walker R. (1995) Examination of the abdomen, *Practice Nursing,* **6**(15), pp. 19–20.

Watson A.J.M. (1993) Diarrhoea. In: Jones D.J., Irving M.H. (eds) *ABC of Colorectal Diseases,* London, British Medical Journal Publishing Group.

Williams C. (1994) Causes and management of nausea and vomiting, *Nursing Times*, **90**(4), pp. 38–41.

Wolfhagen F.H.J., van Neerven J.A.F.M., Groen F.C., Ouwendijk R.J.Th. (1998) Severe nausea and vomiting with timolol eyedrops, *Lancet*, **352**, August 1998, p. 373.

CHAPTER 10

The male reproductive system

Mike Walsh

Introduction

Disorders of the reproductive system, by their very personal nature, tend to cause a great deal of embarrassment. This may be exacerbated if the nurse practitioner is female while the patient is male. A great deal of tact and diplomacy is therefore required in dealing with male reproductive system disorders. Men may present in a variety of ways, such as seeking treatment for an acute problem in the A&E department or at the health centre. In such circumstances they will probably be anxious and/or distressed. Alternatively there may be a chance finding on a routine examination such as a preoperative assessment. It is also possible that the initial contact may be made with the patient's partner, usually female, who might see the nurse practitioner for a range of reasons. In the course of the consultation it may become apparent that the source of her problem is her partner and advice to help him is needed. A wide range of skills will be needed by the nurse practitioner to help men with reproductive system disorders, but good communication skills will always lie at the heart of a successful patient consultation.

Pathophysiology

The penis

As the penis is primarily a sexual organ, it is not surprising that many problems affecting this organ arise as a result of sexual activity. These include a range of sexually transmitted diseases and also trauma. Sexually transmitted diseases that produce obvious lesions include genital herpes, genital warts (condyloma acuminatum) and syphilis. Cancer of the penis may also produce a lesion, commonly under the foreskin. Sexually transmitted diseases frequently do not produce an obvious external lesion; the main presenting symptom may be a urethral discharge,

soreness and discomfort. The common infecting organisms are *Neisseria gonorrhoeae*, *Chlamydia trachomatis*, *Trichomonas vaginalis*, *Ureaplasma urealyticum* and *Candida albicans*.

Trauma may be due to catching the foreskin in a zip, biting in over-vigorous oral sex or damage to the glans, urethra or foreskin as a result of sado-masochistic practices. An emergency condition which may be seen in young males is paraphimosis, where the foreskin has become retracted behind the glans and cannot be pulled back into its normal position. This causes discomfort, oedema and embarrassment, especially as it may occur after an early sexual encounter. A congenital abnormality which occasionally occurs is hypospadias, in which the urethral orifice is located on the ventral surface of the penile shaft.

The scrotum

Testicular cancer is the commonest cancer in young men aged 20–34 with approximately 1000 new cases presenting each year in the UK (Cook 1995). Most cancers arise from the germ cell epithelium lining the testicular tubules and are therefore known as germ cell tumours or GCTs. Early detection and treatment are especially important as the tumour is very responsive to chemotherapy, with a good prognosis if treated early enough. Springhouse (1997) cites 5-year survival rates of 90–100% but, in more advanced cases, the prognosis seriously deteriorates. The main risk factor cited by Cook (1995) associated with testicular cancer is undescended testicle, especially if both are undescended.

Benign swellings may also occur in the scrotum, such as a hydrocele, an accumulation of fluid in the tunica vaginalis, while a spermatocele is a fluid-filled cyst occurring in the epididymis. A distorted knot of veins around the spermatic cord may produce a painful mass known as a varicocele, commonly seen in young men and adolescents.

An inguinal hernia presents as a protrusion of abdominal viscera into the inguinal canal. This may reach as far as the testes in what is known as an indirect inguinal hernia, which usually affects young men. Here the abdominal viscera have slipped through the inguinal ring and followed the spermatic cord. Older men suffer a direct inguinal hernia which results from a weakness in the fascial floor of the inguinal canal (Springhouse 1997). This does not reach the testes. The hernia may be irreducible (incarcerated) or become strangulated. This latter situation is a surgical emergency as part of the intestine has become entangled in the hernia and may have its blood supply cut off, leading to necrosis and intestinal obstruction.

Inflammation may occur within the scrotum: epididymitis is the commonest cause, usually in association with a urinary tract infection. Orchitis or inflammation of the testes is usually seen in mumps and frequently affects only one testicle.

A particularly urgent emergency presentation occurs when a testicle rotates upon the spermatic cord, impairing the blood supply. This occurs in young men and is known as a torsion testes. The result is severe pain, nausea and discoloration of the scrotum with the potential for sterility in the affected testicle if prompt medical intervention is not carried out.

Various skin conditions may involve the scrotum and surrounding areas, including the penis. Psoriasis or dermatitis can present with familiar scaly lesions in this area; there will often be evidence of the problem elsewhere on the body, although in the case of a contact dermatitis the lesions may be localized to the genital area. Fungal infections are also possible; tinea cruris is a common example and may be localized to the groin area, producing an irritating, scaly, erythematous rash which has a well-delineated border. In all these cases the man may be anxious and upset, convinced that he has caught a sexually transmitted disease, which of course he has not.

The prostate gland

Benign prostatic hyperplasia (BPH) affects most men over 60 and causes obstruction to normal urinary outflow from the bladder, resulting in urinary problems. The course of the disease seems very variable, with some men improving over time, while others may experience severe problems and even the distress of acute urinary retention (York Centre for Review and Dissemination 1995). It is likely that many men with BPH are at present unknown to the NHS as they have not presented for treatment, fatalistically accepting urinary problems as part of growing old. Even so, there are around 78 000 new cases diagnosed per year in the UK (Marchant 1995).

Prostatic cancer is the second commonest cause of death in men after lung cancer in both Europe and the USA. No obvious causes are known. It has been found that approximately 32% of men who die aged 60 have histological changes in their prostate gland, whereas only around 4% of 60-year-old men have clinical signs of the disease (Selley *et al.* 1997). It is true therefore that many more men die *with* cancer of the prostate than *of* cancer of the prostate. The initial symptoms are similar to BPH but as the disease metastasizes, the skeleton in particular is prone to secondary deposits, leading to bony pain and pathological fractures. The course of the disease is variable and poorly understood at present.

Inflammation of the prostate (prostatitis) occurs in younger men aged most frequently between 30 and 50. The cause is frequently coliform bacteria and the condition may be acute or chronic. Prostatitis is recognized as sometimes being non-bacterial in origin and various explanations such as autoimmune problems and allergic reactions have been proposed (Donovan and Nicholas 1997). Various routes have been described, including ascending urethral infection after unprotected anal intercourse, backflow of infected urine in urinary tract infection or migration of organisms through the rectal wall (Marchant 1995).

AIDS

Over 90% of AIDS patients in the UK are male and 54% of these men were infected as a result of homosexual activity (Weller and Williams 1995), making AIDS a major health issue which must be addressed in any discussion of male sexual health. The normal pattern of the disease starts with a mild acute infection producing general symptoms of feeling unwell, although in many cases the person may not notice any signs as they are so mild and short-lived. Antibodies usually develop in 2–6 weeks, although in some cases seroconversion may take longer. A chronic infection develops, of which the patient is often unaware. Weller and Williams (1995) point out that the only likely physical sign to be found at this stage is persistent lymphadenopathy, most frequently affecting the cervical and axillary lymph nodes. As the disease progresses, generalized symptoms such as fever, night sweats and weight loss appear together with opportunistic infections affecting the mucous membranes (e.g. oral candidiasis, herpes-zoster). Deterioration in the patient's condition occurs over time with the appearance of various diseases characteristic of AIDS, mainly affecting the respiratory, nervous and gastrointestinal systems. As there is no cure at present, the long-term prognosis is bleak.

Infertility

Infertility in men has historically been much less of an issue than in women, yet the probability of a man alone being the cause of an infertile couple is around 35% – the same as a woman. In the remaining cases it is either a joint problem or no cause can be found (Mason 1993). Male infertility should not be confused with impotence. Most men who are impotent are still fertile, so while impotence can prevent a woman conceiving naturally, it does not mean that the man is sterile. Setting aside impotence, Mason cites a range of causes of male infertility, such as damage to the testicle (e.g. orchitis), hormonal imbalance, undescended testicles and congenital malformations. She points out that, in most cases, there is no known cause, going on to speculate about the importance of psychological factors in sperm production. One other possible condition which may present is priapism, a sustained and inappropriate erection which can become painful as well as embarrassing.

Sexuality

A possible cause of consultation is the young man who realizes he is homosexual. This may be associated with a great deal of confusion and anxiety and it is possible that the nurse practitioner in primary health care may be seen as someone the young man can talk to about his concerns. The fact that the nurse practitioner is likely to be female may encourage such a consultation, as a male would be more threatening. Feelings of transsexuality and/or transvestism may also bring a desperately confused and embarrassed male patient seeking advice from the nurse practitioner particularly if she is female.

Generalized effects

Remember that the conditions discussed above affect the whole person, not just the genital area. Some diseases spread to affect the whole body (e.g. syphilis, AIDS, testicular cancer) whilst others which may be localized physiologically can have a profound psychological effect (e.g. impotence, infertility, BPH). The holistic perspective that characterizes nursing is therefore essential in assessing and managing male sexual and genital problems. Assessment should therefore extend further than simply asking the man to unzip his flies.

History-taking

Absolute privacy is essential to obtain an accurate history. Even then, the patient may be embarrassed and reluctant to talk about his problem. An open and welcoming attitude, showing unconditional regard for the individual, is more important than ever in these circumstances. If the man has had a limited education, expression may be even more difficult and may involve the use of terms the nurse practitioner may consider crude or even obscene; however they may be the only words the man knows and he may be equally embarrassed at having to use them.

Encourage the patient to tell his story in his own words and give him the time and space to explain the problem fully. Beware making jokes to try and lighten the atmosphere as these could go badly wrong in such a sensitive area. The non-verbal aspect of communication is equally important, with special reference to facial expression and body posture on both the part of the nurse practitioner and patient. At all times avoid being judgemental.

Complaints of urethral discharge or lesions on the penis suggest that sexually transmitted disease is the most likely cause. A detailed sexual history is required, covering the following points:

- Details of all sexual partners in last 4 weeks
- Gender of partners
- Use of condoms
- Sexual practices, i.e. oral, anal, etc.
- Overseas contacts

In addition, find out how long the complaint has been present and whether it can be related to a specific incident in the sexual history, such as a casual, unprotected sexual encounter. Ask the patient to describe the nature and quantity of any urethral discharge. A small amount of fluid under the foreskin is normal; however, it should not be sufficient to stain underwear – a pathological sign – nor should there be any smell. Enquire about pain, burning or any itching sensation. Previous sexually transmitted diseases should be enquired about together with medication, including attempts at localized self-medication. This will allow you to assess the probability of a sexually transmitted disease before examination. Intravenous drug use is a key issue if HIV infection is suspected, as this group constitutes the second largest group of HIV-positive individuals (30%, according to Weller and Williams 1995).

In the case of trauma, an accurate account is essential, including mechanism and timing of injury, however embarrassing this may be. The patient may be reluctant to disclose the nature of the practices involved but correct treatment requires knowledge of the cause of injury. A human bite, for example, is extremely infective and antibiotic therapy is essential; such an injury should not normally be sutured (except on the face where the excellent blood supply usually ensures healing without infection). This is clearly a different situation from a zip injury. Rectal trauma could have major implications if associated with unprotected anal intercourse, a high-risk behaviour for HIV. If it was caused by the insertion of objects such as dildoes and no body fluids were involved, the HIV risk is greatly reduced. Health education advice about safer sex is a part of the nurse practitioner role and this requires an accurate history of whatever the patient has been doing in order that advice about, for example, the use of lubricants, condoms and latex gloves (where full-fist insertion is practised) in anal sex can be given. As a final example, the presence of a retained rectal foreign body must be disclosed, before definitive treatment to remove it can begin. These examples show the importance of obtaining an accurate history from the patient, however difficult this may be.

If the patient is complaining of pain in the scrotum, the PQRST system can be used to analyse the symptom. Torsion of the testis produces a sudden onset of pain while epididymitis is more gradual. The pain of testicular cancer may be referred to the pelvic region if metastasis has occurred. In the case of a sports injury, the onset of pain is obviously simultaneous. Referral of pain into the loins suggests renal pathology (e.g. a stone) as the cause of the pain.

If the patient presents with a mass in the scrotum it is essential to find out when he first noticed this mass. Enquire about pain (testicular cancer initially presents as a painless lump), any sensation of heaviness, changes in size of the testis and whether it feels normal or if changes such as irregularities in contour have occurred. Childhood history with regard to undescended testes should be explored. A history of weight loss, coughing, lethargy and fatigue unfortunately suggests an advanced stage of the disease. If the lump is intermittent and can be reduced, this suggests an inguinal hernia as the likely cause, especially if associated with lifting and heavy manual work.

The history suggestive of prostatic disease is usually focused on urinary symptoms. The enlarging prostate causes hesitancy and dribbling on passing urine. The patient may also complain of frequency in wanting to pass urine but of being unable to manage an adequate stream. He may report urgency and, in some cases, urge incontinence. It is important to take the history carefully in order that the patient's urinary problems may be distinguished from incontinence due to other causes. A useful means of assessing the impact of the disorder on the patient's life is to use the American Urological Association symptom index, which consists of a series of statements which can be scored and added up to give a total which gives a more objective measure (Barry et al. 1992). This tool can also be used to measure therapeutic response and progress over time. The patient with prostatic cancer will also present with a history similar to BPH.

The younger man presenting with some prostatic symptoms but also complaining of generally feeling unwell, having a temperature with lumbar or suprapubic pain and/or perineal discomfort is more likely to have prostatitis.

If the patient presents with problems of impotence, the initial history should focus on how long the disorder has been present, medications and other medical history, alcohol and other recreational drug use and psychological factors such as stress and emotional upsets. In the case of infertility, the following areas should be explored in addition to the possibility of impotence:

- Previous children by other women
- Length of time attempting pregnancy, frequency of intercourse and knowledge of the female reproductive cycle
- Are there factors raising scrotal temperature above normal, such as the work environment?
- Medications
- History of undescended testes or any other relevant medical history
- Investigations undertaken on the female partner and her medical history

The man who presents with problems relating to his sexuality should be encouraged to talk about how long he has had these feelings and whether he has felt able to share them with others. It may be that he feels threatened by other men and so prefers to see a female nurse practitioner to discuss his problems. This is particularly true of younger patients who are concerned they may be gay or men experiencing feelings of transsexuality/transvestism. The patient's level of knowledge and experience should be carefully explored, as appropriate referral and advice can only be given when the nurse practitioner has a clear view of his feelings, relevant knowledge, family and social networks.

Physical examination

Discretion and a private area are necessary to carry out a physical exam which should be conducted in as thorough and professional manner as any other. In order to examine the male genitalia, the nurse practitioner should ensure that there is a good light source and s/he is wearing gloves. It is easier to sit and have the patient stand in front of you.

A logical sequence should always be followed, starting away from the genitals and working inwards. The groin area should first be gently palpated to check for any abnormalities such as a hernia or enlarged lymph node. The standing position makes any hernia more obvious, as does asking the patient to cough if a suspicious swelling is felt. If a hernia is identified, the nurse practitioner should see if it can be reduced by gently pushing it and the results noted as reducible/irreducible. An irreducible hernia has the potential to become strangulated, leading to a bowel obstruction. The distribution of pubic hair should also be observed and noted; it is normally absent on the shaft of the penis and scant on the scrotum. Testicular malfunction may lead to a more female pattern of pubic hair distribution.

The penis should be examined next, checking first whether there are any lesions along the shaft (e.g. genital herpes) and if it has been circumcized. The glans must be examined; this requires retraction of the foreskin in an uncircumcized male. The patient should be asked to do this but it is essential to check that it has been fully retracted. If it is necessary for you to perform this manoeuvre, it should be done gently. If the foreskin cannot be retracted in an adult (phimosis), this suggests recurrent infections or inflammation of the glans; this condition is often seen in poorly controlled diabetics. If the patient is a small boy, this is likely to be a congenital problem needing surgical referral for correction by circumcision. The glans should consist of smooth pink tissue with no lesions present; a small amount of fluid (smegma) is a normal finding in an uncircumcized male, it is normally dry in a circumcized male. No odour should be present. Any signs of trauma to the penis should be noted and if nothing has been mentioned in the history, tactful questioning should follow to determine the cause.

The external urinary meatus should be examined, first to ensure that no congenital abnormalities are present (e.g. hypospadias) and second, to check whether there is any urethral discharge. Asking the patient to press his penis between the finger and thumb behind the glans will open the meatus and also express any discharge.

The final logical step is to examine the scrotum. The skin is normally darker than the rest of the body and having the left testicle lower than the right is a normal finding. Swelling and bruising of the scrotum can reach alarming proportions after trauma but will resolve with the aid of ice packs. An inflammatory condition such as orchitis or a torsion testes will lead to the scrotum appearing redder than normal, being oedematous and tender to palpation. After observation, the next step is gentle palpation of each testicle between the thumb and first two fingers. The patient's facial expression should be checked for discomfort during this part of the exam. The testicles should feel equally smooth and have a soft rubbery texture. Any irregularity is abnormal, along with any other swelling or mass felt in the scrotum. If it is possible to feel above such a swelling then that suggests it is confined to the scrotum and not a hernia. A cyst full of fluid (hydrocele) is fluctulant when gently compressed and can be transilluminated by holding a pen torch against the scrotum in a darkened room. A dense mass such as a tumour will not allow light to pass through it and therefore appears opaque as well as feeling solid.

If the history suggests a prostatic problem, then a digital rectal examination is necessary. The patient should lie in the left lateral position with his knees drawn up to his chest. Care should be taken to ensure he does not roll off the couch; an assistant may therefore be necessary who can also act as a chaperone. A careful explanation is needed before a well-lubricated index finger is inserted through the anus, checking for a normal external appearance first. Some initial spasm of the anal sphincter is normal but usually, after relaxation, the index finger can be eased into the rectum. The patient should be asked to contract his anus around the sphincter as a check for normal muscle tone. The walls of the rectum should feel smooth and even. The prostate gland may be palpated through the anterior rectal wall and normally protrudes about 1 cm into the rectum (Seidal *et al.* 1995). It should feel firm and smooth. Irregularities are an abnormal finding and a hard nodular feel suggests malignant changes. A protrusion that feels in excess of 1 cm indicates an enlarged prostate, typically feeling soft or boggy in BPH. The findings should be carefully noted. Secretions may be forced out of the urinary meatus by digital rectal examination. This should be explained to the patient as a normal side-effect and any such secretions wiped away. The patient with prostatitis has an enlarged, indurated and tender prostate, therefore the exam should be carried out with particular gentleness if the history is suggestive of this condition.

Investigations

It is normal practice to refer suspected cases of sexually transmitted disease to a specialist genitourinary clinic for diagnosis and treatment. The patient should be advised to abstain from sexual activity with a partner until he has been to the clinic. A simple test to determine whether the man has an anterior urethral infection is the two-glass test. He should be asked to pass urine into two glasses, 60–100 ml in the first and the rest into the second. If the urine in the first glass is hazy and contains threads but the second glass is clear, this suggests an anterior infection, rather than infection involving the posterior urethra, bladder or kidneys. Confirmation may be obtained by adding 5–10% acetic acid which would clear the urine specimen if the haziness were simply due to phosphates rather than an infection. On referral to the clinic it is helpful to tell the patient not to pass urine for 4 hours before attending as, apart from wishing to carry out a routine 'dipstick' test, the clinic may wish to repeat this two-glass test for anterior urethral infection, particularly if your test was inconclusive due to the man having passed urine too recently. Advise the patient that, in addition to blood samples, swabs of any discharge will also be taken at the genitourinary clinic for diagnostic purposes, therefore he should abstain from any attempts at self-medication.

If a patient presents anxious that he may have contracted HIV and requesting an HIV test, counselling is necessary before the test; the test can only be performed when sufficient time has elapsed from possible exposure for seroconversion to occur. Both these points need careful explanation before referring the man to the genitourinary clinic in order that he may attend with realistic expectations. Counselling is essential before the test so that the man may be helped to work out how to respond to a positive result, as well as to ensure that he understands the basic facts about HIV infection.

Sperm counts can be carried out in cases of suspected infertility. Give the patient a suitable container and plastic bag to place it in with a pathology form clearly indicating the test required. Best results are obtained with a fresh sample which is less than 1 hour old, so if possible he should go directly to the hospital pathology laboratory with a fresh sample, rather than hand in to the health centre a sample which may be 1–2 days old before it reaches the path lab.

Tests for prostate-specific antigen (PSA) in cases of prostatic cancer have become available in the last few years and have aroused considerable controversy. Whilst cancers do produce PSA which can be detected well before any clinical signs become apparent, there are major problems with this approach. Selley *et al.* (1997) cite lack of standardization amongst assay techniques and the lack of sensitivity and specificity of PSA testing as major drawbacks. Many other conditions can lead to abnormal PSA levels. Consequently, Selley *et al.* (1997) recommend that there is no evidence to support the widespread use of PSA testing or population screening at present. Their conclusions can be summed up as follows: 'There is no justification for the routine use of PSA testing in primary care. GPs should be actively discouraged from using PSA tests for the purpose of early detection'.

Differential diagnosis

In men who present with lesions of the penis it is important to differentiate between sexually transmitted disease and other causes such as cancer of the penis. The sexual history will usually make it clear which is the most likely cause.

Testicular torsion can be differentiated from other causes of scrotal pain by the rapidity of onset and the common association of vomiting and loss of appetite. The patient is typically a teenager or in his 20s. The presence of a mass with scrotal pain indicates that a tumour is more likely, while signs of inflammation clearly indicate that an inflammatory process such as epididymitis or orchitis is the problem.

It is important to distinguish between urinary incontinence and a prostatic problem in elderly male patients presenting with urinary problems. Sometimes this may not be possible, as BPH may be one contributory factor amongst others in urinary incontinence. The history, a 'dipstick' urine test, culture and sensitivity of a sterile urine sample to check for a urinary tract infection and a digital rectal examination will all assist in assessing the importance of the prostate in causing urinary problems. Digital rectal examination is notoriously unreliable when it comes to distinguishing between BPH and a prostatic cancer. Referral for specialist medical opinion is urgently needed in such cases.

Treatment

If you suspect a sexually transmitted disease, normal policy is to refer to a genitourinary clinic for investigation, diagnosis and treatment. There are obvious reasons for this policy, such as the need for contact tracing, the extreme confidentiality required and the possible need for specialist counselling, especially in the case of a confirmed HIV infection. Antibiotic therapy begun before referral to the genitourinary clinic and therefore diagnosis of the pathogens involved by microbiology can result in inappropriate, ineffective therapy and increase the risk of developing resistant strains. These reasons should be carefully explained to the patient if he is unhappy about delaying treatment for a day or two and the journey to the general hospital genitourinary clinic. Conditions such as epididymitis or prostatitis may be secondary to a sexually transmitted disease. When such conditions are suspected it is worth checking the local protocols for management with the genitourinary clinic. Before referring on to the genitourinary clinic the patient should be advised to abstain from sex with a partner, with a careful explanation why. If he refuses, he should be urged to use a condom. He should also be asked not to pass urine for 4 hours before attending (p. 142)

Trauma to the penis, such as a zip injury, can provoke a great deal of fear and anxiety. The rich blood supply ensures that any small wound bleeds profusely, increasing the patient's anxiety. Direct pressure will control bleeding and ice packs will reduce swelling. Depending on the location of the wound, i.e. if it is on the shaft, steristrips may suffice to close it. Referral to a hospital A&E department for assessment and treatment is advised if such simple measures are not effective as suture under local anaesthetic may be required. The highly infective nature of a human bite is such that referral is essential in such cases. If the foreskin has become retracted, it may be possible to manoeuvre it back into position after using ice packs to reduce the swelling and with a generous application of lignocaine gel as a lubricant. Otherwise, referral to hospital is needed.

A significant number of conditions affecting the contents of the scrotum have potentially serious consequences, such as reduced fertility (e.g. torsion testes, orchitis) or even death (testicular cancer). An urgent medical opinion is therefore required when such conditions are suspected. The man with orchitis secondary to mumps may be helped by a scrotal support and oral prednisolone 40 mg/day for 5 days for pain relief, but this will have little impact on the risk of a reduction in fertility. A patient with suspected torsion testes needs an immediate surgical referral as an emergency admission.

The nurse practitioner has a valuable role to play in educating men about testicular self-examination. Many men display depressing ignorance about their genitals and you should be prepared for initial resistance in undertaking health education in this field. Reactions may vary from embarrassment to defence mechanisms such as denial and trivialization of the whole issue. However, persevere, as eventually the message will get through to some male patients. This is particularly important given the high success rates achieved by treatment when an early diagnosis is made.

Basic guidelines for testicular self-examination are as follows (Cook 1995):

- Self-examination should be carried out monthly, preferably after a bath, as the scrotal sac is more relaxed
- Initially the man should aim to become familiar with the normal feel and weight of his testicles. (Taboos about 'playing with yourself' and masturbation may need to be overcome at this juncture)
- Roll each testicle between the thumb and fore-finger to ensure there is a smooth feel with no irregularities or bumps
- Check for the normal feel of the epididymus, which lies posterior to the testicle, in order that this is not confused with any new growth

If anything abnormal is detected, he should report to the surgery at once.

BPH is commonly managed by surgical referral and transurethral resection of the prostate (TURP) or transurethral incision of the prostate (TUIP) in cases where the prostate is less enlarged. This latter procedure produces equal benefits but fewer complications (York Centre for Review and Dissemination 1995). Many men have mild symptoms which can be managed without surgery, using a combination of health education and community support to achieve lifestyle modification supplemented by drug therapy. Alpha-blocking agents improve symptoms in BPH by relaxing smooth muscle, improving flow rates and reducing obstruction. Examples include alfuzosin, indoramin, prazosin and terazosin (*British National Formulary* 1999). An alternative approach is provided by the drug finasteride which has been shown to produce significant improvements in symptoms by inhibiting testosterone metabolism and thereby reducing the size of the prostate, although side-effects include impotence and reduced libido. The York Centre for Review and Dissemination (1995) points out that there is no evidence from any large randomized controlled trial to support the use of natural remedies or alternative therapies in treating BPH.

The course of the disease is uncertain and significant numbers of men experience substantial improvements in their urinary symptoms and even complete remission. The regular use of the American Urological Association symptom scale (Barry *et al.* 1992) allows the nurse practitioner and patient to monitor progress and assess the effect of simple health education advice about the timing and quantities of fluid to drink. This watchful waiting approach may be the most cost-effective option for many men with mild to moderate symptoms, whilst surgical intervention is reserved for those with more serious symptoms. The nurse practitioner has a key role as s/he is the ideal person to manage the patient with mild symptoms in the community. Should symptoms become worse, it is important that the patient makes an informed decision about whether to opt for surgery and if so, what type of surgery (TURP or TUIP). It is no longer acceptable for the patient to be put on a surgical waiting list and undergo TURP as a matter of routine without playing any part in the decision-making process or considering alternatives. The primary health care nurse practitioner has a key role in assisting the patient to make an informed choice about surgical treatment by spending time explaining the different procedures available and the risks and benefits associated with each. In this way the patient will be better equipped to discuss treatment with the surgical team at the hospital. Of course, it is possible that his first point of contact at the hospital may be another nurse practitioner, specializing in this field, permitting a full exploration of the available options.

Whilst the benefits of surgery in moderate to severe cases of BPH are well-proven, the same cannot be said of cancer of the prostate. The course of the disease is poorly understood and uncertain. Selley *et al.* (1997) in a major review concluded that the evidence concerning the effectiveness of different treatments (radical prostatectomy, radiotherapy or conservative management) is poor and inconclusive. They therefore conclude that: 'In the absence of evidence from randomized controlled trials (RCTs) concerning the relative benefits of treatments, informed patient choice should be a major consideration'.

This statement underlines the importance of the nurse practitioner spending time with the patient, allowing him to talk through the options together with the possible benefits and side-effects. This will help the patient when he sees the medical specialists to decide on the course of treatment that he feels happiest with.

If acute prostatitis is suspected, rapid medical referral is needed as intravenous antibiotic therapy is required. Treating chronic prostatitis is difficult as the drugs (such as penicillin) which will be effective against the usual pathogens involved penetrate prostatic tissue poorly. There is also considerable debate about the treatment of non-bacterial prostatitis – all of which makes this a condition which is perhaps best referred for a medical opinion, whatever form is suspected.

The adolescent or young man who has problems associated with sexuality may need specialist counselling to help him deal with potentially complex issues. Give the man time and space to talk about his feelings, remembering that this may be the first time he has felt able to do so. The issue of homophobic bullying at school received a great deal of attention at the Royal College of Nursing Congress in 1998. The discussions that took place there emphasize the need for the nurse practitioner to be aware that teenagers may be experiencing a great deal of distress as they try to come to terms with their emerging sexuality. They need a reassurance that there is nothing wrong in being gay and that there are many gay men and women in society. There are obvious issues of sexual health to be discussed and the young man should be made aware of the risks of contracting sexually transmitted disease, of which HIV is only one. Schools find themselves in a difficult situation when having open discussions about gay sexuality because current legislation prevents them from doing anything which may be interpreted as promoting gay lifestyles. The nurse practitioner may be the only professional source of information to which a youngster can turn.

A key area to explore is how the young man's family may react to the news that their son is gay, as family acceptance can significantly improve his quality of life. Confidentiality should be ensured at all times however. This is particularly important in small communities away from large urban areas where attitudes towards gays are less tolerant and where people know much more about their neighbours' business.

It may be that the chance to confide in a trusted person coupled with reassurance is all the young man needs. It would be helpful if the nurse practitioner had the phone number of the local gay switchboard or self-help group to pass on. If there are problems with bullying at school, the nurse practitioner should seek his permission to take the matter further, preferably involving the family and school nursing service, as well as the school. The potential for a ruined life ending in suicide is all too real.

The issues of transsexuality and transvestism are complex and their long-term solution clearly lies beyond the scope of a single nurse practitioner consultation. If a man does present with such problems, as is possible, you should have a strategy to try and help. Many of the points made in the discussion about a youngster with emerging gay sexuality are equally valid (non-judgemental approach, awareness of fear and embarrassment on the part of the man, confidentiality, etc.) but remember that many transvestite men are not gay and transsexuals see themselves as fundamentally of the wrong gender, which is not the same as being gay either. Transsexuals and transvestites as a group constitute a broad spectrum and vary considerably in behaviour and motivation. Many would argue that they are two separate groups but there is a grey area where a clear distinction is not possible. Reassurance that he is not the only person in the world to feel like this and that there is nothing inherently wrong about such feelings may help the man feel a little better about himself. Practical help ranges from referral to a counsellor specializing in such problems through to the phone number or address of a self-help group, of which there are many in the UK (Northern Concorde, PO Box 258, Manchester M60 1LN is one such group; if contacted by a nurse practitioner, they would probably be able to pass on a local contact number or address, depending on the area of the UK concerned).

Summary

Women's health has received a great deal of attention in recent years, and men's health is equally important. The attitude that many men have towards health is unhelpful and must change if the trend for men to die younger than women is ever to be reversed. The nurse practitioner has a major role to play in promoting health amongst men in many areas not covered in this chapter. The topics covered in this chapter are perhaps the most sensitive as they focus directly on the man's genital tract. Sadly, many men know more about the workings of the offside trap than they do about their own genitalia, and find discussing football a lot less embarrassing. Nurse practitioners must overcome these barriers with tact, diplomacy and perseverance if they are to make their potentially beneficial contribution to the nation's health. Many problems must be referred promptly to a medical practitioner for treatment (sexually transmitted diseases, testicular cancer, torsion testes) and the nurse practitioner can fulfil a valuable role in prompt diagnosis and referral. A great deal of health education work can take place, whether in the context of safer sexual practices or testicular self-examination, whilst a common chronic disease such as BPH is eminently suitable for nurse practitioner management in the community. The use of therapeutic communication skills with men having problems of sexuality can be beneficial. The nurse practitioner can achieve a great deal in helping men with problems relating to their reproductive systems.

References

Barry M.J., Fowler F.J., O'Leary M.P. (1992) The American Urological Association symptom index for benign prostatic hyperplasia, *Journal of Urology*, **148**, pp. 1549–1557.

British National Formulary (1999) London, British Medical Association/Royal Pharmaceutical Society of Great Britain.

Cook R. (1995) Teaching and promoting testicular self-examination, *Nursing Standard*, **9**(5), pp. 38–41.

Donovan D., Nicholas P. (1997) Prostatitis: diagnosis and treatment in primary care, *Nurse Practitioner*, **22**(4), pp. 144–156.

Marchant R. (1995) *Diseases of the Prostate*, London, Office of Health Economics.

Mason M. (1993) *Male Infertility*, London, Routledge.

Seidal H., Ball J., Dains J., Benedict G. (1995) *Mosby's Guide to Clinical Examination*, St Louis, CV Mosby.

Selley, S., Donovan J., Faulkner A., Coast J., Gillatt D. (1997) Diagnosis, management and screening of early localised prostate cancer, *Health Technology Assessment*, **1**(2).

Springhouse (1997) *Handbook of Medical Surgical Nursing*, 2nd edn., Springhouse, PA, Springhouse Corporation.

Weller I., Williams I. (1995) AIDS. In: Adler M. (ed.) *ABC of Sexually Transmitted Diseases*, London, British Medical Journal.

York Centre for Review and Dissemination (1995) Benign prostatic hyperplasia. *Effective Health Care Bulletin* **2**(2).

CHAPTER 11

The female reproductive system

Alison Crumbie and Lesley Kyle

Introduction

In many clinical settings nurse practitioners have been introduced to enhance the diversity of health care services available to the local population. Whilst not all nurse practitioners are female, there has often been an underlying added advantage to introducing a female into a practice or clinical setting, as it has enhanced women's choice in who they might consult with to discuss issues of women's health. Barbara Stilwell's practice was analysed over a 6-month period in 1982 and the results showed that 71.6% of patients seen by the nurse practitioner were women. Most were under the age of 40 (Stilwell 1985). Salisbury and Tettersell (1988) compared the work of a nurse practitioner with that of a general practitioner and found that 63.4% of the nurse practitioner's consultations were with women and the general practitioner's consultations with women were at a similar rate of 63.6%. More recently, Shirley Reveley (1998) reported that the nurse practitioner in her study recorded 71.7% consultations with women compared with the general practitioner's 64.2%. It is clear that women consult frequently with nurse practitioners and it is therefore necessary to have an in-depth understanding of the major issues relating to women's health. Whilst it is clear that it is not possible to cover family planning advice, management of the menopause and the whole gamut of women's health problems in one chapter, this chapter aims to cover the major types of clinical presentation of women's health problems in practice, the important aspects in taking a focused history from women who present with clinical problems and the essentials of physical examination related to the female reproductive system. The management and patient education relating to a selection of women's health problems will be covered to offer guidance for nurse practitioners who are dealing with women in their practice setting.

Pathophysiology and clinical presentations

A woman may choose to consult with a nurse practitioner because a clinical problem has developed, because she needs advice on a completely normal process in her life or she may present for screening. The normal development of puberty, the menstrual cycle and the menopause will be discussed here, followed by clinical presentations of breast disease and of genital tract disease.

Puberty

The transformation from childhood to adolescence is known as puberty and this occurs between 8 and 13 years for girls; the average age of the menarche is 12.5 years (Epstein *et al.* 1997). At this time there is a rapid growth spurt and development of sexual characteristics and sexual arousal. Puberty involves growth in a number of body systems and development in one part of the body may not necessarily coincide with development in another part (Jones 1991). Development can be assessed using Tanner's staging (Tanner 1973; Figures 11.1 and 11.2). Pubertal milestones such as the presence of breast buds and the appearance and growth of pubic hair have been divided into five stages by Tanner and provide a useful guide for assessing development.

The developmental changes that occur during puberty are the product of hormonal influences. Gonadotrophin-releasing hormone (GnRH) is a small polypeptide which is produced by the hypothalamus. GnRH secretion is inhibited until puberty. GnRH release causes the release of luteinizing hormone (LH) and follicle-stimulating hormone (FSH) in the pituitary gland, which in turn stimulates the gonads. The hormonal influence of the gonads results in the development of the reproductive system, the development of secondary sexual characteristics and

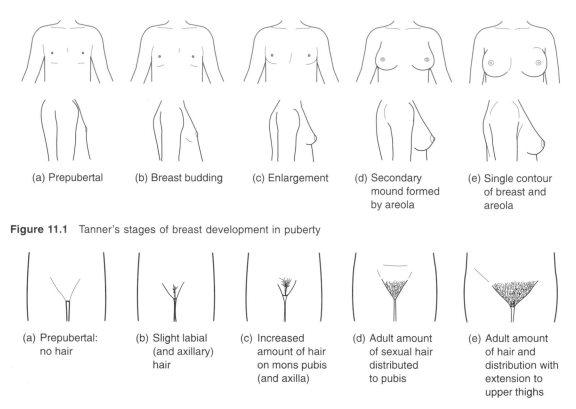

Figure 11.1   Tanner's stages of breast development in puberty

(a) Prepubertal

(b) Breast budding

(c) Enlargement

(d) Secondary mound formed by areola

(e) Single contour of breast and areola

(a) Prepubertal: no hair

(b) Slight labial (and axillary) hair

(c) Increased amount of hair on mons pubis (and axilla)

(d) Adult amount of sexual hair distributed to pubis

(e) Adult amount of hair and distribution with extension to upper thighs

Figure 11.2   Tanner's stages of pubic hair development

the menstrual cycle becoming established. It is usual for the female's first menarche to be anovulatory. The first ovulation may be up to 2 years after the first menstruation (Jones 1991). Eventually the endocrine system and the brain mature so that the LH surge is sufficient to cause the first ovulation.

Menstrual cycle

In order to understand some of the problems of menstruation it is important first to review the normal menstrual cycle. The purpose of the menstrual cycle is to release a single egg from the ovary and prepare the uterus to receive an embryo after fertilization occurs. When fertilization does not occur, the lining of the uterus degenerates and is expelled from the body at menstruation. Currently this process occurs in women who are on average between the ages of 13 and 51 years (Thomas and Rock 1997) and the length of cycles averages between 25 and 35 days (Jones 1991). Jones points out that only 10–15% of menstrual cycles are exactly the length of a lunar month and younger women tend to have longer cycles than older women.

The physiology of the menstrual cycle is summarized in Figure 11.3. GnRH is produced by the hypothalamus and its release is controlled by neurotransmitters and by feedback of oestrogen and progesterone from the ovary. GnRH flows through the hypophyseal portal system to the anterior pituitary and stimulates the secretion of LH and FSH.

LH and FSH stimulate the formation of a few selected dormant follicles in the ovary. Only one follicle usually matures to the point of ovulation (Epstein *et al.* 1997). Under the influence of LH and FSH, the follicle secretes increasing amounts of oestrogen and grows to a preovulatory size of approximately 2–3 cm. In mid-cycle there is a surge of LH and FSH which is thought to trigger the follicle to rupture and expel the ovum from the ovary. The ruptured follicle changes into the corpus luteum which secretes progesterone. By about the 23rd day of the cycle, if no pregnancy has occurred the corpus luteum begins to degenerate, progesterone levels fall, allowing FSH to start to rise again and, following vasospasm in the arterioles which feed the superficial layers of the endometrium, the lining of the uterus becomes necrotic and is finally expelled from the uterus through the vagina.

The menstrual cycle is divided into three phases: the menstrual, proliferative and secretory phases. The cycle begins with the onset of menses and the degeneration of the endometrial lining (Martini 1995a). In the proliferative phase the epithelial cells of the uterine glands multiply and spread across the endometrial surface. This occurs at the same time as the follicles in the ovary enlarge and is also

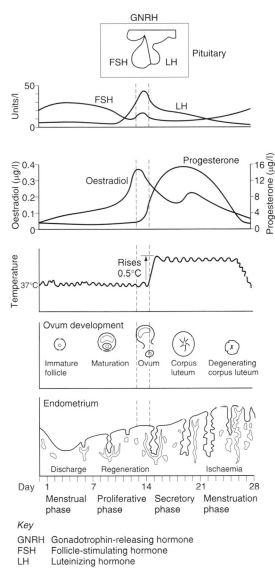

Key

GNRH Gonadotrophin-releasing hormone
FSH   Follicle-stimulating hormone
LH   Luteinizing hormone

Figure 11.3 Physiology of the menstrual cycle

Source: Adapted from Epstein *et al.* (1997)

known as the preovulatory or follicular phase of the cycle. This phase is stimulated and sustained by oestrogen secreted by the developing follicles. At ovulation the corpus luteum secretes progesterone and this, in combination with the continuing effects of oestrogen, is responsible for the secretory phase. During the secretory phase the endometrial glands enlarge and the arteries elongate. This is also known as the postovulatory or luteal phase of the menstrual cycle. The granulosa cells of the corpus luteum have receptors for LH which are also capable of binding with human chorionic gonadotrophin (hCG). hCG is secreted by fetal tissue and therefore in the absence of fertilization hCG does not appear and the corpus luteum begins to atrophy, progesterone levels fall and a new cycle begins with the onset of menses.

The secretory phase usually lasts for 14 days and therefore the date of ovulation can be estimated by counting backwards 14 days from the first day of menses.

Climacteric and the menopause

The menstrual cycle continues until approximately 45–51 years of age. It is common for women who have problems with menopausal symptoms or who are anticipating the onset of the menopause to seek help and advice from the nurse practitioner. The climacteric begins when the number of functional oocytes in the ovary has fallen to the point where the synthesis of sex hormones is reduced (Epstein *et al.* 1997). FSH levels initially increase in an attempt to stimulate follicular ripening and gradually the cycles become more irregular and anovulatory. As the ovarian follicles become less sensitive to circulating hormones, the follicular phase shortens and it is not uncommon for women to experience shortening of the menstrual cycle to 18–24 days before the cycle lengthens, with gaps of amenorrhoea and finally cessation of menstruation. The final cessation of menstruation is due to the loss of the hormonal feedback system and this results in measurably high serum levels of FSH and LH. At the menopause oestrogen production decreases and this results in atrophy of the breasts, genital organs and bone.

Symptoms of the menopause

The symptoms of the menopause can be spilt into physical and psychological symptoms. Physical symptoms include flushes, sweats, dizziness, palpitations, migraine headaches, atrophic vaginitis, urethral symptoms, joint pain, stiffness and dyspareunia. Psychological symptoms include loss of libido, mood changes, depression, panic attacks, agoraphobia, poor concentration, tiredness and loss of self-esteem (Wright 1998). The flushes associated with the menopause are associated with vasodilation of the blood vessels of the face, neck and hands. Hot flushes may occur as often as every 10 minutes and result from a more active sympathetic nervous system. Coope (1993) states that depression at the menopause is caused by many factors. It is important to measure the depth of the depression using an appropriate scale such as the Beck Depression Inventory (France and Robson 1986) and to refer suicidal patients appropriately. Coope (1993) also reports that perimenopausal patients respond better to oestrogen treatment than postmenopausal women and this may be due to the large swings in hormone levels which occur during the transition stage.

Clinical presentations of breast disease

Breast cancer is the commonest form of cancer in

women in the UK. One in 12 women will develop breast cancer at some stage of their life (Austoker and Sharp 1993) – 26 000 women are diagnosed and almost 16 000 women die each year of the disease (Cancer Research Campaign 1991). In recent years increased awareness and media coverage of breast cancer have heightened women's anxiety who have then felt the need to seek help and reassurance from health care professionals. Most consultations regarding breast symptoms in general practice are for benign breast disease. The nurse practitioner may encounter many women in planned consultations as well as opportunistically and therefore a detailed understanding of breast disease is vital.

The main role for the nurse practitioner is to encourage women to be breast-aware by informing and educating them as well as stressing the importance of the National Breast Screening Programme for women aged 50–64 which commenced in the UK in 1988. This screening programme uses mammography, which is the only effective method to detect and screen breast tumours and this has been supported by various randomized controlled trials (Day 1991). Breast self-examination carried out as a monthly routine is now regarded as ineffectual as several studies have shown that it does not affect breast cancer mortality (Austoker and Sharp 1993). Health professionals used a variety of techniques and methods to encourage women to carry out breast self-examination and this caused confusion and anxiety in some women, who then felt reluctant to touch and examine their own breasts as they were worried about using an incorrect technique. Breast awareness for women in all age groups is now being encouraged (Austoker and Sharp 1993). This involves teaching women what is normal and abnormal, educating them to recognize changes in their breasts and encouraging them to report changes at the earliest possible opportunity. This results in more appropriate referral to specialist breast services.

Women who are experiencing breast problems consult with health professionals as they need a clear diagnosis and the reassurance, if possible, that they do not have cancer. For the purpose of this section there will be a brief overview of the physiology of the breast with discussion of breast lumps, breast pain and nipple discharge.

The female breast

The female breast is composed of glandular tissue arranged in lobes around the nipple, supportive fibrous tissue and fat which surrounds the breast. Cooper's suspensory ligaments are fibrous and link the skin with fascia under the breast. It is the glandular tissue that produces milk following a pregnancy; each lobe is drained by a lactiferous duct opening out on to the nipple. The proportions of glandular tissue, fibrous tissue and fat vary with age, pregnancy, nutritional status, use of hormones such as hormone replacement treatment (HRT) or oral contraceptives as well as other factors. Figure 11.4 shows the normal breast.

For descriptive purposes the breast may be divided into four quadrants – the upper outer, the upper inner, the lower outer and the lower inner – and the tail of Spence, which extends towards and into the axilla (Epstein *et al.* 1997); (Figure 11.5).

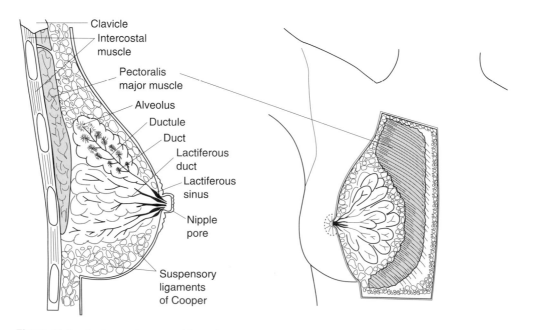

Figure 11.4   Anatomy of a normal breast

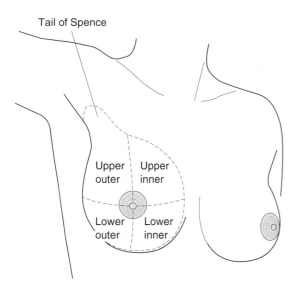

Figure 11.5   Four quadrants of the breast and tail of Spence

Lymphatic drainage is important as breast cancer can spread to regional lymph nodes. Of particular note is the fact that the internal mammary chain drains towards the opposite breast and abdomen (Figure 11.6). The axillary nodes are arranged in five groups to drain the outer breast and the internal mammary chain which drains the inner breast (Figure 11.7).

Breast lump

The commonest causes of breast lumps in women will be one or more of the following: cyst, abscess, fibroadenoma, fibroadenosis, lipoma or carcinoma of the breast.

Cysts

Cysts are inflamed lobules or fluid-filled sacs found in the glandular tissue which develop and enlarge over a short period of time. The commonest age of presentation is 40–50 years. They are usually found in the upper outer quadrant and 50% of women present with multiple cysts. Cysts are usually round and mobile, clearly defined from other tissues and feel soft or firm. They may appear in one or both breasts and may be tender due to leakage of fluid into the surrounding tissues. The pain associated with a cyst is unrelated to the menstrual cycle and there is normally no retraction of the nipple or tethering of the skin (Austoker and Sharp 1993).

Abscesses

Abscesses most commonly occur as mastitis during breast-feeding when one of the ducts becomes blocked. The skin is inflamed, red and may be hot to touch as well as extremely painful. The most common causative organism is *Staphylococcus aureus*. Treatment involves antibiotics and emptying the breast by expression to reduce the overall pressure on the tissue of the breast. An additional reason for carrying out expression of milk with these women is to help them maintain lactation. A small number of women will not respond to this treatment and will require surgical drainage of the abscess.

Fibroadenoma

Fibroadenoma are benign tumours which are more common in puberty and younger women between the ages of 18 and 30. They may be round, disc-shaped or lobular in one or both breasts and feel

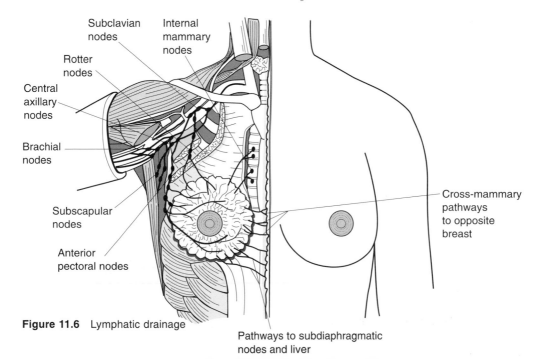

Figure 11.6   Lymphatic drainage

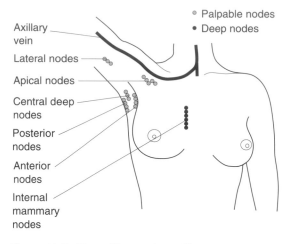

Axillary vein
Lateral nodes
Apical nodes
Central deep nodes
Posterior nodes
Anterior nodes
Internal mammary nodes

° Palpable nodes
• Deep nodes

Figure 11.7   The axillary node positions

firm or rubbery. They are usually extremely mobile and non-tender with no retraction of the nipple or tethering of the skin. They may grow slowly in size but most regress with age as they are uncommon in women over the age of 30. Diagnosis is normally via referral to the specialist breast clinic where clinical examination, ultrasound and fine-needle aspiration will confirm the benign nature of the disease. Some women prefer to have the lump excised and this can be performed under local anaesthetic. Fibro-adenosis or 'lumpy breasts' is often bilateral and related to the hormonal influences of the menstrual cycle, causing pain during the premenstrual and menstrual phases. A lipoma may occur in the breast and, like its occurrence in other parts of the body, it tends to be benign and fatty. A pseudolipoma may occasionally be the earliest sign of ductal carcinoma (Baum 1996).

Cancer

Cancer of the breast is often due to a primary tumour and most commonly affects women over the age of 40, and this continues to be a problem for women in the later years. Despite early diagnosis it may not be possible to confine the disease within the breast as there may already be lymph node involvement. However, this is less likely when the lump or cancer is 2 cm or less: early detection and diagnosis are important as this influences the survival rate. A lump associated with breast cancer is often hard, irregular and painless but is more likely to be fixed to underlying tissues or skin. This may cause dimpling or puckering of the skin due to pectoral contraction when the lump is attached to the skin and fascia. This may be diagnosed during the physical examination when the woman raises her arms or places them on her hips. The lump may be single, although there may be other nodules present and it is more commonly found in the upper outer quadrant of the breast.

Some women may have always had retracted nipples and this should be established during the history-taking process. Recent retraction of the nipple and areola may suggest an underlying cancer which is near the centre of the breast. It is essential to ensure that you examine the breast thoroughly over this area. All women with suspected breast cancer must be referred urgently to the specialist breast clinic for assessment and treatment.

Risk factors for breast cancer are varied and some remain controversial. An assessment of family history is important and should be assisted by completing a genogram to help distinguish between familial and hereditary breast cancer. Familial breast cancer can be defined by two or more family members who have had breast cancer; hereditary is associated with the autosomal dominant transmission of the disease and is found in women who have the disease before the age of 45 years (McCance and Jorde 1998). Several factors are associated with the development of breast cancer and therefore the aetiology of this disease is complicated. Table 11.1 summarizes the most common risk factors.

Table 11.1   Risk factors for breast cancer

Genetic history
Previous breast cancer
Previous ovarian, colon, thyroid or endometrial cancer
Early menarche (before age 12)
First pregnancy over the age of 35
Nulliparous
Late menopause (over the age of 55)
Increasing age
Ionizing radiation

Austoker and Sharp (1993) state that some women may be anxious about exposure to radiation in mammographic screening. However, the potential benefit of screening far outweighs the risk of exposure to radiation.

Nipple discharge

In women who have never been pregnant any discharge is regarded as abnormal. This presents more commonly with a lump but may be spontaneous. The discharge can be milk, blood-stained or coloured.

Milk

The most common discharge is milk, either after pregnancy or in endocrine abnormalities, causing a rise in prolactin level. This is known as galactorrhoea and may be due to a pituitary tumour or, more commonly, as a side-effect of medication such as phenothiazines or metoclopramide.

Blood-stained fluid

Blood-stained fluid may be associated with benign

or malignant disease. The cause should always be investigated. Possible diagnoses are duct papilloma, epithelial proliferation or cancer (Baum 1996).

Coloured discharge

Duct ectasia is a benign but painful condition in which the terminal lactiferous ducts become dilated and the surrounding tissues are inflamed. It is most common in postmenopausal women and often presents as a thick multicoloured discharge from multiple ducts. This is due to cellular debris from the epithelial lining forming in the ducts. A hard indurated lump may then be felt close to the areola and hopefully this resolves within a few weeks. Cystic disease may cause a green or yellow discharge which can be swabbed for culture and sensitivity. Pus is usually associated with acute mastitis which is accompanied by inflammation or abscess.

Breast pain

Hormonal influences are the commonest cause of breast pain. Other causes include pregnancy, cracked nipple, cyst, abscess, trauma, anxiety state, angina and herpes-zoster (Baum 1996). Cyclical breast pain with or without nodularity is usually bilateral and most commonly occurs in the week preceding the woman's period. For most women this is not a problem as it resolves following menstruation. For some women the pain is more prolonged and more painful during the luteal or secretory phase of their cycle, which can lead to anxiety and insomnia. This may be due to prolactin causing a hypersensitive reaction in the duct epithelium (Baum 1996) or an abnormality in the secretion of gonadotrophins (Austoker and Sharp 1993). The oral contraceptive pill and HRT preparations may also be related to breast pain due to the hormonal influences of these medications. Non-cyclical pain is unrelated to the menstrual cycle, is often localized in one breast and is most common in women over the age of 40. Symptoms often resolve without treatment.

If a woman presents with a breast lump, nipple discharge or breast pain she should be fully assessed for the presence of all three symptoms as they are often related and one symptom may obscure the presence of another.

Clinical presentations of genital tract disease

Adnexae

The adnexae include the fallopian tubes, ovaries and the pelvic fascia and ligaments. There are a variety of problems associated with these structures, including salpingitis, pelvic inflammatory disease, ectopic pregnancy, ovarian cysts and prolapse. Figure 11.8 shows the normal female pelvic anatomy.

Salpingits and pelvic inflammatory disease

Several sexually transmitted diseases and other organisms such as *Streptococcus*, *Staphylococcus* or *Escherichia* can invade the uterus and eventually the fallopian tubes, resulting in salpingitis. This inflammation may cause lower abdominal pain, fever and vomiting in the patient and may result in scarring which may eventually be the cause of an ectopic pregnancy. If the infection spreads beyond the fallopian tubes, the pelvic organs may become involved, resulting in pelvic inflammatory disease, which can be a serious and life-threatening condition. Pelvic inflammatory disease can be acute or chronic. The acute presentation produces tender bilateral adnexal areas, the patient may guard on palpation and often cannot tolerate bimanual examination. Chronic pelvic inflammatory disease tends to produce irregular tender areas.

Ectopic pregnancy

Ectopic pregnancy is more common in women who have been sterilized, women who have had a previous abortion, multiparous or older women, or those women who have experienced pelvic inflammatory disease or endometriosis. In a normal pregnancy implantation occurs on the posterior wall of the uterus. The pregnancy is termed ectopic if implantation occurs outside the uterus. This most often occurs in the fallopian tubes and is extremely dangerous, as the embryo is growing in a restricted area, exerting pressure on the thin vascular walls of the tubes. The patient presents with lower abdominal pain and, if the condition has been allowed to develop unchecked, the woman will eventually haemorrhage, resulting in a serious risk to life. A woman who presents with unilateral tenderness and an adnexal mass should be assessed for tachycardia and shock as ruptured ectopic pregnancy is an emergency and must be treated surgically.

Ovarian cysts

There are two major kinds of ovarian cysts – cystic follicles which are large, fluid-filled sacs formed from unovulated follicles and luteinized cysts, which are solid masses filled with luteal cells. Both are common and can disappear spontaneously. In some cases the cysts persist and secrete abnormal amounts of steroid hormones, resulting in complications with fertility. These cysts must be removed surgically. In some women the ovaries may contain many cysts – a condition known as polycystic ovarian syndrome (Jones 1991). A ruptured ovarian cyst can mimic the symptoms of tubal pregnancy; intact cysts tend not

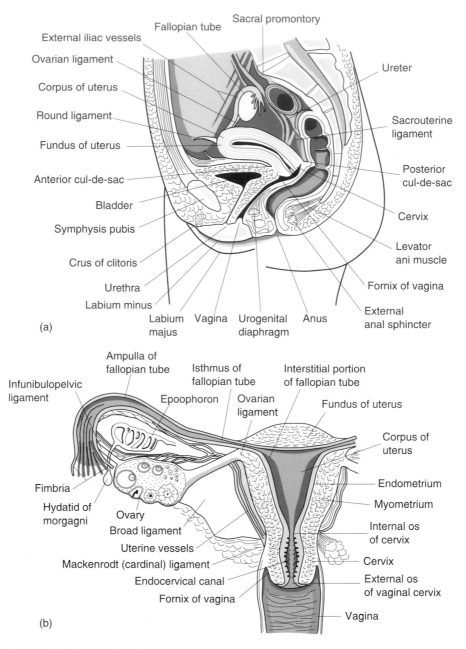

Figure 11.8 Normal female pelvic anatomy

to be tender. On palpation, a cyst is smooth and sometimes compressible, whereas tumours feel more solid and nodular (Seidel *et al.* 1995).

Prolapse

The ligaments of the pelvis span laterally, connecting the cervix and upper vagina to the bony pelvis. These are known as the cardinal ligaments. The uterosacral ligaments pass posteriorly and backwards from the posterolateral cervix to the sacrum. If the pelvic ligaments become lax and the muscular floor of the pelvis weakens, the pelvic organs may drop and

prolapse (Epstein *et al.* 1997). There are several causes of genitourinary prolapse (Jackson and Smith 1997). Those associated with childbirth include large babies, long labours, assisted delivery and poor postnatal exercise regimens. Other causes of prolapse include hysterectomy, increased intra-abdominal pressure associated with obesity, chronic respiratory disease and pelvic masses which may have the same effect, and connective tissue disease which may also weaken the supporting structures of the pelvis.

The patient may present with a variety of clinical problems (Table 11.2).

Table 11.2 Presenting symptoms of genitourinary prolapse

Cystourethrocele	Urinary stress incontinence, urinary retention, recurrent urinary tract infection
Uterine prolapse	Backache, difficulty inserting and keeping tampons in, ulceration if procedentia
Rectocele	Constipation
Any prolapse	Lump coming down, difficulties with sexual intercourse

Uterus

Abnormal patterns of uterine bleeding

Problems with uterine bleeding may present as oligomenorrhoea, amenorrhoea or dysfunctional uterine bleeding, including intermenstrual or postmenopausal uterine bleeding.

Oligomenorrhoea and amenorrhoea

Oligomenorrhoea is the term used to describe infrequent or scanty menstrual periods. Dealy (1998) defines oligomenorrhoea as irregular bleeding episodes that occur at intervals of more than 42 days. This pattern may be a normal feature of the climacteric or of menarche before a regular menstrual pattern develops. In some women this pattern persists for life and it is therefore worthwhile taking a thorough history of the woman's experience of menstruation to determine how abnormal this pattern is for her. If this pattern presents as a definite change from the woman's normal experience of menstruation then it should be treated in the same way as amenorrhoea, as the causes are generally the same (Rees 1993).

Amenorrhoea can cause great distress to a woman as the absence of the normal pattern of menstruation has implications for her femininity and her overall general health and well-being. Tothill (1998) states that all women who present with amenorrhoea should be considered pregnant until proven otherwise and that they should all be advised to continue with a reliable form of contraception as amenorrhoea does not necessarily indicate subfertility. There are numerous causes of secondary amenorrhoea and oligomenorrhoea, which are summarized in Table 11.3. Primary amenorrhoea results from genetic disturbances such as Turner's syndrome when the woman will never menstruate and the reproductive tract never matures fully.

Dysfunctional uterine bleeding

Dysfunctional uterine bleeding can be defined as painless irregular vaginal bleeding which originates from the endometrium and may be excessive, prolonged or irregular (Jaffe and Jewelewicz 1991).

Table 11.3 Causes of secondary amenorrhoea and oligomenorrhoea

Ovarian, uterine and vaginal disorders
Polycystic ovarian disease
Ovarian failure
Ovarian tumour
Severe acute illness
Chronic infections or illness
Autoimmune disease

Hormonal disorders
Thyroid hormone deficiency or excess
Pituitary tumours
Adrenal tumours
Post oral contraceptive pill

Psychological
Anorexia nervosa
Depression
Fear of pregnancy
Stress or anxiety

Physiological
Pregnancy
Lactation

Dealy (1998) defines five terms related to abnormal uterine bleeding:

- Hypomenorrhoea: decreased uterine bleeding that occurs at regular intervals
- Intermenstrual bleeding: episodes of uterine bleeding between regular menstrual periods
- Menorrhagia: uterine bleeding at the usual time of menses that is excessive in either duration or flow
- Menometrorrhagia: frequent irregular bleeding that may be excessive in amount or of prolonged duration
- Metrorrhagia: uterine bleeding that occurs at regular intervals and may range from spotting to a menses-like flow

The unusual pattern of bleeding can be related to an underlying systemic or local lesion but most often in young women it is related to anovulation. Dysfunctional uterine bleeding can be divided into three categories: cyclical abnormal uterine bleeding, cyclical bleeding superimposed with abnormal uterine bleeding and non-cyclical. These categories can help the nurse practitioner make decisions about the probable causes of the bleeding pattern and make appropriate treatment and management decisions. For example, cyclical bleeding superimposed with abnormal uterine bleeding may have an organic pathology such as trauma, uterine polyps, congenital malformations, cervical haemangiomas or infections (Dealy 1998). The list of potential diagnoses for women who present with dysfunctional bleeding is extremely lengthy. Some possible causes are listed in Table 11.4.

Table 11.4   Possible causes of abnormal bleeding

Vaginal/cervical	Cervical polyps
	Cervical erosions
	Cervical cancer
	Infection, *Chlamydia*,
	trichomoniasis, gonorrhoea
	Vaginal trauma
	Atrophic vaginitis
Ovarian/uterine	Intrauterine devices
	Endometrial polyps
	Retained tampon
	Uterine fibroids
	Ovarian cancer
	Uterine cancer
Hormonal	Ovulation
	Oral contraceptive pill
	Hormone replacement therapy
Pregnancy	Incomplete or missed abortion
complications	Threatened abortion
	Molar pregnancy
	Ectopic pregnancy
Medications	Phenytoin
	Warfarin
	Hormonal contraceptives
	Phenobarbitone
Blood dyscrasias	Leukaemia
	Pernicious anaemia
Hypothalamic	Stress
anovulation	Eating disorders
	Chronic disease, for example,
	hypothyroidism, diabetes
	mellitus
	Excessive exercise

Intermenstrual and postmenopausal bleeding require a special mention here as it is particularly important to maintain a high level of suspicion with these women and to take a thorough history followed by a thorough physical examination with investigations to rule out the possibility of malignant causes of the problem. Diseases of the uterus and cervix may present in this way, so it is worth considering disorders of the mucosa, such as endometritis, carcinoma or endometrial polyps, or submucosa, such as fibroids or submucosal leiomyomas. Postcoital bleeding usually indicates local cervical or uterine disease such as cervical polyp, cervicitis, or erosion; it may also indicate carcinoma.

Dysmenorrhoea

Painful menstruation may be classified as primary or secondary dysmenorrhoea and is a common reason for missing school, work or leisure activities (Tothill 1998). Primary dysmenorrhoea appears 6–12 months after the menarche and in general is not associated with pelvic pathology. Secondary dysmenorrhoea can present at any time and may be associated with other pelvic disease (Rees 1993). In primary dysmenorrhoea the patient may complain

of discomfort in the first 2 days of menstruation. The pain may be described as lower abdominal cramps and backache and there may be associated diarrhoea and vomiting. Dysmenorrhoea has been found to be associated with uterine hypercontractility resulting in ischaemia as the contractions reduce endometrial blood flow and produce colicky-type pain (Rees 1993). It has been found that this hypercontractility is related to increased prostaglandin production and raised vasopressin levels, although the stimulus for their production remains unknown.

Secondary dysmenorrhoea is associated with endometriosis, pelvic inflammatory disease, endometrial polyps, the use of an intrauterine device and adenomyosis. The patient may present with a change in intensity or timing of pain; it may be associated with discomfort before the bleeding begins and may last for the whole of the menstruation. Any such changes or presentations which occur several years after the onset of menstruation should be thoroughly investigated to rule out possible pelvic pathology.

Dyspareunia

Dyspareunia is pain occurring during sexual intercourse. The pain may be superficial and localized or deep and experienced as a sensation of discomfort deep inside the pelvis. The history-taking process and symptom analysis using PQRST (as described in Chapter 2) is extremely useful in this situation as it will help differentiate between the various causes of dyspareunia. If the patient describes a sensation of pain at the entrance to the vagina, this may be due to vaginismus (vaginal spasm), failure of the vagina to lubricate, irritation or damage to the clitoris, inflammation of Bartholin's glands or a vaginal infection. If the pain is described as dull and deep it may be due to lack of arousal and consequent absence of ballooning in the inner vagina, which results in the cervix being buffeted during sexual intercourse and produces an uncomfortable sensation in the pelvis. Deep pain can also be related to a retroverted, displaced or prolapsed uterus or other pelvic pathology such as chronic salpingitis, fibroids or endometriosis. In an older postmenopausal woman it may be necessary to consider atrophic vaginitis as the vulva and vagina become dry after the menopause, resulting in discomfort on intercourse. Whatever the cause of the pain, it is likely to be associated with a great deal of anxiety and therefore it is essential that the woman is treated with sensitivity and care. It may be that she simply needs advice about lubrication, sexual arousal or positioning during intercourse to help reduce discomfort or in the case of pelvic pathology it will be necessary to investigate the problems further.

Vagina

Vaginitis is a common presenting problem in general practice. There are a number of causes, including bacterial vaginosis, candidiasis and trichomoniasis.

Bacterial vaginosis

Bacterial vaginosis was previously known as non-specific vaginitis (Thomas and Rock 1997) and results from high concentrations of anaerobic bacteria such as *Gardnerella vaginalis*. Contributory factors in the development of this disease include retention of a diaphragm or tampon, recent intrauterine device placement, administration of antibiotics and multiple sexual partners.

Candidiasis

Candidiasis tends to present as vaginal itching and burning. Predisposing factors for the development of *Candida* include diabetes mellitus, pregnancy, vaginal trauma, antibiotics and tight-fitting synthetic underwear.

Trichomoniasis

Trichomoniasis is the third commonest cause of vaginitis and is one of the most common sexually transmitted diseases. Symptoms vary enormously between patients. In about 15% of women there are no symptoms while in others there may be acute inflammatory disease. Most commonly there is a copious yellow-grey or green malodorous discharge and vulvovaginal irritation. The condition is caused by the organism *Trichomonas vaginalis* and diagnosis is confirmed with a fresh wet slide for mobile flagellated organisms. Occasionally diagnosis may be established as a result of a report following a cervical smear.

Each of these three conditions may cause the woman great discomfort and irritation. They are often associated with discharge. There are several other causes of vaginal discharge, summarized in Table 11.5.

Genital herpes

Genital herpes may be caused by herpes simplex virus 1 (HSV1) or 2 (HSV2). Infection with HSV1 is the same virus responsible for cold sores on the mouth. In all, 80–90% of genital herpes cases are caused by an infection with HSV2 (Martini 1995b). The presentation of this condition is extremely painful: itchy, ulcerated lesions appear on the external genitalia and may also appear on the cervix. Sometimes these lesions produce a serous discharge which may be swabbed for viral cultures. The ulcers gradually heal in 2–3 weeks. The initial infection is extensive but recurrent infection tends to be localized on the vulva, vagina, perineum or cervix. This

Table 11.5   Causes of abnormal vaginal discharge

Vaginal causes
Candida
Trichomoniasis
Gardnerella
Genital warts
Genital herpes
Atrophic vaginitis
Bacterial infection caused by retained tampon
Irritants and allergic reactions

Cervical causes
Gonorrhoea
Cervical polyp
Cervical erosion
Herpes
Intrauterine contraceptive device

condition is sexually transmitted and recent research has indicated that transmission may occur during acute episodes and even in the latent phase of the disease (Patel *et al.* 1997).

Chlamydia

Chlamydia is a further cause of vaginal discharge. The discharge is mucopurulent and originates from the cervical os. It is a sexually transmitted bacterium responsible for 50% of pelvic inflammatory disease. Women who have this infection often have few, if any, symptoms. If left untreated it may go on to cause scarring of the fallopian tubes, leading to infertility. If symptoms are present these may include intermenstrual postcoital spotting and there may be a discharge from the Bartholin's glands. An area of the cervix may appear hypertrophic, oedematous and friable and the patient may have asymptomatic urethritis. Swabs must be taken from the endocervical canal of the cervix.

Vulva

Women may present with complaints of vulval swelling, itching, discomfort or pain, soreness, bleeding or purulent discharge from the vulva. It is not uncommon for women to be unaware of problems in this area of their body and the nurse practitioner may notice a lesion during a routine examination for a smear or for other pelvic problems. The vulva is a common site of thrush, boils, genital warts and cysts and it may also be the site of a carcinoma. A vaginal discharge due to *Candida* or *Trichomonas* can result in excoriation of the vulva or may result in *Candida* spreading to the labia and upper thighs. The patient may present with a painful swelling on the vulva which may be a furuncle (a deep staphylococcal follicular pustule). Cysts tend not to be tender on palpation and present as firm round, yellow lesions.

Genital warts

A crop of small painful perianal pustules and vesicles may suggest herpes infection. The patient may also present with multiple genital warts which may extend into the vagina and posteriorly may extend on to the perineum. The warts may coalesce to form irregular tissue masses and most often are caused by the human papillomavirus. The presence of genital warts is linked to the development of cervical intraepithelial neoplasia and this should therefore heighten your suspicion for the possibility of a positive smear test.

Inflamed Bartholin's glands

A further cause of vulval discomfort is inflamed Bartholin's glands. This condition may present as an acute or chronic problem and is commonly but not always caused by gonococcal infection. The acute inflammation causes hot, red and tender swelling which may drain pus and the chronic condition may result in a non-tender cyst on the labium.

History-taking

It is essential during the history-taking process to build up a rapport with the woman as most often examination of the most intimate parts of the woman's body will follow and if the woman is relaxed the examination will proceed more smoothly. An anxious patient will have tense muscles and the examination will be traumatic for both patient and nurse practitioner. It is therefore essential that you consider the history taking process to be an integral part of the whole consultation and that one of the underlying purposes of the communication at this stage of the consultation is to relax the patient and to gain her confidence.

In many consultations with women for problems associated with the female reproductive system it will be important to enquire about family history. Incidence of genetic disorders in the family is important, as is the incidence of breast cancer. It is useful to enquire about the patient's mother's and, if appropriate, sister's experience of the menarche and menopause as this is likely to have an impact on the patient's expectations. As systemic disorders such as diabetes and thyroid disease can have an effect on menstruation it is worth enquiring about the incidence of these problems in the family.

Past medical history is important to discover any incidence of surgery such as dilatation and curettage, cone biopsy, hysterectomy or a repair of prolapse, for example. It is also useful to ask the woman about previous pregnancies and methods of delivery as trauma at the birth such as prolonged labour or a large baby may account for the presenting symptoms of the current problem. Termination of pregnancy is an extremely sensitive issue which should only be addressed with a woman if it is deemed to be an important aspect of the examination and history-taking process with regard to the presenting clinical problem.

Other generally important aspects of history-taking include current medications, particularly those which might affect the menstrual cycle. It may be useful to ask about numbers of sexual partners and to what extent the presenting problem is affecting the patient's lifestyle. Methods of contraception in the past and at present should also be addressed. It is useful not only to ask the patient whether she has been sterilized but also whether her partner has been sterilized, as this has implications for the development of ectopic pregnancy.

A general history from any woman should also include her smear status. This will provide an excellent opportunity to follow up patients who have slipped through the screening net or those who may need encouragement and education relating to the process of screening for cervical cancer. It is almost always necessary to enquire about the woman's last menstrual cycle and whether she considers that this was a normal period or if it was different in some way. The timing of the last menstrual cycle is necessary before smear-taking, discussing contraception, assessing a woman in abdominal pain and many other likely presenting clinical problems associated with the female reproductive system.

Focused history for problems associated with the breast

The most common symptoms will relate to breast lump, breast pain or nipple discharge. Some women may present with one, two or all three symptoms and the most useful starting point for the assessment is using the mnemonic PQRST, adapted according to the presenting problem (Chapter 2).

Table 11.6 is a summary of the questions you might choose to explore with the patient.

Past medical history

This should include any previous breast problems and investigations undertaken with dates and results, any gynaecological problems or investigations and previous pregnancies, including complications. The presence of chronic illness such as thyroid disease, diabetes or other endocrine abnormalities may also be relevant.

Family history

Genetic risk factors associated with breast cancer are discussed above (p. 152). It is essential to enquire about a family history of breast cancer.

Personal and social history

Occupation, including exposure to radiation,

Table 11.6 History-taking for breast lumps, pain and nipple discharge

Breast lump
- Identify when the patient first became aware of the problem and how it was detected
- Was the onset sudden or gradual?
- Describe the quality and quantity of the lump or lumps
- What size is the lump? Has it grown or changed in any way?
- Is it smooth, soft, hard, irregular, mobile, attached?
- In one breast or both?
- Single or multiple?
- Ask the patient to identify on a diagram the exact location
- Is it painful? How severe is the pain, using an appropriate scale?
- How often do you notice the lump? Is it present constantly or does it vary?
- Is the nipple retracted? Is this permanent or transient?

Breast pain
- What causes the pain? Does anything relieve or provoke it?
- Is it related to your menstrual cycle?
- How would you describe the pain?
- How often do you experience the pain?
- Where is the pain? Is it in both breasts?
- Is the pain localized or diffuse? Is there any radiation?
- How severe is the pain using an appropriate pain scale?
- When did you first notice the pain?

Nipple discharge
- What provokes the discharge? What reduces it?
- Is it spontaneous? Does it need to be expressed?
- Is the discharge from single or multiple ducts?
- How much discharge is there? What colour is it?
- Is there an odour present?
- How often do you have the discharge? Is it constant?
- Are there any skin lesions or crusting around the nipple?
- Are both breasts affected or only one?
- Is it related to your menstrual cycle?
- Do you experience pain with the discharge?
- When did you first notice the discharge?

chemotherapy, heavy lifting or trauma to breasts, should be explored. It is important to discuss current medication, including oral contraceptive, HRT, antidepressants, opiates or tamoxifen. If the woman reports that she has recently experienced stress, this is an important issue to discuss further. It is also worthwhile exploring her values and beliefs in relation to breast disease.

Focused history for problems associated with the genital tract

Menstrual cycle

Important questions to ask a woman who presents with problems with the menstrual cycle include age of menarche and development during puberty. As a baseline it is important to establish the woman's normal pattern of menstruation, length of cycle, days of blood loss, number of tampons or pads used each day, presence of blood clots and any recent changes. It is also useful to determine if the woman is using the contraceptive pill or HRT. Recent changes in appetite or weight and general health and psychological well-being will help identify the possibility of stress-related causes for change in menstruation. It is clearly important to discuss contraceptive methods used and any possibility of contraceptive failure resulting in pregnancy.

Dysfunctional uterine bleeding

Fisher and Glenn (1998) state that it is essential to ask the patient to describe what she thinks is a normal menstrual cycle and normal quantity of bleeding before eliciting a history relating to the current problem. Women vary enormously in their perception of what is normal and abnormal and it is therefore worth attempting to quantify the problem before making a judgement about its extent. The patient can be asked to report the number of tampons or pads used with each episode of bleeding and this will help you gain an idea of how heavy the blood loss is. Thomas and Rock (1997) state that the patient can be asked if she floods the bed at night, as this is a good indicator of the amount of blood loss. Ask the patient how long it has been since her pattern of bleeding was normal if she has had an episode of irregular bleeding before, and whether she has a history of sexually transmitted disease. It is also useful to ask the following:

- Do you experience premenstrual syndrome?
- Do you have any menopausal symptoms?
- Have you been sterilized?
- Have there been any episodes of dysmenorrhoea?
- What is your usual form of contraception?

The patient should be asked if she has an intrauterine device, if she is taking the oral contraceptive pill and if she is on HRT. In addition it is worth exploring whether she has noticed any bruising or bleeding elsewhere on her body and if there is any history of other illness or family history of bleeding disorders. Ask the patient to tell you when her last period was and to describe if it was normal and whether the bleeding occurs after sexual intercourse.

Vaginal discharge

Ask the woman to describe the colour and consistency of the discharge, whether it is blood-stained and if it has an odour. It is useful to explore how long the discharge has been present and if there has been any associated itching or burning of the vulval area. Ask the woman to quantify the amount of discharge by describing if it is scanty and whether or not she needs to use protective pads.

Physical examination

Examination of the female genitalia may occasionally cause embarrassment and anxiety not only for the patient but also for the nurse practitioner. It is important to recognize these feelings and to make the environment as safe and relaxed as possible. In addition to the embarrassment of being exposed for the examination, some women may have psychological difficulties associated with past traumatic experiences or possibly sexual abuse. It is therefore important to appear calm and relaxed yourself, to let the patient know that the examination will take place in a private room where no one else will be expected to interrupt during the examination and that you will make every effort not to cause any discomfort or pain. This explanation should take place before the patient has undressed, including a full discussion of what to expect during the examination.

Ask the patient to empty her bladder and assist her into a comfortable position, with a blanket or sheet covering the areas of her body which do not need to be exposed. It is useful to ask the woman to lie in a supine position with her head and shoulders slightly elevated and arms resting beside her. This helps the woman relax and specifically helps to relax the abdominal muscles. Any instruments used should be warmed to the appropriate temperature and the patient should be kept informed of the progress throughout the examination so that she can equally inform you if the exam becomes uncomfortable in any way.

Before commencing with the specific examinations associated with the female reproductive tract, it is useful to carry out a general inspection of the patient. There may be signs of anaemia which could be associated with menorrhagia. Signs of thyrotoxicosis, hypothyroidism, anorexia nervosa or other chronic diseases might be clues to presenting problems with the menstrual cycle. Signs of hirsutism or thinning hair may be a clue to a hormonal imbalance. As with all physical examinations, a general inspection is vital to inform your decision-making process and the rest of your examination.

Examination of the breasts

It is essential to ensure that you are fully competent to carry out breast examination when required to do so. Breast examination should not form a routine part of a well-woman check but may be necessary if a woman consults with you because she is experiencing a problem with her breast or breasts. As with all physical examinations, it is essential to ensure that you are operating within the scope of professional practice (United Kingdom Central Council 1992) and that you are working within local guidelines and protocols.

A full explanation regarding the examination is necessary to reduce anxiety and embarrassment. The room should be warm and private as the woman will need to undress to the waist. There should be a good light source available.

Inspection

The patient should be sitting on the couch or in a chair with her arms by her side. Observe the breasts for size and symmetry. Look at the contour, lumps, skin changes and nipple retraction. Note redness, ulceration, oedema and an abnormal venous pattern. Have the patient raise her arms above her head to observe mobility. Ask her to place her hands on her hips and lean forwards to assess tethering to the serratus anterior muscles.

Palpation

Always examine the unaffected breast first if only one breast is involved.

With the patient lying down flat on the couch, a pillow is inserted under the shoulder and the arm placed above the head on the side to be examined. This will help relax the pectoral muscles and allow the breast to 'float' on the chest wall.

The breast is palpated with your fingers flat against the breast, using a circular motion, applying gentle pressure and then firm pressure, compressing the tissues against the chest wall. Each quadrant is examined systematically as well as the areola and tail of Spence well into the axilla. Alternatively the breast can be assessed using a concentric circular pattern from the periphery, ensuring the axillary tail is included, inwards towards the nipple. The nipple and retroareolar tissue is palpated between the index finger and thumb. Further palpation will be necessary if an abnormality is detected. Bimanual palpation may be necessary if the breasts are pendulous.

Examining the axilla is part of the examination of the breasts and the patient should be asked to sit up for this. To examine the left axilla you will need to support the weight of the patient's left arm in your left hand. Using your right hand, palpate the anterior lymph nodes by pressing against the muscles and fascia of the anterior wall (Figure 11.9a and b). To palpate the apical and medial lymph nodes, cup your fingers and press upwards and inwards into the apex of the axilla and then move downwards over the medial wall, continuing to apply pressure (Figure 11.9c and d). In order to examine the posterior and lateral nodes it is necessary to stand behind the patient (Figure 11.9e and f). The procedure is then repeated for the right axilla using your left hand (Lumley and Bouloux 1994).

Examination of the female genital tract

If a woman presents to the nurse practitioner in

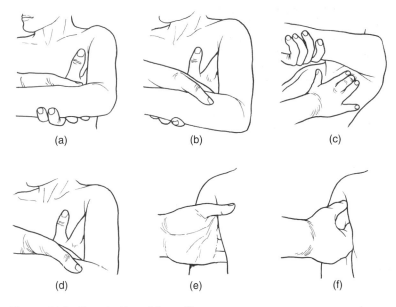

(a)   (b)   (c)

(d)   (e)   (f)

Figure 11.9 Examination of the axilla

severe lower abdominal pain you should consider the differential diagnoses of salpingitis or ectopic pregnancy and the possible harmful effects of carrying out a physical examination. In some cases it may be necessary to scan the woman or to take swabs and send them for culture and sensitivity before carrying out an examination. The physical examination may cause discomfort and harm and yet it would be unlikely to have an impact upon your management plan. If a woman presents with lower abdominal pain it is important to consider referral to a medical colleague for advice and assistance.

In other presentations of problems with the genital tract a full abdominal examination should precede examination of the vulva and vagina. An overview of the abdominal examination can be found in Chapter 9. It may be possible to identify abnormalities associated with the uterus and adnexae just above the pubis. Ovarian tumours or cysts may fill the abdomen and an ectopic pregnancy or a normal pregnancy may appear as a large mass which is dull to percussion. Ascites may be present; this tends to have a central resonance and dullness in the flanks on palpation. An added advantage of starting the examination of the external genitalia with the abdominal examination is that you have placed your hands on the patient and the subsequent examination of the vulva, vagina and cervix will appear a little less intrusive.

External genitalia

Position the woman on the couch in the supine position with hips and knees flexed. The heels may be placed close together or slightly apart, depending upon the patient's comfort and your own personal preference, and this should allow the legs flop

outwards. Ensure that you have a good source of light that shines directly on the area and can be adjusted if necessary as you inspect the area.

Inspect the mons pubis, labia and perineum. It is particularly useful to look for excoriations, and to observe the pattern of hair distribution which confirms the sexual maturity of the woman. Gently separate the labia with the fingers of your gloved hand and inspect the clitoris, urethral meatus, vaginal introitus and the labia minora (Figure 11.10). Palpate the length of the labia majora, which should feel smooth and fleshy. If there are any noticeable lesions, palpate them, noting tenderness and any signs of ulceration or swelling. The Bartholin's glands can be checked by inserting your finger into the vagina near the posterior end of the introitus while the thumb palpates the outer surface of the labia majora posteriorly (Figure 11.11). A normal Bartholin's gland is not palpable; however, these glands may become acutely or chronically infected, producing great discomfort and swelling.

If the patient has presented with a history which makes you suspect urethritis you can milk the urethra from inside out by placing your index finger into the vagina and gently palpating anteriorly and moving downwards. Note any discharge and collect a sample for culture and sensitivity.

Examination of the vagina

Separate the labia to expose the vestibule. Ask the patient to 'bear down' and observe the area for bulges and swellings. If the pelvic floor muscles are lax or damaged, it may be possible to see the posterior bladder wall prolapsing along the anterior vaginal wall (cystocele or urethrocele) or the rectum

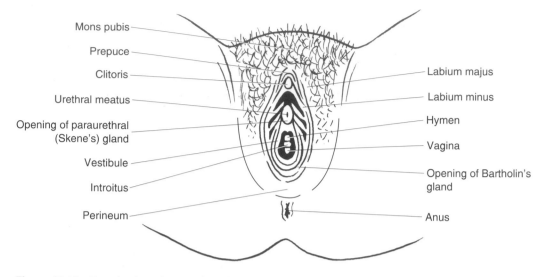

Mons pubis
Prepuce
Clitoris
Urethral meatus
Opening of paraurethral (Skene's) gland
Vestibule
Introitus
Perineum

Labium majus
Labium minus
Hymen
Vagina
Opening of Bartholin's gland
Anus

Figure 11.10 Examination of external genitalia

prolapsing into the posterior vaginal wall (rectocele). Examination of the vagina continues with the insertion of a speculum, allowing inspection of the walls of the vagina.

Internal examination

A bivalve speculum (Cusco's) is the instrument which is most commonly used to inspect the vagina. Specula are available in a variety of sizes and can be obtained in either disposable plastic or reusable metal. Selection of an appropriate size for the woman is important and paediatric or virginal specula are available for women with small vaginal openings. Familiarize yourself with both types of specula and

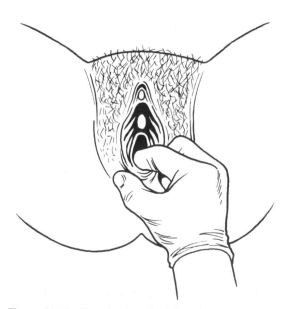

Figure 11.11 Examination of the Bartholin's gland

check the use of the thumbscrew and how to open and shut the blades.

Insertion of the speculum can be assisted with water to lubricate the instrument. Other lubricants should not be used as they might interfere with subsequent cytological studies or swabs for bacteriology or viral cultures. Insertion of the speculum is assisted by you inserting your index and middle fingers inside the vaginal introitus and applying a slight pressure downward. You can then feel when the muscles are relaxed and you can gently slide the speculum into the vaginal opening over your fingers at a 45° downward angle (Figure 11.12a). Slide the speculum into the vagina, rotating it in a clockwise direction until the blades run along the length of the anterior and posterior vaginal walls (Figure 11.12b). Remove your fingers and open the blades of the speculum by pressing on the thumb piece of the instrument. If you have directed the blades in the downward direction on insertion the cervix will come into view as you sweep the speculum slowly upward on opening the blades. Once the cervix is visualized, manipulate the speculum a little further so that the cervix is well exposed between the blades and lock the blades into place. If you are unable to find the cervix it may be necessary to withdraw the speculum and to reinsert it on a more horizontal angle. Ensure that you have a good source of light and then you can carry out a thorough inspection of the cervix.

Inspect the cervix for colour, size, position, discharge, size and shape of the os, presence of polyps and surface characteristics. In early pregnancy the cervix may be a bluish colour, which indicates increased vascularity; a pale cervix may indicate anaemia and erythema may be associated with exposed columnar epithelium from the cervical canal

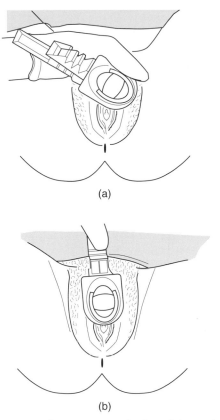

Figure 11.12   Speculum examination of the vagina

– commonly known as an erosion. There are many causes of erythema on the cervix and this should always be considered as an abnormal finding until proven otherwise.

During the speculum examination you may wish to take a smear or swabs for culture and sensitivity. You should familiarize yourself with local guidelines on cervical screening and national standards for the methods of obtaining samples for cytology. If obtaining smears is part of your role in clinical practice you should ensure that you have received adequate training and regular updates on cervical cytology. The purpose of cytology is to detect premalignant cells to allow early detection and give a higher successful cure rate.

Before proceeding with the smear you should ensure that your equipment is prepared and that you have a labelled slide ready to collect the sample. You may use an Aylesbury spatula, a Cervex brush or a cytobrush for the collection of the specimen. The Aylesbury spatula collects cells from the ectocervix, the cytobrush collects endocervical cells only and the Cervex brush is used to collect both ectocervical and endocervical cells at the same time. Dey *et al.* (1996) found that there was no difference in the adequacy rates of smear tests when comparing the Aylesbury spatula with the Cervex brush. Clearly

your choice of instrument will depend on the purpose of your investigation.

You should always carry out the smear test before taking any other swabs for culture. Place the tip of the Cervex brush or spatula in the cervical os and, whilst maintaining gentle pressure, rotate the brush or spatula by rolling the handle between the thumb and the forefinger three to five times to the left and to the right. It is essential that you cover the whole 360° surface of the cervix when collecting your specimen so that you do not miss any of the vital cells which may assist in the diagnosis of premalignant disease (Figure 11.13). Withdraw the brush and transfer the specimen to a slide. With two single paint strokes, apply first one side of the spatula or brush and then the other (with the cytobrush you will need to roll and twist the brush across the slide). You need to be gentle but firm when applying the cells to ensure that the cells can be visualized in the laboratory and have not been damaged in the process of application to the slide. Apply fixative to the specimen immediately and arrange for transfer to the laboratory.

If you need to take further swabs, do so before withdrawing the speculum. Unlock the speculum and, as you withdraw the instrument, rotate it slowly and gently to inspect the vaginal walls. Note the colour, any lesions and any discharge. You may find that there will be a pool of discharge on one of the blades after withdrawal and, if you have not already done so, you may wish to take a swab from this and send it for culture and sensitivity. Always ensure that you dispose of the speculum appropriately and that reusable specula are sterilized before use with the next patient.

Bimanual palpation

You may now wish to carry out a bimanual examination of the woman's genital tract. Using gloved hands and plenty of lubricant, insert the index and middle

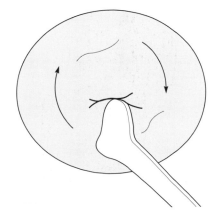

Figure 11.13   Cells are collected by rotating the spatula 360° around the cervix

finger into the vagina. The thumb should remain abducted and the ring and little finger should be flexed into the palm (Figure 11.14). Pressure should be exerted posteriorly rather than anteriorly as this avoids causing discomfort by exerting pressure on the sensitive urethra. The flexed fingers should press inward towards the perineum as this causes little or no discomfort. It is useful to be in a standing position to perform this procedure. Palpate the vaginal walls, which should be supple, moist and slightly rugose. Note any nodularity or tenderness. Locate the cervix and note its position. Palpate it for regularity, shape and consistency. The cervix should normally be slightly mobile without causing the patient any discomfort. Pain on movement of the cervix is known as cervical excitation and, together with discomfort in the adnexae, may be due to pelvic inflammatory disease.

Place the palmar surface of your second hand on the abdomen about midway between the umbilicus and symphysis pubis. The fingers of the pelvic hand elevate the cervix and uterus and you attempt to capture the uterus by gently apposing the fingers of both hands (Figure 11.15). This allows you to assess the size, shape and mobility of the uterus and to identify any tenderness or masses. Your pelvic hand can also be placed in the anterior fornix and this may allow you to palpate the anterior surface of the uterus with your pelvic hand; the posterior surface may be palpated by the hand on the abdominal wall. It is quite normal to feel nothing on bimanual palpation of the pelvis and only regular practice will make you confident in your technique.

If you are checking for a prolapse it may be necessary to turn the woman on to her left side with her lower arm placed behind her in a similar location to the recovery position. Using a Sims speculum to inspect the vaginal walls, ask the woman to cough or bear down and observe for signs of a rectocele, cystocele or urethrocele.

When you have completed your examination, explain to the woman that she may experience some spotting associated with the disturbance of the cervix. You may wish to provide her with a small protective pad and to advise her that this is a completely normal occurrence, particularly after a smear test. Allow her the time and privacy to put her clothes on and then you may wish to conclude your consultation with a report of your findings and your plan for follow up and investigation. This may be the appropriate moment for you to offer education and advice on a particular subject to help inform her of what to expect and how her particular problem may be managed.

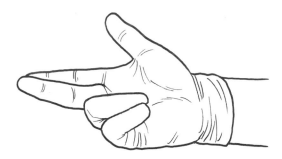

Figure 11.14   The thumb and finger positions for a vaginal examination

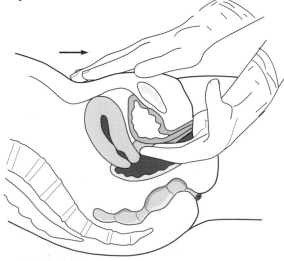

Figure 11.15   Examination of the anterior surface of the uterus

Patient education

Women may consult with nurse practitioners for a whole variety of reasons and will need education and management according to their presenting problem and individual needs. Refer to the specialized texts for more detailed advice. We have chosen to focus on the management of breast disorders here as there are clear national guidelines in operation to help guide your practice.

Breast care remains a sensitive area in women's health and is still the cause of considerable anxiety and embarrassment for some women. The psychological impact of discovering a breast lump and experiencing breast pain or nipple discharge can be very disturbing and should not be underestimated. Nurse practitioners will need to use their communication skills effectively to establish a safe and therapeutic environment to explore the woman's concerns. Social factors are important and should be discussed to establish if there is a family member or friend who can offer support should referral be necessary.

The NHS has issued guidelines for the referral of patients with breast problems (Austoker and Mansel 1999). The guidelines cover breast lumps, nipple discharge and breast pain.

Breast lump

Cysts are usually managed in the specialist clinic by fine-needle aspiration by the nurse specialist or medical staff. If the fluid is blood-stained, then a sample will be sent for cytology but otherwise the woman should be advised that the cyst may refill or recur elsewhere in the breast (50% may recur)

and to reconsult as necessary. See Figure 11.16 for NHS guidelines.

Nipple discharge

The woman should be assessed as described earlier in the history-taking section and then should be managed according to the guidelines shown in Figure 11.17.

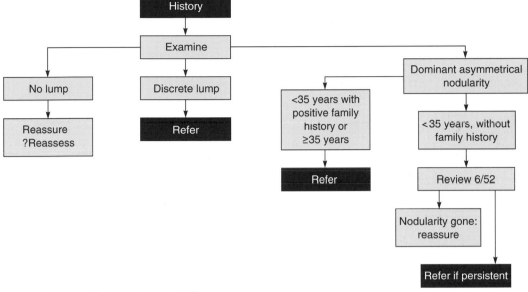

Figure 11.16   NHS breast lump guidelines
Source: Austoker and Mansel (1999), NHS Breast Screening Programme. Reproduced with permission

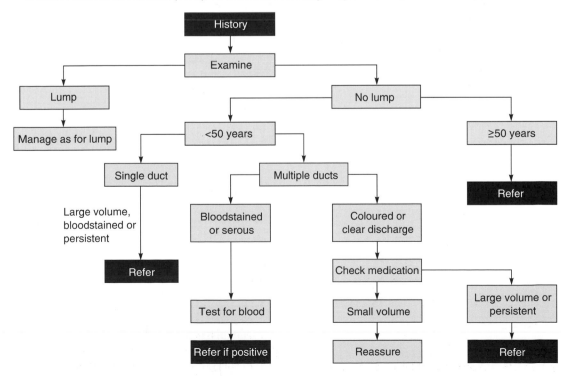

Figure 11.17   NHS nipple discharge guidelines
Source: Austoker and Mansel (1999), NHS Breast Screening Programme. Reproduced with permission

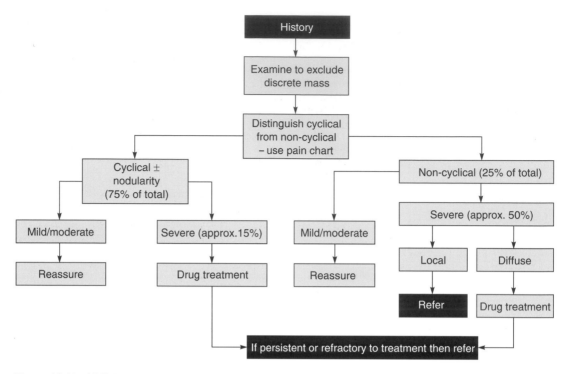

Figure 11.18 NHS breast pain guidelines
Source: Austoker and Mansel (1999), NHS Breast Screening Programme. Reproduced with permission

Breast pain

Figure 11.18 summarizes the NHS guidelines for the management of breast pain. After completion of a pain diary, cyclical pain can be managed with mild analgesics and reassurance that the pain is physiological rather than due to cancer. Women taking the oral contraceptive or HRT may need their medication altered to ensure that the lowest dose of oestrogen is used. The nurse practitioner, although unable to prescribe, can give advice regarding methods of contraception and of HRT as well as discuss alternative approaches that may be appropriate to the individual.

Referrals from nurse practitioners to a specialist breast clinic need to be negotiated locally with the hospital trust and primary care teams. This varies according to locality, although a woman with a suspicious lump or needing urgent referral will ideally be assessed as soon as possible to minimize anxiety. Any woman consulting with the nurse practitioner for health checks and cytology should be educated in breast awareness and leaflets are available to reinforce this message.

Nurse practitioners have a great deal to offer women who consult with them. The research shows that women consult more frequently with health care professionals than men (Stilwell 1985; Salisbury and Tettersell 1988; Reveley 1998) and it is therefore worthwhile developing your skills of history-taking and physical examination for women. These skills, in conjunction with the more generic communication and holistic assessment skills of the nurse practitioner, can help provide a service to the individual and unique needs of women.

References

Austoker J., Sharp D. (1993) Breast cancer and benign breast disease. In: McPherson A. (ed.) *Women's Problems in General Practice,* 3rd edn., Oxford, Oxford University Press.

Austoker J., Mansel R. (1999) *Guidelines for Referral of Patients with Breast Problems,* 2nd edn., Sheffield, NHS Breast Screening Programme.

Baum M. (1996) Breast lumps, breast pain, nipple abnormalities and nipple discharge. In: Bouchier I., Ellis H., Fleming P. (eds). *French's Index of Differential Diagnosis,* 13th edn., Oxford, Butterworth-Heinemann.

Cancer Research Campaign (1991) *Facts on Cancer,* CRC fact sheet 6, London CRC.

Coope J. (1993) Menopause. In: McPherson A. (ed.) *Women's Problems in General Practice,* 3rd edn., Oxford, Oxford University Press.

Day N.E. (1991) Screening for breast cancer, *British Medical Bulletin,* **47,** pp. 400–415.

Dealy M. (1998) Dysfunctional uterine bleeding in adolescents, *Nurse Practitioner,* **23**(5) pp. 12–23.

Dey P., Collins S., Desai M., Woodman C. (1996) Adequacy of cervical cytology sampling with the Cervex brush and the Aylesbury spatula: a population based randomised controlled trial, *British Medical Journal,* **313,** pp. 721–722.

Epstein O., Perkin G.D., deBono D.P., Cookson J. (1997) *Clinical Examination,* 2nd edn. London, Mosby.

Fisher P., Glenn K. (1998) Intermenstrual bleeding, *Practice Nursing,* **9**(17), pp. 39–42.

France R., Robson M. (1986) *Behaviour Therapy in Primary Care: A Practical Guide,* Kent, Croom Helm.

Jackson S., Smith P. (1997) Diagnosing and managing genitourinary prolapse *British Medical Journal,* **314**, pp. 875–880.

Jaffe S., Jewelewicz R. (1991) Dysfunctional uterine bleeding in the paediatric and adolescent patient *Adolescent Pediatric Gynecology,* **1**(4), pp. 62–69. Cited in: Dealy M. (1998) Dysfunctional uterine bleeding in adolescents *Nurse Practitioner,* **23**(5), pp. 12–23.

Jones R.E. (1991) *Human Reproductive Biology,* London, Academic Press.

Lumley J.S.P., Bouloux P.M.J. (1994) *Clinical Examination of the Patient,* Oxford, Butterworth-Heinemann.

Martini F. (1995a) *Fundamentals of Anatomy and Physiology,* 3rd edn., London, Prentice-Hall.

Martini F. (1995b) *Fundamentals of Anatomy and Physiology. Applications Manual,* 3rd edn. London, Prentice-Hall.

McCance K.L., Jorde L.B. (1998) Evaluating the genetic risk of breast cancer *Nurse Practitioner,* **23**(8), pp. 14–27.

Patel R., Cowan F M , Barton S.F. (1997) Advising patients with genital herpes, *British Medical Journal,* **314**, pp. 85–86.

Rees M.C.P. (1993) Menstrual problems. In: McPherson A. (ed.) *Women's Problems in General Practice,* 3rd edn., Oxford, Oxford University Press.

Reveley S. (1998) The role of the triage nurse practitioner in general medical practice: an analysis of the role, *Journal of Advanced Nursing,* **28**(3), pp. 584–591.

Salisbury C.J., Tettersell M.J. (1988) Comparison of the work of a nurse practitioner with that of a general practitioner, *Journal of the Royal College of General Practitioners,* **38**, pp. 314–316.

Seidel H.M., Ball J.W., Dains J.E., Benedict G.W. (1995) *Mosby's Guide to Physical Examination,* 3rd edn., St Louis, Mosby.

Stilwell B. (1985) Opportunities in general practice, *Nursing Mirror,* **161**(19), pp. 30–31.

Tanner J.M. (1973) *Growth at Adolescence,* 2nd edn., Oxford, Blackwell Scientific Publications. Cited in: Jones R.E. (1991) *Human Reproductive Biology,* London, Academic Press.

Thomas E.J., Rock J. (1997) *Benign Gynaecological Disease,* Abingdon, Health Press.

Tothill S. (1998) Diagnosis and treatment of menstrual problems, *Prescriber,* **19**, pp. 91–95.

United Kingdom Central Council (1992) *Scope of Professional Practice,* London, UKCC.

Wright J. (1998) Older women's experience of the menopause, *Nursing Standard,* **12**(47), pp. 46–48.

CHAPTER 12

The musculoskeletal system

Mike Walsh

Introduction

Problems with the musculoskeletal system are most likely to manifest themselves as pain or a decrease in function. These are the type of symptoms that patients are least likely to ignore, consequently the primary health care nurse practitioner may expect to see a significant number of patients with back pain, rheumatological and other disorders. In addition, the nurse practitioner working in a minor injuries or A&E department may expect to manage many patients with minor – although still painful – joint injuries and bruises and will be the first point of contact for many other patients with fractures and dislocations. The management of serious injuries clearly lies in the medical field and the nursing care of such patients can be found in other A&E nursing texts. Consequently this chapter will focus on the kind of injury that the nurse practitioner may reasonably be expected to manage.

Pathophysiology

This section will initially consider some orthopaedic conditions affecting the whole body before introducing the more common localized disorders and traumatic conditions which you may be involved in diagnosing and/or managing. It is not a substitute for a textbook on orthopaedics, to which you should refer if you wish to know more.

Osteoarthritis

Osteoarthritis (OA) is mostly found in older people and rarely in those under 40. It is more common in women and typically begins to appear around the age of 50. Disease of the knee and hip causes most disability. Obesity is a major risk factor for knee disease and Spector (1996) estimates that for every extra 5 kg in weight, the risk of a woman over 50

developing OA of the knee increases by 30%. Any abnormal localized factor affecting wear and tear on the joint also predisposes the person to develop OA over a period of years. This may be termed secondary OA, to distinguish it from primary OA which has no known cause. Secondary OA may be caused by excessive lifting and bending affecting the hip (well-documented in farmers) and the effects of trauma such as meniscectomy or fracture disrupting the normal contours or weight-bearing characteristics of a joint.

The disease affects synovial joints and involves loss of articular cartilage and a consequent reaction in the surrounding bone. After the breakdown in articular cartilage, irritation of the synovium occurs and attempts at repair lead to the formation of new bone, including fragments known as osteophytes. These tend to be located towards the edges of the joint and will limit joint movement. Eventually the joint surface may be eroded down to the bone, causing severe pain and stiffness. Callus formation in response to the trauma leads to the development of dense sclerotic bone, further deformity and eventual disorganization of the joint (Dandy 1993). Diagnosis by radiography is therefore a reliable method; in fact, many patients whose radiographs show changes indicative of OA may not be complaining of any symptoms at that time. The disease is usually more advanced when pain and disability bring the patient to the health centre. OA is not the inevitable, degenerative disorder that was once thought.

Osteoporosis

This term refers to any loss of bone and occurs most commonly in postmenopausal women. Lack of oestrogen leads to a reduction in collagen and consequently the bone becomes thin and porotic. Other risk factors include early menopause, low body weight, smoking and being of European descent.

Osteoporosis can also occur as a side-effect of large doses of steroids or prolonged immobilization.

The obvious effect of osteoporosis is to make the person more prone to fractures. The most serious fractures involve the femoral neck area and this is likely to happen to one in four women living to the age of 85, and carries a high mortality rate of around 25%. Weakening of the spinal vertebrae leads to chronic backache and the possibility of a vertebra collapsing (pathological fracture). A fall on the outstretched hand which in earlier life would probably have produced nothing worse than a few bruises now leads to a fracture of the distal radius, often with significant posterior displacement (Colles fracture) or a fractured neck of humerus.

Spector (1996) estimates that of a typical general practice list of 2000 adults, osteoporosis will affect some 65 patients, of whom 50 will be women. Falls are the leading cause of death as a result of trauma in the elderly. Over 85% of fatal falls in the home are in people aged over 65 and fractures account for 40% of deaths from injury (York Centre for Review and Dissemination 1996). Statistics such as these show the serious effect of osteoporosis on the elderly.

Rheumatoid arthritis

This condition can occur at any age but is most common between 30 and 50 years, affecting women more than men, particularly in the younger age groups. Both genetic and environmental factors seem to be involved in causing the disease and Spector (1996) estimates that, of those patients referred to a specialist clinic, approximately one-third will be suffering moderate or severe disability within 10 years. In addition to its disabling effects, rheumatoid arthritis causes increased mortality due to the systemic effects of pericardial disease, interstitial lung disease and systemic vasculitis (Ross 1997).

The disease usually has an insidious beginning, affecting peripheral joints first. Both small and larger joints may be involved simultaneously. Pain and signs of inflammation are present initially and if the disease is not controlled there will be serious joint damage and deformity such as the characteristic ulnar deviation that affects both hands. Tendons can also become involved, adding to the deformity and disability the patient suffers. The disease can affect other parts of the body, producing rheumatoid nodules, small blood vessel disease and ischaemic skin ulcers, eye problems and neurological complications as peripheral nerves become involved. The disease may have periods of remission followed by active flare-ups. The side-effects of the drugs used to manage the condition can be serious.

Other rheumatoid disorders

There are several other rare rheumatoid diseases which occur in a handful of patients in each general practice. Polymyalgia rheumatica and giant cell arteritis are two closely related conditions which mostly affect the over-50s and women more than men. They present as a syndrome of pain and stiffness in the neck, shoulders and pelvis associated with generalized symptoms such as weight loss and tiredness. A low-grade pyrexia may be present and there is an increased erythrocyte sedimentation rate.

Another important but rare autoimmune condition is systemic lupus erythematosus. This is a complicated syndrome that is nine times more common in women than men and, similarly, nine times more common in Asians and Afro-Caribbeans than Europeans. The major features include generalized pain and stiffness in the joints, a characteristic butterfly rash on the face after exposure to the sun (not to be confused with acne rosacea: p. 25), hair loss and fatigue. Major organ involvement may occur, with potentially fatal outcome.

Malignant disease

This is most likely to occur to be due to secondary deposits from primary growths in the lung, breast or prostate. Primary tumours can occur, most commonly involving bone marrow (e.g. myeloma or Ewing's sarcoma) but fortunately are rare.

Other conditions

Of course many other diseases affect the skeleton. Metabolic disorders associated with vitamin D deficiency produce diseases such as rickets (in children) or osteomalacia (in adults). Paget's disease is the commonest of the diseases which disrupt bone architecture, mostly affecting older people. Its cause remains unknown. There are a whole range of diseases affecting children (Perthe's disease, juvenile arthritis, etc.) which are beyond the scope of this chapter. The reader is referred to orthopaedic texts should s/he wish to learn more about the generalized pathophysiology of the musculoskeletal system.

Disorders affecting the spine

In addition to osteoporosis and OA, the spine may be affected by a range of other conditions. Abnormal spinal curvature may develop (Figure 12.1) and Bates (1995) suggests that the following are most likely to be encountered:

- Kyphosis – a rounded thoracic convexity due to the ageing process, especially amongst women
- Lordosis – where the normal lumbar curve is accentuated, usually to compensate for serious obesity or for pregnancy
- Scoliosis – lateral curvature of the spine. It is best seen when the patient bends forward as in the

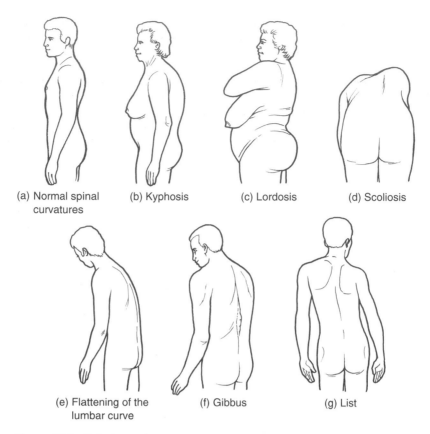

(a) Normal spinal curvatures   (b) Kyphosis   (c) Lordosis   (d) Scoliosis

(e) Flattening of the lumbar curve   (f) Gibbus   (g) List

Figure 12.1   Spinal curvatures

vertical plane compensation may have occurred; when the patient stands upright that the gluteal cleft lies directly below the first thoracic vertebra. A list may be observed with the patient standing upright, where the spine is tilted to one side and no compensation has occurred

- Flattened lumbar curve suggests ankylosing spondylitis in men, although it may be due to a herniated lumbar disc

Low back pain is a serious chronic problem that affects many individuals, not least nurses. In 1993 there were 14 million GP consultations for back pain and a further 480 000 A&E attendances. It is estimated that treating low back pain cost the NHS £480 million and the DSS paid £1.4 billion in benefits as a result of back pain (Clinical Standards Advisory Group 1994). The CSAG report notes that the incidence of low back pain seems to have been increasing steadily since the 1950s, as has the amount of time off work for back problems. Some 50% of attacks of back pain will have settled within a month, although 15–20% will continue to report symptoms for a year or more (CSAG 1994).

Risk factors identified for low back pain include low social class, poor educational achievement, smoking, low job satisfaction and depression;

incidence is about equal in men and women. As social class is usually determined by occupation, low social class is another way of saying manual labourer, hence it is not surprising to find a higher incidence of low back pain in this group. Educational achievement also links to social class, as does smoking behaviour, whilst any chronic disabling condition might be expected to produce depression. The significance of this sort of epidemiological data is therefore debatable.

In trying to understand the origins of low back pain it is best to differentiate between a localized mechanical and a systemic cause. In mechanical pain the problem lies at the articulation of one lumbar vertebra with another and usually involves the intervertebral disc: degeneration of the nucleus pulposus within the disc is the most likely candidate (Jenner and Barry 1996). The pain experienced by the patient stems from the interaction of the diseased disc with the surrounding structures. This may take the form of classic sciatica, where a protruding disc presses against the nerve root, but alternatively may involve the ligaments surrounding the spine or the joint facets.

Non-mechanical causes of back pain include the possibility of secondary growths that have metastasized from a malignancy affecting the prostate or breast, bad posture and lifting practice, unequal leg lengths, narrowing of the spinal canal in older people due to degenerative disease and ankylosing spondylitis. This last disorder is an inflammatory disease involving joints, especially in the spine, and usually affects young men aged under 30. In some patients no physical cause can be found. In the USA it is estimated that in nearly 80% of patients presenting with low back pain no discernible cause can be demonstrated (Jones 1997). It is possible therefore that psychological factors may be at work in a significant number of patients. Abnormal findings may also be present on examination which do not relate to organic pathology. There is evidence that the longer a person is off work with back pain, the less likely s/he is even to return to work. This suggests some form of learned sick-role behaviour (Jenner and Barry 1996).

The lower part of the back is not the only region affected by disease. Disc problems can affect any part of the spine, including the cervical region, and compression of a cervical nerve root by a protruding disc may occur. Spondylosis is a degenerative disease which occurs around intevertebral discs and may also involve the cervical as well as lumbar regions. Cervical spondylosis typically produces a dull pain across the shoulders and into the upper part of the arm which is worse on movement. Torticollis describes acute and often severe neck pain which is usually caused by muscle spasm, causing the patient to hold the neck rigid and often to one side. Care needs to be taken to exclude any more serious pathology such as an acute disc prolapse.

Common disorders affecting the hand and wrist

The tendons which connect the bones of the hand to the muscles of the forearm are prone to localized problems in the wrist region. Tenosynovitis refers to inflammation of tendons and most commonly occurs as a result of repeated twisting movements involving the extensor pollicis brevis and abductor pollicus longus tendons (involved in thumb movements) where they run adjacent to the radial styloid. Movement becomes painful as the inflamed tendons swell and a soft creaking sound may be heard on movement. Friction and inflammation can also affect the flexor profundus longus tendon leading to trigger finger (or thumb), a condition in which the finger becomes locked in the flexed position for several hours until the soft-tissue swelling subsides, allowing normal tendon movement to be resumed.

Carpal tunnel syndrome is caused by compression of the median nerve as it enters the hand through the restricted space of the carpal tunnel. Overuse of the wrist is the most likely cause of compression, although fluid retention associated with pregnancy can also cause this condition. The effect is paraesthesia in the median nerve distribution (see below) which may even disturb sleep. In time pain and even numbness may develop.

Both the radial and ulnar nerves may suffer from compression in the arm. Radial nerve compression is most commonly caused by sustained pressure on the inner aspect of the upper arm where the radial nerve winds over the surface of the humerus. Poor technique in the use of axillary crutches is a possible cause. The result is the development of wrist drop: due to motor nerve damage the person cannot extend the wrist properly. The ulnar nerve is closely involved in the anatomy of the elbow and therefore susceptible to damage in this region, especially when the elbow is flexed and therefore stretching the nerve over the medial epicondyle of the humerus. The symptoms of numbness and tingling will be confined to the ulnar nerve distribution of the hand (Figure 12.2).

Conditions affecting the elbow and shoulder

Damage can occur to the muscle or tendon which

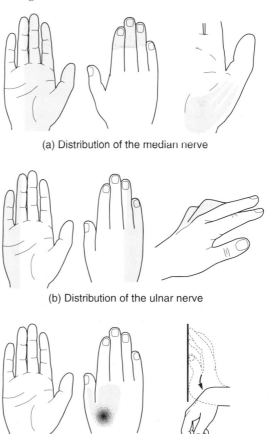

(a) Distribution of the median nerve

(b) Distribution of the ulnar nerve

(c) Distribution of the radial nerve

Figure 12.2   Peripheral nerve distributions in the hand

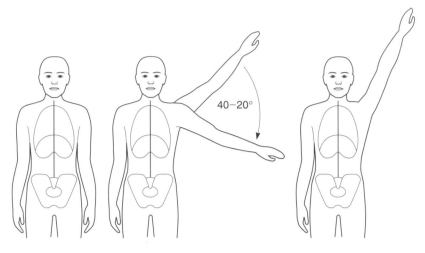

Figure 12.3 Painful arc syndrome

inserts into the lateral epicondyle of the humerus as a result of sharp flexion of the wrist. Although called tennis elbow, this disorder can occur as a result of other activities such as gardening and lifting. The patient usually presents with a painful elbow exacerbated by gripping or twisting movements. Tenderness is found over the lateral epicondyle: if the patient attempts to extend the wrist against resistance this will produce pain.

Inflammation of the olecranon bursa (olecranon bursitis) can lead to a hot and painful elbow with restricted movement. The cause may be infection but may also be associated with rheumatoid arthritis, gout or minor trauma.

The tendons of the shoulder joint can become inflamed. Several tendons combine to form the rotator cuff, one of which is the supraspinatus tendon. This is prone to inflammation, giving rise to the painful arc syndrome (Figure 12.3). In this situation the supraspinatus tendon becomes inflamed where it crosses the humeral head, leading to swelling just below the acromion (Figure 12.4). As the arm is abducted, this swelling comes into contact with the acromion but, when the arm reaches more than 60° of abduction, it slips out from below the acromion. The result is little pain when the arm is at rest against the side of the body or abducted out beyond about 60° but in the arc between 30 and 60° of abduction, the patient experiences considerable pain; hence the name painful arc syndrome.

One other common condition is frozen shoulder (adhesive capsulitis). The patient finds it painful and difficult to rotate the arm externally at the shoulder joint, consequently s/he cannot comb the hair at the back of the head or, if female, fasten her bra. Typically the patient at first finds it painful and difficult to move the shoulder in all directions. Several months later the pain disappears but the stiffness remains and it may be over a year before a large

degree of normal movement returns. The cause of this problem remains unknown.

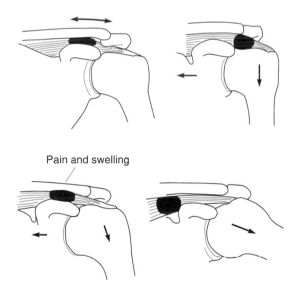

Figure 12.4 Painful arc syndrome. Note how inflamed supraspinatus tendon is released from below the acromion at 60° of abduction and hence the pain is relieved

Disorders of the foot and ankle

The big toe is the source of many foot problems. A frequent complaint is that of a bunion. This term is often used loosely to refer to any bump or lump on the foot. It is more accurate to restrict the term to describe a bursa occurring over the first metatarsal head. This may become infected and involve the metatarsophalangeal joint. The first metatarsophalangeal joint is also the classic site for gout. This condition involves the deposition of urate crystals in and around the joint. It can occur at any age and the result may be exquisitely painful. Pseudogout is similar but the deposits consist of crystals of calcium pyrophosphate.

The big toenail is notorious for developing as an ingrowing toenail. This is because toenails are curved and consequently the medial edge can dig into the soft tissue of the toe, leading to a painful lesion which in turn may become infected.

Hallux valgus is the final problem associated with the big toe. This deformity leads to the big toe pointing laterally and consequently the second toe underlies or overlies the big toe. Dislocation of the second metatarsophalangeal joint may occur as a result of this deformity and an inflamed bursa develops over the protuberance at the first metatarsal head. Dandy (1993) points out that there is a strong familial tendency, the condition often occurs in young adults and may also occur in the elderly due to degenerative changes. There is no evidence to implicate fashionable footwear in the origins of this condition.

Conditions affecting the knee

The prepatellar bursa may become inflamed, infected or injured as a result of minor trauma leading to the accumulation of fluid within the bursa. This is the classic housemaid's knee of old, although today it is other groups such as carpet-fitters who spend a great deal of time kneeling, who are prone to the disorder.

Adolescent girls are prone to recurrent dislocation of the patella due to laxity of the ligaments holding it in place and a smaller bone structure compared to boys. A twisting mechanism is sufficient to cause the problem and ice skating and playing netball are frequent causes. Anterior knee pain is a common problem in adolescent girls but usually no obvious cause is found and the problem resolves with time. It may well be associated with the growth spurt found in adolescence and the mechanical strains this puts on the lower limbs. Dandy (1993) cautions against the use of the term chondromalacia patellae as a synonym for anterior knee pain in young girls. This term means softening of the articular cartilage of the patella which can occur in young girls and is only one possible cause of knee pain in this group.

Trauma

This chapter is only concerned with patients who have minor injuries which the nurse practitioner might be expected to manage or for whom s/he would be the first point of contact. The following section excludes serious injuries such as fractures of the femur, tibia and fibula, pelvis and major spinal injuries, as these patients will be taken to an A&E department and after immediate triage become the responsibility of the medical staff.

The spine

The problem of low back pain has already been discussed. The other type of spinal injury you may encounter is commonly known as whiplash or post traumatic neck injury. The patient is sitting in a car when it is hit from behind, causing an extension–flexion injury to the neck. Often symptoms do not appear for 6–12 hours after the accident. When they do, the patient typically complains of pain and stiffness in the neck and shoulders, sometimes dysphagia and transient neurological symptoms such as numbness and tingling. Unfortunately many patients continue to suffer symptoms for lengthy periods after the accident, even though there are no obvious accompanying physical signs, which has led to suggestions of malingering, particularly where compensation claims are involved.

A study by Mayou and Bryant (1996) of a sample of 74 consecutive adults attending A&E in Oxford who were diagnosed with post traumatic neck injury revealed that, of the 63 patients who could be followed up, 54% subsequently attended their GP with neck problems. The average age of the group was 31 years old and they were predominantly female, as has been found in other studies. Almost half the group (49%) reported neck complaints 1 year later, which they attributed to the accident. There was no association between physical symptoms and psychological characteristics or compensation proceedings in this group. A quarter of the group reported considerable impairment in their everyday life. These findings should be compared with an Australian study by Landy (1998), who reported that 70% of patients had settled within a few weeks but that for 30% there remained considerable pain and discomfort for lengthy periods of a year or more. His view is that excessive introspection due to lengthy legal proceedings and courses of physiotherapy leads to the prolongation of symptoms in some patients.

The hand and wrist

The hand is prone to injuries for obvious reasons and, as it has a good nerve supply, not only are injuries painful but they may involve damage to the nerve fibres themselves. The hand is usually in a dependent position, therefore gravity will exacerbate any soft-tissue swelling occurring as a result of injury. Finally, such is the peripheral nature of the hand that the blood supply can easily be compromised in trauma. These obvious fundamentals should be borne in mind whatever injury to the hand is involved.

Crush injuries to the tip of the finger are common and painful. These may involve fracture of the distal phalanx; however, the soft-tissue injury is more important than the fracture and the focus should be on successfully healing the wound without infection. Closed fractures of fingers are painful but usually involve little or no displacement. If fingers are immobilized for any period of time, stiffness rapidly becomes a major problem and 3 weeks should be considered the absolute maximum time for any finger to be immobile. Stiffness is less of a problem if the fingers are immobilized in extension and the metacarpophalangeal joints in flexion (Crawford Adams and Hamblen 1992), but the 3-week rule should still apply.

Dislocation of an interphalangeal joint in the finger is a common problem, especially in sporting injuries. It is usually caused by forced hyperextension and may have already been reduced at the scene of the accident by a sharp pull. Chronic strain of the interphalangeal joint capsule may occur due to forced lateral movement of the joint. This can cause pain lasting for several weeks, even though no bony injury has occurred. The patient may present with the tip of their finger flexed and unable to straighten it. This is known as mallet finger and is due to a rupture of the extensor tendon where it inserts into the distal phalanx or an avulsion fracture at the insertion of the tendon (Figure 12.5). An avulsion fracture means that the tendon (or ligament) has pulled a small piece of bone off the bone to which it normally attaches.

Fractures of the metacarpals are usually confined to the fifth metacarpal, just below the head. This is known as a boxer's fracture (perhaps a weekend fracture might be a more appropriate term given the usual time such individuals present) and is usually caused by punching. There may be significant

angulation of the fracture and, if in excess of 30°, this requires manipulation by an orthopaedic surgeon.

Injuries involving the thumb are particularly serious as, without the thumb, a large part of the function of the hand is lost. A fracture may run across the base of the first metacarpal or, in the case of a Bennet's fracture, run through the base of the first metacarpal and involve the joint (Figure 12.6). As we have already seen, fractures involving joints are significant due to the long-term possibility of OA caused by disruption of the normal joint structure.

The carpal bones of the wrist are all at risk of fracture due to a fall on the outstretched hand, although conventional wisdom states it is usually the scaphoid which fractures. However, this injury is notorious for failing to show on radiography, which prompted Brown (1995) to carry out bone scans on 36 patients who clinically had a fractured scaphoid with no evidence of a fracture on the initial X-ray. He found 18 fractures amongst these 36 patients, but only 3 involved the scaphoid. Nine involved other carpal bones and a further 6 patients had fractures of the distal radius. Complications arising from an untreated scaphoid fracture include delayed union, malunion, avascular necrosis of the scaphoid and osteoarthritic changes in the wrist.

Injuries affecting the arm

A fracture of the distal 2–3 cm of the radius is a common injury after a fall on the outstretched hand and in the classic Colles fracture involves a posterior

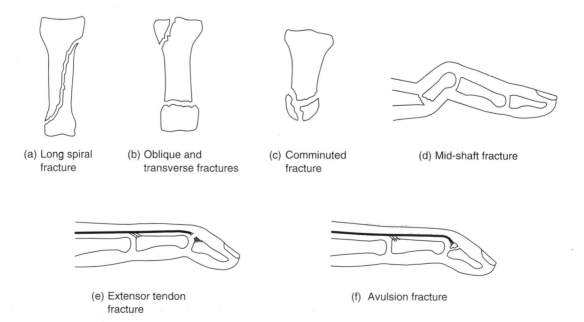

(a) Long spiral fracture

(b) Oblique and transverse fractures

(c) Comminuted fracture

(d) Mid-shaft fracture

(e) Extensor tendon fracture

(f) Avulsion fracture

Figure 12.5   Fractures affecting the phalanges

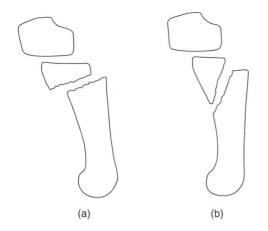

(a)   (b)

Figure 12.6 Fractures of first metacarpal: (a) through the base of the metacarpal, and (b) involving carpal–metacarpal joint (Bennet's fracture)

displacement of the lower fragment. The fracture may also be impacted and typically occurs amongst late middle-aged and elderly patients.There are several complications of a Colles fracture, including median nerve compression due to the swelling involved, subluxation of the inferior radioulnar joint and rupture of extensor pollicus longus 4–8 weeks after the injury which leaves the patient unable to extend the thumb at the interphalangeal joint. The reverse injury – anterior displacement of the lower fragment – is called Smith's fracture and results from a fall on a clenched hand such as might happen to a cyclist. This injury is notoriously unstable and prone to displace in a simple cast.

Young children falling on an outstretched arm can also fracture the distal radius, frequently involving the epiphysis, which has potentially serious implications for fracture healing as deformity may result unless the fracture is correctly managed by orthopaedic surgeons. The current fascination with roller-blading has led to what has been described as an epidemic of distal radius fractures by some authors. O'Farrell *et al.* (1997) saw 110 children aged 4–14 with falls from roller-blading in a 6-month period: 68 sustained fractures, 49 of which were of the distal radius. Similar findings were reported by Spicer *et al.* (1996) whose sample included adults seen at a central London hospital. In 12 weeks, 29 patients were referred from A&E to the orthopaedic department with 23 fractures and 2 dislocations. In 14 cases the injuries involved the wrist and distal radius. Both O'Farrell *et al.* and Spicer *et al.* are severely critical of the ineffectiveness of expensive protective equipment sold as part of the roller-blading kit when it comes to preventing arm injuries.

A considerable degree of violence is needed to sustain a fracture of the shaft of the radius and ulna, so much so that if one bone is fractured, either the other will also be fractured or there will be disruption of the superior or inferior radioulnar joint. A fracture of the radial head may occur after a fall on an outstretched hand in a younger adult. The injury usually consists of a longitudinal crack running into the elbow joint with bleeding into the joint (haemarthrosis) which is painful and restricts the movement of the elbow.

Injuries involving the elbow can range from a simple fracture of the olecranon caused by a fall on to the point of the elbow to childhood injuries, usually associated with falling off walls or out of trees. A supracondylar fracture of the humerus is a likely result of such a fall and involves the lower fragment being displaced and tilted backwards. A range of serious complications may ensue from this injury, including median nerve damage and brachial artery occlusion in the immediate short term and deformity and loss of function in the long term associated with epiphyseal damage. The child may also fracture the lateral epicondyle of the humerus – an injury which may not be visible on X-ray due to the immature state of the child's skeleton and the involvement of epiphyseal cartilage. This too can lead to long-term deformity if not managed properly.

Fractures of the shaft of the humerus may be pathological in origin due to metastatic deposits or occur as a result of high-energy trauma. A more likely scenario that the nurse practitioner will encounter is the elderly woman who has fallen and suffered a fracture of the neck of humerus. Osteoporosis plays a major part in this injury, which may be a day or more old by the time you see the patient. This delay may be partly due to social factors and also may be attributed to the fact that a significant number of these fractures are impacted so that the arm may still move as one unit. Such old injuries have a characteristic pattern of bruising over the outer part of the upper arm below the fracture site.

Reference has already been made to chronic shoulder problems; acute injuries are common. Dislocation of the shoulder usually occurs as a result of a fall and is most frequently an anterior dislocation – the head of the humerus is displaced forwards and downwards through a tear in the joint capsule. The shoulder appears flattened and angular, having lost the normal rounded contour which is due to the head of the humerus. Damage to the axillary nerve can occur. Posterior dislocation is rare but can happen due to a severe epileptic fit, an electric shock or a violent force driving the humeral head backwards (Crawford, Adams and Hamblen 1992). The appearance is less striking than the usual anterior dislocation but the key sign is that the patient cannot externally rotate the arm even to a neutral position.

Violence to the shoulder such as a heavy fall can cause a subluxation (partial dislocation) or dislocation of the acromioclavicular joint. A fracture of the clavicle may result from a heavy fall, but usually this is an indirect injury as the person has managed to break the fall with an outstretched hand. A fracture of the scapula may occur due to direct violence but this is a rare injury.

Injuries affecting the leg and foot

Foot trauma usually involves the toes and is frequently a crush injury or the result of a longitudinal force (stubbed toe). The comments concerning finger injuries are equally valid for toe injuries (p. 173). Fractures of the metatarsal bones are usually due to heavy objects being dropped on them. Although painful, they are usually stable injuries and require little active intervention to promote healing.

An extremely common problem you will encounter is the sprained ankle. A sprain is simply a tear in some of the ligament fibres holding the joint together followed by an inflammatory response, hence the pain and swelling. The ankle joint has four sets of ligaments: anterior, posterior, medial and lateral, any of which can be damaged depending upon the mechanism of the injury. The most common injury involves inversion (adduction) which the patient describes as 'going over on my ankle' and this results in pain and swelling on the lateral aspect of the ankle. In a more severe injury the possibility exists of an avulsion fracture as the stretched ligament pulls a fragment of bone away from the lateral malleolus (Figure 12.7). It is possible in a high-energy accident for all of the lateral ligament to be ruptured, leading to a dislocation of the ankle, with the

possibility of coexisting fractures of the lateral and medial malleoli. The lateral malleolus can also be fractured by a direct blow.

A complex range of ankle injuries is possible with increasing force as various combinations of ligament rupture and malleolar fracture may occur, leading to disruption of the ankle joint and the risk of neurovascular impairment. More serious accidents such as these tend to occur as a result of road traffic, agricultural and industrial accidents. The risk of serious ankle injury in low-energy accidents has been shown to increase if the patient is seriously overweight (Spaine and Bollen 1996). In the study of Spaine and Bollen a serious injury was defined as joint disruption with more than one malleolar fragment requiring either internal fixation or manipulation under anaesthetic.

Patients who fall a distance of up to a few metres but land on their feet may suffer a compression fracture of the calcaneum. In falls from a greater height, the whole ankle joint may be disrupted. Alternatively the patient may suffer a compression fracture of a spinal vertebra.

The knee is prone to a complex array of possible injuries, of which dislocation of the patella has already been discussed (p. 173). Dislocation of the knee itself is a serious high-energy injury that should never be confused with dislocation of the patella. The patella may however be fractured by a direct blow.

A tear of the meniscus in the knee joint (semilunar cartilage) occurs as a result of a twisting injury with the knee flexed. This is a typical sporting injury,

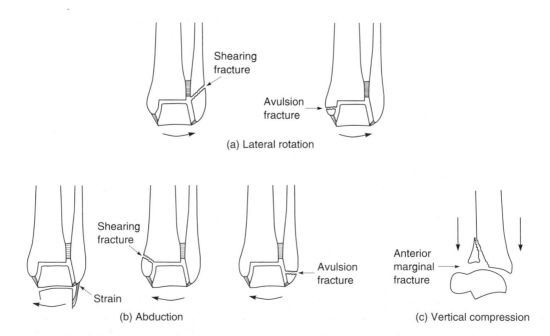

Figure 12.7 Fractures involving the ankle joint

especially in football. The medial meniscus is much more commonly injured than the lateral. It is accompanied by an effusion of synovial fluid. The individual finds it impossible to extend the knee fully and carry on with activity. The knee is painful and within 24 hours has become swollen. Subsequently the patient has further episodes of locking when s/he cannot fully extend the knee.

Knee ligaments can also be damaged. The injury may be a partial tear (sprain) or a complete rupture in more severe cases. It is usually the medial ligament which is sprained as a result of a force which abducts the tibia under the femur, the reverse injury produces a sprain of the lateral ligament. The joint is stable as the ligaments are grossly intact but, like the ankle, there will be localized pain and swelling. If violence is sufficient to rupture a medial or lateral ligament leading to a haemarthrosis, it may also tear the cruciate ligaments. A severe force pushing the tibia backwards relative to the femur may rupture the posterior cruciate ligament. A force acting in the opposite direction, hyperextension of the knee joint or the effects on the weight bearing knee of suddenly changing direction (typically a sporting injury) can rupture the anterior cruciate ligament.

A less dramatic knee injury is known as jogger's knee and is due to a combination of natural degeneration of the articular cartilage within the knee due to ageing and the repeated stress of jogging and road running. Not surprisingly, this affects people over 30 who do a lot of running on hard surfaces.

Tendons and muscles are prone to injury as a result of sporting activity. The Achilles tendon may rupture as a result of a sudden dorsiflexion of the ankle, making it a common injury in racket sports such as squash. There is a sudden sensation of being kicked in the back of the leg followed by pain. This injury is more common in men than women (M:F ratio 3:1) and typically occurs in the late 30s to early 40s age group (Levi 1997). The quadriceps tendon can be ruptured just above the patella by a forced flexion injury of the knee, such as falling on to a flexed knee. Muscles may also be damaged. Usually there is a tearing injury with the possibility of haematoma formation within the damaged muscle. Swelling and tenderness quickly occur and bruising becomes apparent after 24 hours. A common tearing injury involves the gastrocnemius muscle in the calf.

Taking a focused history

The patient's initial description of the presenting condition should in most cases make it clear whether this is a traumatic or non-traumatic problem. Occasionally the patient may complain of an injury aggravating a problem s/he has had for some time.

Where the patient presents with a non-traumatic condition, it is usually possible to focus on whether the problem involves joints, muscles or bones and, in cases of trauma, the patient will be able to indicate which structures are involved.

If the patient is complaining of a non-traumatic joint problem, the history should try and ascertain exactly which joints are involved as the pattern of joint involvement can be a key finding (e.g. in rheumatoid arthritis). How the condition affects the joints should be ascertained next. Important symptoms include pain, stiffness, swelling, redness and the effects on activities of daily living. The PQRST symptom analysis tool provides a useful framework and the list below shows some typical questions which could be asked about any joint symptom the patient mentions:

- Provocation/palliation: What brings on the symptom? (strenuous activity, work, repetitive movements) What relieves the symptom? (rest, heat, ice packs, elevation) OA tends to produce pain which is constant even at rest
- Quality: Is there redness, swelling or inflammation around the joint? How does the symptom affect function? Do you need a walking stick? How easy is it to stand up from a sitting position? Describe the sensation, is it tingling, numb, pins and needles?
- Radiation/region: Exactly which joints are affected? Does the pain radiate anywhere else? Does the funny sensation you describe in your wrist affect your fingers or go up your arm? If so, exactly where?
- Severity: How severe is the pain on a scale of 0–5? How much limitation in function is there? How far can you walk before walking becomes a problem? Does the symptom disturb your sleep and wake you up?
- Time: How long have you had the problem? Is it worse in the morning? At the end of the day? How long does it take for the symptom to wear off?

Joint stiffness is found in both inflammatory and degenerative joint disease while swelling around a joint strongly suggests an inflammatory disease process. Inflammatory disease such as rheumatoid arthritis is associated with a marked daily variation in symptoms which are worst first thing in the morning and last thing at night. A localized inflammatory lesion such as gout also produces severe throbbing pain which can prevent sleep and interfere with joint movement as a result of protective muscle spasm. Degenerative diseases such as OA do not show the classic diurnal pattern of rheumatoid arthritis. The pain and stiffness may be worst early in the morning, but they are present all day, even at rest and so will disturb sleep. Function gradually deteriorates over time.

A similar approach can be used if the patient is complaining of a more general skeletal problem such as backache. Pain associated with spinal nerve root disorder may be felt over a wide area of the body and the distribution should be carefully checked. For example, cervical lesions involving the C6 and C7 nerve roots typically result in pain affecting the whole chest wall: the patient should be asked to describe the distribution of low back pain. The onset of back pain is a key indicator as acute herniation of a disc produces pain of sudden onset, often while the patient is lifting or bending. OA and degenerative disc disease pain develop gradually over time.

The patient should be asked whether there are any problems with walking, pain on movement, unusual sensations or if any changes in body shape and contour have been noted. In the case of a woman, she should be asked whether she is postmenopausal in order to assess the risk of osteoporosis.

General questions about whether the presenting problem is confined to a joint(s) or is skeletal in nature include:

- Current medication: drugs such as steroids and hormone replacement therapy have a direct bearing on musculoskeletal problems, together with other non-steroidal anti-inflammatory drugs (NSAIDs) that the patient may be taking without a prescription. Diuretic therapy can also precipitate gout
- Past medical history: key points include known orthopaedic disease such as osteoporosis or OA, previous trauma and skeletal deformities
- Family history: the presence of conditions such as rheumatoid arthritis, OA and ankylosing spondylitis in the family should be established
- Social history: occupational hazards can predispose to certain conditions such as back pain (poor posture, lifting) whilst sporting activities may predispose to others (e.g. jogger's knee). Diet, weight and exercise levels should be checked, together with tobacco and alcohol use. These areas are particularly important when dealing with OA and osteoporosis

It is possible that the history presents a bizarre picture of generalized joint and back pains which are constant or rapidly changing, do not fit any logical pattern and are unassociated with other objective signs such as joint stiffness and swelling. This raises the possibility of psychological problems rather than organic disease.

In traumatic conditions it is important to obtain a clear history of the mechanism of the injury and the forces involved, as well as the time since the injury. It may require a little coaxing to obtain this history and possibly the assistance of an eye witness, as the accident will probably have happened suddenly and when the patient's attention was on other things, such as where to pass the ball in the case of a sporting injury. By reconstructing the strength and direction of the forces involved, the nurse practitioner can obtain a good idea of the injury and its severity. For example, someone walking along the pavement and stumbling over an uneven paving stone is likely to have sustained much less of an injury to the ankle than a footballer running headlong into a crunching tackle.

Patients with ankle injuries will sometimes mention hearing or feeling a crack at the time of the accident. Some may interpret this as evidence of the bone breaking. A study of 464 patients by Reid et al. (1996) showed that there was no association between patients reporting a cracking sound or sensation and any increased probability of fracture. A report of hearing a cracking sound is of no significance in taking the history from a patient with a low energy injury of the ankle.

Pain and swelling are common features and the patient should be carefully questioned concerning these symptoms, together with others such as alteration in sensation which might suggest peripheral nerve involvement. This is particularly true if the injury is not fresh. The PQRST approach will be useful, as this tool directs the nurse practitioner initially to find out what caused the injury and what has been done by way of first aid and subsequent symptom relief. The nature of the pain/swelling, the affected area, severity and time since the accident naturally follow on in this sequence. Loss of function after the injury should also be assessed. It is important to relate this to function before the accident to gain a clear picture of the impact of the injury. This is especially important in elderly people.

The history should include significant medical history, including allergies, and note any medication. This is essential: for example, advice about analgesia for minor injuries must take into account the risks of taking NSAIDs if the patient is asthmatic or has a history of peptic ulceration. If the patient happens to be an insulin-dependent diabetic, this should be taken into consideration in the care provided whilst any allergies to plasters should be determined *before* the patient with a finger injury has the fingers strapped together!

Social and occupational history should also be noted as treatment may present significant problems. A cast for a Colles fracture may make walking with a zimmer frame difficult for an elderly patient, whilst a single mother with a young child, a self-employed window cleaner or mechanic may be unimpressed with advice about the need for initial rest and elevation in dealing with a sprained ankle. A more realistic, negotiated approach will be needed – see later in the treatment section.

Physical examination

General principles

The examination begins when the patient is first met. Observe the patient's posture, manner and gait for any obvious clues. Although the patient history may focus on one particular joint or limb, such is the generalized nature of many conditions that you should ensure a thorough physical examination has taken place focusing on inspection and palpation, testing range of joint movements and carrying out other procedures to test the functioning of associated structures such as ligaments, nerves and tendons. In cases of trauma the examination should include the whole limb as there may be more than one injury. Injuries elsewhere to the body must also be excluded once the injured limb has been examined if for no other reason than good medicolegal practice. In non-traumatic conditions, the examination should assess whether there are any other systemic effects of the disease process, checking for example whether the patient is pyrexial or has circulatory problems. When carrying out the exam you should remember that many orthopaedic conditions and injuries are extremely painful. Palpation, range of movement assessment and other tests should therefore be carried out with great care.

Inspection should reveal whether there are any swellings, signs of inflammation, deformities, skin changes, nodules or other abnormalities. Palpation helps to identify swelling and inflammation (warm feel) and will also pinpoint areas of tenderness. Localized bony tenderness is the cardinal sign of a fracture and, if present, should be assumed to indicate a fracture until proved otherwise. Range of movement should be assessed when performed actively by the patient and then passively by the nurse practitioner.

A goniometer is useful for accurate measurements and movements should be recorded from the neutral positions described in the classical anatomical position, except that the hands should rest by the side with the palms against the thigh and the feet firmly placed on the ground at 90° to the leg (Munro and Edwards 1995). If any joints have a restricted range of movement, *gentle* passive movements may be performed whilst palpating the joint for any unusual sensations or evidence of crepitus, which usually indicates roughened articular cartilage (OA) or, if felt over tendons, inflamed tendon sheaths.

Palpation may reveal the presence of osteophytes around a joint as a hard swelling. A soft, warm, generalized swelling indicates synovitis and a synovial effusion within the joint capsule may coexist with the inflamed synovial membrane. If palpation elicits tenderness, try and be as specific as possible in placing the tenderness as this indicates which structures are involved – a bursa, tendons, intra-articular structures or the bone itself, indicating osteomyelitis or a fracture.

In carrying out passive joint movements, pay particular attention to the feel of the joint when the maximum range of movement is achieved. A hard end feel, i.e. an abrupt stop, indicates bone disease affecting the joint (OA) whereas a soft end feel, i.e. an elastic end to the range of movement, indicates soft-tissue problems such as a cartilage or other intra-articular structure. If a joint capsule or ligament has been sprained it will be painful to both active and passive joint movements which stretch the damaged ligaments and movement will be restricted by the pain. Movement which relieves the tension on the damaged ligament will be possible. Tenderness will be found over the swollen area and a joint effusion is likely if the joint capsule is intact. A dislocated joint due to trauma will be painful and have little movement.

If the tendon sheath is involved (tenosynovitis), the inflammation and swelling will cause limitation of active movement and possibly crepitus over the sheath. Passive movement will still be possible. Rupture of a tendon (e.g. Achilles) will mean that the patient cannot carry out active movement, although passive movement remains possible. In muscle injuries, any contraction of the muscle, with or without movement, causes pain.

Regional examination

The spine

Ask the patient to remove all clothing from the upper half of the body and trousers or a skirt to permit a full examination of the spine. Privacy is essential. Spinal posture and alignment should first be viewed with the patient upright and then bending forward, attempting to touch the toes. Asking the patient to bend forward not only allows assessment of flexion but makes a scoliosis more apparent. Range of movement in the neck can be tested by asking the patient to look right and left (rotation) then to tilt the head forward, trying to touch chin on chest and then tilt backwards while finally moving the head from side to side to test lateral movement. Loss of lateral movement is most likely to occur in cervical disease and may indicate degenerative changes such as OA. Sit behind the patient, stabilizing the hips with your hands and ask the patient to bend sideways to left and right (lateral movement), then backwards (extension) and finally to rotate about the hips by twisting first the left and then the right shoulder forwards. OA and ankylosing spondylitis are most likely to cause a reduction in the range of movement of the spine. Any scars from previous surgery or other spinal abnormalities should be noted at this stage.

The spinous processes and bony contours of the spine should then be palpated with the thumb, checking for tenderness and abnormal protrusions. If none are detected, the spine may be percussed by gently thumping with the ulnar aspect of the fist. This may identify tenderness associated with osteoporosis or malignancy not apparent on palpation. This should be followed by palpating the paravertebral muscles. If palpation identifies tenderness between L4 and L5 or L5 and S1, this suggests a herniated intervertebral disc, while tenderness over the sacroiliac area is associated with ankylosing spondylitis.

If the history involves low back pain, the patient's ability to straight-leg raise should then be tested (Figure 12.8). S/he should lie on a couch and raise each leg in turn as far as it will comfortably go. The nurse practitioner then repeats the movement passively for the patient, dorsiflexing the foot at the end of the manoeuvre. If the patient experiences sharp pain radiating down the leg in an L5 or S1 distribution, this indicates that a herniated lumbar disc is probably compressing the relevant nerve root as the leg is raised. Dorsiflexion of the foot increases the pain under these circumstances. The patient may

also experience pain in the affected leg when the other leg is raised. This is a positive crossed straight-leg raising sign (Bates 1995).

If there is doubt about the authenticity of a positive straight-leg raising test, the patient may be asked while lying flat to sit upright to permit examination of the back. This manoeuvre is only possible if there is no sciatic nerve root irritation. Alternatively the patient can be asked to sit on the side of the couch with legs over the side to test knee jerk reflexes. If the knee is extended in this position as if to test ankle jerk reflexes, this is the equivalent of a straight-leg raise; consequently the patient should experience pain and lean backwards to relieve the tension on the nerve root. Failure to respond in this way suggests that the individual is malingering (Munro and Edwards 1995).

If there is L5 and S1 nerve root irritation, a range of neurological signs will be present. These include inability to walk on the heels (L5) and loss of ankle jerks plus inability to walk on tiptoe (S1). These may be tested for if nerve root irritation is suspected as a cause of low back pain.

It is possible that a lumbar disc may have prolapsed at a higher level (L2–L4) which will affect the femoral

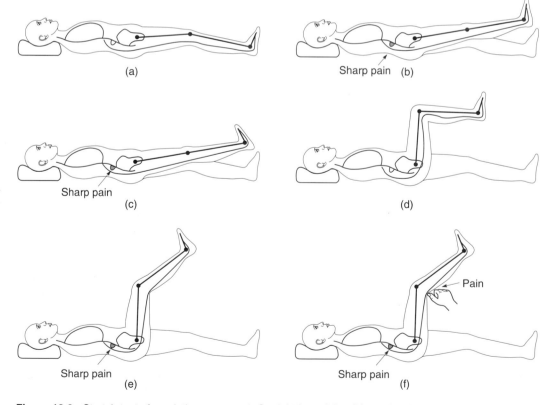

Figure 12.8 Stretch tests for sciatic nerve roots. Straight leg raising (b) restricted by pressure of prolapsed disc on nerve root, made worse by dorsiflexion of foot (c). Flexion of knee (d) relieves pressure but subsequent extension (e) increases pressure causing pain radiating to back. Pressure over centre of popliteal fossa exacerbates pain in back and causes localized pain (f)

nerve. This may be tested by asking the patient to lie face-down on the couch (prone), gently flexing each knee in turn and then extending the hip with the knee still flexed. The test should stop as soon as the patient reports any pain (Figure 12.9).

It should be remembered that, for many patients with a history of back pain, no obvious cause can be found on examination.

The upper limb

The patient's history should act as a guide to ensure that the examination is concise and relevant. It is a useful principle in examining either the upper (or lower) limb always to examine the unaffected side first for comparison. The basic stages of inspection, palpation and assessing movement apply whichever area of the upper limb is involved.

Inspection of the hand and wrist should be guided by the history and presenting complaint. It should also document the metacarpophalangeal and inter-phalangeal joints, noting any abnormalities such as ulnar deviation of the fingers or swan-neck deformity (flexion of the metacarpophalangeal, extension of the proximal interphalangeal and flexion of the distal interphalangeal joints) found classically in rheumatoid arthritis. Any areas of redness, swelling or abnormal alignment of the fingers should be noted (e.g. mallet finger). The swelling and deformity of a displaced fracture of the distal radius are obvious but there may be little to see with a scaphoid fracture.

Palpation will demonstrate the hard, small bony fragments (osteophytes) characteristic of OA which are found at the interphalangeal joints or the soft,

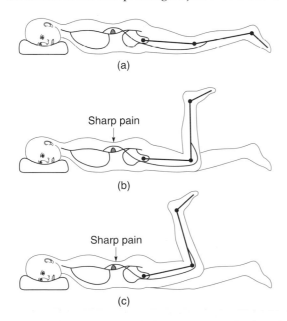

(a)

Sharp pain

(b)

Sharp pain

(c)

Figure 12.9 Stretch tests for femoral nerve. Flexion of knee (b) or flexion of knee and extension of hip (c) cause pain as femoral nerve roots are tightened.

rubbery joint swelling that indicates synovitis. Tenosynovitis frequently produces palpable swelling over the affected area. The wrist bones and distal radius should be carefully palpated for localized bony tenderness if the patient's history indicates a fall on an outstretched hand. The scaphoid can be palpated in the anatomical snuff box – the hollow at the base of the thumb just distal to the end of the radius. The ulnar styloid should also be palpated where a distal fracture of the radius is suspected, as this may also be involved.

The ability to reach 90° of flexion or extension of the wrist joint may be assessed by asking the patient to place the backs of the hands together and then raise the arms or the palms of the hands together and lower the arms respectively. Gross finger movement can be assessed by asking the patient to make a tight fist and then open out the hand, fanning out the fingers and thumb. Arthritis, tenosynovitis or Dupuytren's contracture (fibrosis of the palmar fascia) all prevent the patient from being able to make these movements. When asked to hold out the fingers, the patient may show a pronounced droop of the ring and little fingers, indicating rupture of the respective extensor tendons. This is a complication of rheumatoid arthritis.

The median nerve is prone to compression, due to its passage through the narrow carpal tunnel (carpal tunnel syndrome). If the history is suggestive of carpal tunnel syndrome, the patient should be asked to press the backs of the hands together (flexing the wrists to 90°) and hold this position (Phalen's test). This compresses the median nerve and is positive if numbness and tingling develop over the distribution of the median nerve.

The motor branch of the median nerve supplies the thenar muscles, allowing abduction of the thumb, while the ulnar nerve permits adduction. The effectiveness of the motor branch of the median nerve can be tested by asking the patient to place the thumb across the palm of the hand and then abduct it against resistance (compare with the unaffected hand). The motor branch of the ulnar nerve can be tested by asking the patient to hold a card between the thumb and the radial side of the second fingers. In the normal hand the thumb will be held straight but in the abnormal hand the thumb will flex at the metacarpophalangeal and interphalangeal joints due to weakness of the adductor muscle. The ability to elevate the thumb into the hitch-hiking position depends on having a patent extensor pollicus longus tendon. Inability to perform this manoeuvre suggests a problem with this tendon. Rupture occurs as a later complication of a Colles fracture or rheumatoid arthritis.

The sensory distribution of the median, radial and ulnar nerves in the hand is described on p. 173. Any suggestion of numbness or tingling associated with an injury to the wrist or arm should be checked by assessing pinprick sensation in both hands with the patient's eyes closed. The motor branch of the radial nerve permits wrist extension, therefore a wrist drop would suggest damage to this nerve. The ulnar and median nerves have been discussed above.

Examination of the elbow should pay particular attention to the olecranon, noting whether there is any swelling suggestive of olecranon bursitis or signs of inflammation. The arms should be examined from behind with both the elbows fully extended as this will reveal any deformity in the elbow joint. Palpation may reveal tenderness over one of the epicondyles, suggesting tennis elbow or synovitis and a joint effusion within the elbow, depending on the history. It may also detect any nodules within an olecranon bursa, other irregularities associated with the joint, or the localized bony tenderness indicative of a fracture. The radial head in particular should be carefully palpated after a story of falling on an outstretched hand as it may be fractured.

The normal elbow may show slight hyperextension beyond the neutral position and should be capable of 150° of flexion. The patient should then be asked to hold the elbows by the sides flexed at 90° and then required to demonstrate full pronation and supination of the forearm. Restricted movement indicates probable arthritic changes within the joint.

Serious injuries of the elbow should always be assessed for evidence of neurovascular compromise before referral on for medical management. Assess sensation in the ulnar, median and radial nerve distributions and check that there is a good radial pulse.

The shoulder is a complex joint and inspection should include comparison of both shoulders to assist detection of any visible abnormality. There may be muscle wasting caused by lack of use due to arthritis or frozen shoulder syndrome or, conversely, the shoulder may appear enlarged as a result of swelling associated with synovitis and joint effusion. Dislocation alters the contour of the shoulder, leading to a flattened appearance (p. 175). Bruising after a fractured neck of humerus may become obvious some 24 hours later and track down the upper arm over the next few days.

Palpation should include the acromioclavicular and sternoclavicular joints. It may reveal a soft, boggy tender area characteristic of synovitis or the hard irregularities of OA (osteophytes). Supraspinatus tendinitis (leading to painful arc syndrome) causes localized tenderness over the shoulder tip and in the subacromial space. If the axillary nerve is damaged in a dislocation, it will produce a paralysis of the deltoid muscle and a small area of anaesthesia on the outer part of the upper arm. This area should always be checked for sensation in suspected dislocations.

The shoulder is capable of a wide range of movements so a structured approach is necessary to test range of movement. Initially ask the patient to raise the arms straight above the head, then lower them to touch the back of the head; then drop the arms to the sides and touch the back between the shoulder blades. If this is pain-free the patient may be asked to hold the arm by the side with the elbow flexed at 90° and rotate the upper arm outwards to test rotation within the shoulder joint. Failure to get beyond half the normal range of rotation indicates a frozen shoulder. The patient should be able to swing the arm forward parallel to the body up to at least 90°. Osteoarthritic changes will restrict movement, particularly in this latter direction, and also in abduction. Painful arc syndrome has already been discussed (p. 172) and will be apparent when the patient attempts to abduct the arm away from the side of the body (see Figure 12.3 on page 172). If the patient is unable to initiate abduction at all, this indicates complete rupture of the supraspinatus tendon. This may be confirmed if the arm is passively elevated to about 45° from the side as, from this position, due to the mechanics of the shoulder, the patient will be able to continue abduction unaided.

The lower limb

The patient's gait, observed as s/he walks into the consulting room, may reveal significant information. Two common abnormalities due to musculoskeletal problems are:

- Pain-relieving hip gait, usually seen in OA: the patient only takes short steps when weight-bearing on the affected side and leans the body over to that side in order to reduce the load on the painful hip
- Trendelenburg gait: this rolling gait is caused by either an unstable hip joint or inadequate abductor muscles. The Trendelenburg test will be positive at every step (p. 186)

There are other abnormal gaits, such as the scissor gait of cerebral palsy where the abductor spasm makes the legs cross over each other. Drop-foot gait is due to a nerve palsy or a lumbar root lesion causing the toes to point downwards and the person therefore has to raise the knee unusually high to compensate. The nurse practitioner will be familiar with the gaits of individuals who are hemiplegic or who have parkinsonism.

After observing the gait for any abnormalities, the feet and ankles should first be inspected for deformities, lesions such as bunions or signs of localized pressure indicated by callus formation. Attention should be focused on the toes and metatarsal heads in particular. Palpation over the metatarsophalangeal joints may demonstrate tenderness, indicating synovitis (tenderness on compression of the metatarsophalangeal joints is an early sign of rheumatoid arthritis) whilst a tender, inflamed area over the first metatarsal head indicates gout. Palpation of the injured ankle should attempt to distinguish between a tender swollen area indicative of a sprain and the localized bony tenderness of a fracture, usually involving the medial or lateral malleolus. If there is extensive swelling, this may be difficult. The history will act as a guide towards the possibility of a fracture, depending on how much force was involved, together with the weight and age of the patient. The Ottawa ankle rules are a useful guide in deciding whether radiography is indicated after clinical examination and are discussed on p. 188.

The active and passive range of movements of the ankle (tibiotalar joint) should be noted (normally dorsiflexion 20° and plantar flexion 45° (Figure 12.10). The subtalar joint should also be tested by stabilizing the ankle with one hand (hold firmly the lateral and medial malleoli) whilst inverting and everting the foot by moving the heel with the other hand. Restricted and/or painful movement in any of these four directions will indicate which part of the joint is damaged. For example, sprained lateral ligaments cause pain on inversion as the injured ligaments are stretched but are pain-free on eversion as they are relaxed in this position. An arthritic ankle joint will be painful whatever direction it is moved in. The joints of the midfoot can be tested by stabilizing the heel with one hand and moving the rest of the foot by holding the metatarsophalangeal joints with the other.

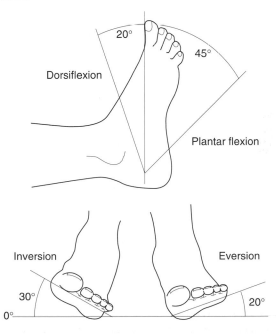

Figure 12.10 Range of ankle movements for normal ankle

The calf-squeeze test is a reliable method of diagnosing a ruptured Achilles tendon. Ask the patient to kneel and squeeze the calf just distal to its maximum circumference. Plantar flexion of the foot should occur in response; if it does not, the tendon is ruptured. If this test does produce plantar flexion of the foot accompanied by localized tenderness in the calf, this suggests injury to the gastrocnemius muscle (avulsion of the medial head) rather than the Achilles tendon.

The knees should be inspected looking for evidence of quadriceps muscle wasting or swelling as revealed by loss of the normal hollows that surround the patella. Swelling adjacent to the patella is likely to indicate an effusion in the joint or thickening of the synovium whilst tenderness and redness suggest synovitis. OA tends to be associated with a non-tender swelling whilst prepatellar bursitis leads to a more localized swelling in front of the patella. A dislocated patella is obvious as the bone is displaced laterally and the knee is usually held in flexion.

Palpation of the knee must be performed carefully to detect one of several possible problems. Initially place a hand some 10 cm above the patella, spanning the leg with the thumb on one side and the second and third fingers on the other, gently compressing the leg and feeling the soft tissue. Gradually moving towards and over the patella will allow palpation of the suprapatellar pouch which should be checked for tenderness, softness or excess warmth, all of which indicate synovitis. A loose body may be detected at this stage of the examination: localized tenderness along the joint line of the knee suggests intra-articular pathology.

Palpate the tibiofemoral joint with the knee flexed at 90° and the patient's foot on the examining table. Palpation is best done by pressing with both thumbs along the tibial margin, starting at the patellar tendon and working outwards and around the joint. Tenderness within the joint indicates intra-articular pathology. The menisci are most likely to be damaged. Tenderness over the collateral ligaments suggests that one or the other has been injured. The patella should also be palpated.

Excess fluid in the knee joint (an effusion) may be tested for with the bulge sign. This involves asking the patient to extend the knee and then 'milking' the medial aspect upwards three times and tapping the lateral aspect of the patella. The effect of this procedure is to cause any excess fluid to return rapidly to the hollow area which lies medial to the patella. This backflow is clearly visible to the observer (Figure 12.11).

The range of movement in both knees should be assessed; normal is 0–150°. Quadriceps weakness may prevent the patient from fully extending the knee actively, indicating a long-term knee problem.

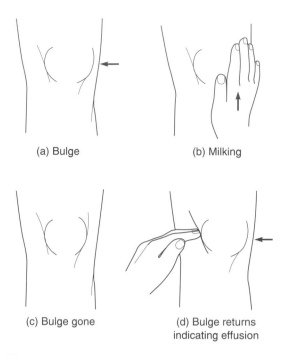

(a) Bulge   (b) Milking

(c) Bulge gone   (d) Bulge returns
                               indicating effusion

Figure 12.11   Bulge sign indicating an effusion in the knee joint

If there is a block to full extension (flexion deformity), this suggests an intra-articular problem such as a torn cartilage. Even full passive extension can be blocked in such a situation if the torn cartilage becomes displaced.

After the general knee examination described above, any of the following tests may be carried out if the history indicates they are necessary.

McMurray's test may be performed if a torn cartilage is suspected (history of knee-locking and/or injury associated with twisting on a flexed knee). The patient should lie on the couch with the hip and knee both flexed to 90°. If right-handed, the nurse practitioner should stand on the right side of the couch and grasp the heel with the right hand whilst steadying the knee with the left. The tibia should be externally rotated and the knee gradually extended whilst the left hand palpates the joint line. Repeat this with the tibia in internal rotation. If there is a torn cartilage the patient will experience some pain and a clunking sensation will be felt with the left hand as the cartilage is suddenly displaced. The patient should be warned in advance that this may be painful, as s/he should for the next two tests, described below.

Two other important tests for knee stability will examine the cruciate and collateral ligaments. The first is the drawer test for damaged cruciates (Figure 12.12). A history of a sudden change of direction on a weight-bearing knee, which is a common sporting injury, suggests anterior cruciate damage. Unfortunately this injury is often missed by doctors

carrying out initial examinations, despite a positive drawer test result. Bollen and Scott (1996) studied a sample of 119 patients with demonstrably deficient anterior cruciates who attended outpatient clinic and found that only 9.8% had been diagnosed by their doctors on initial examination, despite all having unequivocal physical signs and 90% having a typical history for this injury. This led to an average delay in diagnosis of 21 months. The test involves the patient lying down flat with the knee flexed and the examiner sitting on the patient's foot to anchor it to the couch. Check that the hamstrings are relaxed and then attempt to draw the tibia forward from the femur – this will test the anterior cruciate – and then push it backwards to check the posterior cruciate. No significant movement should be possible in either direction in a normal knee. Both knees should be compared in this way. Any abnormal laxity suggests damage to the anterior or posterior cruciate.

The collateral ligaments may be tested by lying the patient flat on the couch and wedging his or her ankle between the nurse practitioner's elbow and side (Figure 12.13). With one hand just below the knee and the other just above (on opposite sides of the leg), you should then attempt to abduct and adduct the femur by a sideways movement. Both legs should be tested and little or no movement should be possible. Laxity indicates damage to the appropriate ligament. Both the drawer test and the collateral ligament test should be painless, but if there has been injury to the ligaments, these manipulations can be painful. The nurse practitioner should therefore be careful when carrying them out and note the site of any pain reported by the patient.

One final test which should be used if the history is suggestive of patellar instability involves laying

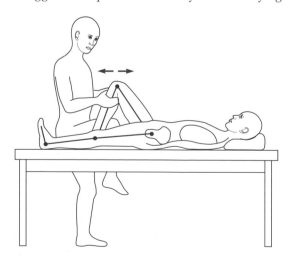

Figure 12.12   Testing cruciate ligaments. The examiner sits on the patient's right foot and draws the tibia forward (anterior cruciate) then attempts to push the tibia backwards (posterior cruciate). Compare the degree of movement of both knees. Hamstrings need to be relaxed for a valid test

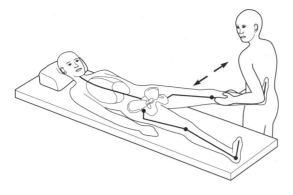

Figure 12.13   Testing collateral ligaments. Attempt abduction and abduction of femur while keeping the knee straight

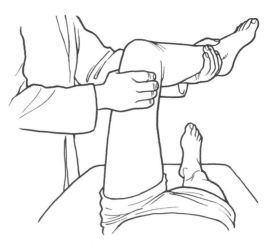

Figure 12.14   Testing external rotation of hip. The lower leg is swung medially while the thigh is held still. Reverse the test for internal rotation. Restricted movement indicates hip disease, especially arthritis

the patient flat and applying a gentle but firm pressure against the medial edge of the patella. The knee should then be gently flexed by the nurse practitioner up to about 30° while maintaining pressure. If there is patellar instability, abnormal laxity will be felt at the start of flexion. The patient's facial expression will indicate discomfort and a sensation that it is about to dislocate again. For this reason this is known as the patella apprehension test!

Inspection of the hip joint rarely shows anything of significance about the joint, although one leg may look shorter than the other. Measurement of limb length is essential as shortening may be apparent due to hip deformity rather than actual loss of bone length. If the patient is elderly and has a history of falling, particular attention should be paid to the injured limb. A fracture of the proximal femur usually produces shortening by about 2 cm and external rotation of the limb. Palpation will reveal tenderness associated with the fracture, although it may be the pelvis that has fractured rather than the neck of femur. The classic shortening and external rotation will not then be present.

If the person has normal hips, s/he should be able to pull each knee (flexed) up to the chest wall to demonstrate normal hip flexion. Restricted internal rotation of the hip is a strong indicator of OA and may be tested by asking the patient while lying on the back to flex both hip and knee joints to 90°. The nurse practitioner should hold the leg firmly just above the knee and grasp the ankle with the other hand. By swinging the lower leg medially, this tests external rotation of the hip, while swinging it laterally tests internal rotation (Figure 12.14). Abduction and adduction should be tested as these will also be restricted by OA. This is best done with the patient lying flat and the pelvis immobilized by holding down the opposite iliac crest to the one being tested. Abduction of 45° is normal and some 20° of adduction beyond the midline should be possible.

If OA is present the hip may have developed a fixed flexion deformity. This may not be apparent when lying the patient flat as s/he will adjust by arching the back to make the position more comfortable and therefore lying the leg flat on the couch. This will conceal the hip flexion deformity.

The nurse practitioner should therefore fully flex the opposite hip and knee which will restore the pelvis to its correct position, making the flexion deformity of the arthritic hip apparent (Figure 12.15).

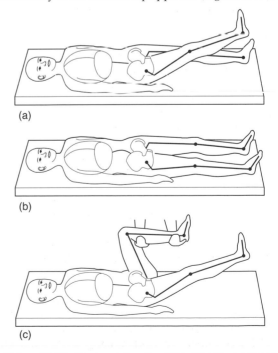

Figure 12.15   Flexion deformity of the right hip. Lordosis of lumbar spine may hide this (b) but full flexion of left hip (c) makes this apparent as lordosis is corrected

This is Thomas' test and will work even if both hips are affected. Thomas' test should be carried out if the history indicates OA of the hip.

Trendelenburg's test is a general assessment of hip function. Ask the patient to stand unsupported on one leg. This is only possible if the hip on the side off the ground is stable and has normal muscles surrounding it. Drooping of the pelvis on the side off the ground, which is apparent from the rear, indicates joint instability and/or muscle wasting (Figure 12.16).

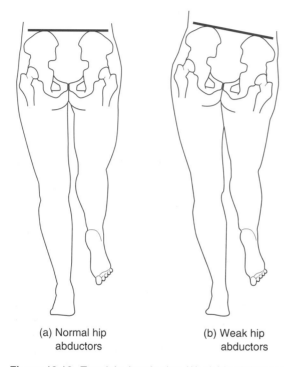

(a) Normal hip   (b) Weak hip
abductors   abductors

Figure 12.16 Trendelenburg's sign. Weak hip abductors mean that when the patient stands on one leg, the pelvis tilts down on the non-weight-bearing side

Differential diagnoses

A common problem is a patient complaining of a painful joint or joints. To differentiate between OA and rheumatoid arthritis, the guide shown in Table 12.1 will be useful.

Back pain is another common problem that may have several different causes. It will be helpful to differentiate between a mechanical cause (prolapsed intervertebral disc), postural problems and other organic causes.

A mechanical origin for the pain will be characterized by a history of sudden onset, previous recurrent episodes, unilateral distribution of symptoms and the pain will usually be eased by rest (Jenner and Barry 1996). True sciatica will produce neurological symptoms in the distribution of the affected lumbar nerve root.

Postural back pain tends to be more chronic with no obvious sudden onset and no neurological signs or symptoms. The history will give clues to poor posture.

Ankylosing spondylitis tends to be found in young men aged 15–30. The patient complains of back stiffness and pain that is worse first thing in the morning and it may be reported as moving from side to side. Chest expansion is restricted to less than 5 cm.

Systemic back pain suggests secondary deposits affecting the spine and therefore in addition to generalized symptoms such as malaise and weight loss there may be evidence of a primary affecting the breast or prostate.

Spinal stenosis affects people aged over 60 and is associated with pain on walking which is relieved by leaning forward.

One other important differential diagnosis lies between gout and an infection such as a septic arthritis as their appearance is similar. In either case the patient may be pyrexial and have a raised erythrocyte sedimentation rate as part of the generalized inflammatory response. A history of trauma, especially a penetrating injury such as a thorn or nail, tends to suggest infection as the diagnosis, whereas gout can be confirmed by microscopy of synovial fluid or tissue which will reveal the presence of urate crystals.

Investigations

Bloods

A patient suspected of having rheumatoid arthritis can have bloods taken for a range of tests, including rheumatoid factors (anti-immunoglobulins). However, as Akila and Amos (1996) point out, approximately 20% of patients with clinical disease are seronegative. The inflammatory nature of the disease leads to an elevated erythrocyte sedimentation rate. The drugs used in treatment tend to cause anaemia and therefore bloods to monitor the red cell count and haemoglobin levels should be taken regularly; this will usually be done by the clinic managing the patient.

An elevated erythrocyte sedimentation rate is a non-specific finding present in other inflammatory disorders such as gout. An elevated blood urate cannot be relied upon to confirm a diagnosis of gout (Snaith 1996).

In patients with suspected osteoporosis, bloods should be taken for serum calcium, phosphate and alkaline phosphatase and creatinine.

Radiography

Radiographic examination is a major component of

Table 12.1   Differential diagnosis of rheumatoid arthritis and osteoarthritis

Rheumatoid arthritis	Osteoarthritis
Usually affects younger patients under 40	Patient likely to be over 50
Affects multiple joints, usually in a symmetrical pattern, starting with swelling, stiffness and pain in the small joints of the hands and feet	Asymmetrical; larger joints affected
Joint shows signs of inflammation and is tender and boggy	Joint usually cool; osteophytes may be palpated (bony enlargements) and crepitus may be present
No relationship between weight and onset of disease	Obesity is a major risk factor for osteoarthritis of the lower limb
Stiffness and pain worse in the morning	No obvious relationship with time of day. Use
Pain present at night and at rest	causes pain in weight-bearing lower limbs; rest reduces pain. Affected upper limb is relatively free from pain as non-weight-bearing
ESR may be elevated	ESR usually normal
Constitutional symptoms such as fatigue, malaise and anorexia	No constitutional symptoms

ESR = Erythrocyte sedimentation rate

the diagnosis in OA, rheumatoid arthritis and, together with bone densitometry, in osteoporosis. The hospital orthopaedic clinic will usually be responsible for these investigations.

Radiography is highly important in the diagnosis of fractures and joint injuries and, now that progress is being made towards allowing nurses to order radiographs, the nurse practitioner needs to be aware of the basic rules to follow. (Chapter 13). In order to avoid unnecessary radiographs, most departments have protocols, but the presence of localized bony tenderness as the cardinal sign of a fracture should underpin decision-making in this field.

This is illustrated by the introduction of the Ottawa ankle rules (Figure 12.17). When trialled in eight Canadian hospitals on a total of 12 777 adults, they resulted in a major reduction in ankle radiography, reduced treatment times by an average of approximately 30 minutes and lowered costs by $90 (Canadian) per patient (Stiell *et al.* 1995). These rules can be successfully implemented by nurses, as has been shown by Salt and Clancy (1997). In their study an experienced A&E nurse was taught the Ottawa rules and saw a total of 324 ankle injury patients. The nurse sent 238 to X-ray and 48 of these patients were then shown to have a fracture. Of the 86 patients not sent for X-ray, none had a fracture, even though medical staff felt it necessary to X-ray 19 of them. Similar protocols can be developed for other common injuries.

Treatment

Rheumatoid arthritis and other inflammatory conditions

If you suspect that a patient has rheumatoid arthritis or some other inflammatory rheumatoid condition such as ankylosing spondylitis, a rapid medical referral should be made. A multidisciplinary approach is essential for the management of patients with these conditions and hospital-based clinical nurse specialists in rheumatology have made a major contribution towards such teams. The nurse practitioner in primary care always has a key role to play in terms of patient education and should be on the look-out for side-effects and drug interactions involving the sometimes powerful medications that may be prescribed by hospital specialists for the management of rheumatoid arthritis.

The patient should be encouraged to maintain the exercise programme prescribed by the physiotherapist (range of movement, muscle strengthening) and advised that weight-bearing exercise is beneficial, rather than something to be avoided (Ross 1997). The valuable role of the occupational therapist should be emphasized to the patient, particularly with regard to activities of daily living. Whatever subsequent consultations the nurse practitioner has with the patient, the rheumatoid arthritis should always be borne in mind when discussing care and every effort made to reinforce the work of the multidisciplinary team.

Gout will usually settle itself and an acute attack will probably only last a week or two. However, it is a painful and disabling condition, so treatment with NSAIDs is required. Snaith (1996) recommends naproxen or indomethacin as the drugs of choice. The side-effects must be reviewed carefully with the patient and, if gastric complications are a problem, colchicine should be used as an alternative. Aspirin should never be used in the treatment of gout. Snaith (1996) also advises that, as gout is often associated with heart disease and hypertension, the opportunity to review the patient's cardiac system should not be lost.

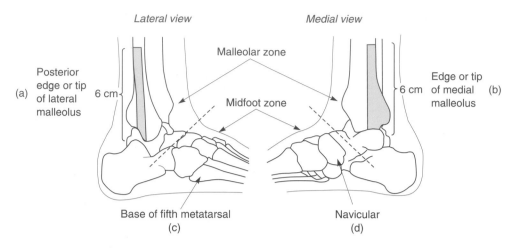

Figure 12.17   Ottawa ankle rules. Ankle X-rays are needed only if there is pain in the malleolar zone and any of the following: bone tenderness at (a) or (b); inability to bear weight both immediately and in A&E.
Foot X-rays are needed only if there is pain in the mid-foot region and any of the following: bone tenderness at (c) or (d); inability to bear weight both immediately and in A&E

Shoulder problems associated with rotator cuff disorders such as painful arc syndrome usually respond to rest and NSAIDs. If necessary, a mixture of local anaesthetic and corticosteroids can be injected into the subacromial bursa by a medical practitioner to achieve symptom relief. The same approach can be used with elbow problems such as tennis elbow. Frozen shoulder will usually respond to NSAIDs during the painful phase but a course of oral steroids may be needed if the pain is severe. Gradual mobilization and exercise will help recover function subsequently when stiffness is a major problem.

Osteoarthritis

This is another condition where a medical referral is required if you suspect its presence in a patient. Even after referral for surgery, the patient may experience considerable pain and disability while awaiting operation. The health education role of the nurse practitioner comes to the fore as every effort should be made to get the patient in the best possible condition for surgery and relieve symptoms as far as possible while on the waiting list. Pain management with paracetamol is preferable to NSAIDs as there are fewer side-effects. Weight loss and improved fitness are obvious targets in the obese as this will reduce wear and tear on all lower limb joints and also improve postoperative recovery. Weight loss is likely to reduce the risk of serious ankle fracture in all obese individuals in the event of a fall. Smoking cessation will be beneficial while waiting for surgery.

The psychosocial dimensions of care are important as isolation and depression are common problems. Efforts should be made to arrange for social support and to stress the positive side of things to the patient.

Nurse practitioners are developing in the specialist field of orthopaedics and they can have a major beneficial impact upon patients with OA, especially in preparing them for surgery.

Osteoporosis

The primary health care nurse practitioner has a major role to play in the management of patients with this condition. Treatment should always begin with prevention. Although it may not be easy to persuade a teenage girl to relate to a health problem that may not affect her for 40 years, there are real benefits to be gained from health education aimed at this age group. General health-promoting activities such as a healthy diet rich in calcium and vitamin D, weight-bearing exercise, avoiding smoking and discouraging an unhealthy obsession with weight loss and dieting will all help build up a stronger skeletal structure which will protect against osteoporosis in later life.

The menopausal woman may consult the nurse practitioner about hormone replacement therapy. This has a strong antiresorptive action and therefore preserves bone mass and density. Treatment with oestrogen for at least 5 years is necessary for real benefits, although there is a slightly increased risk of endometrial cancer (countered by progestogen) if treatment is continued for over 10 years (*British National Formulary* 1999). There is also a slightly increased risk of breast cancer. There are other benefits, such as reducing menopausal symptoms and the risk of cardiovascular disease and, as a result, the benefits outweigh the risks. In older postmenopausal women, oral calcium (800 mg daily) or a combination of calcium and vitamin D will help reduce the rate of bone loss. The York Centre for Review and Dissemination (1996) cites evidence showing that high-dose supplementation with vitamin D is effective in reducing fractures amongst the elderly with or without calcium supplements.

Treatment to reduce the rate of loss of bone mass should be combined with a strong health education message to ensure that women understand the benefits of calcium supplements in order to gain cooperation with the medication regime. Steps should also be taken to avoid falls. This requires reducing the risks in the environment, such as ensuring good footwear and avoiding obstacles such as rugs which could be tripped over. There is evidence that exercise such as balance training and home visits to assess and modify the home environment are effective in reducing the number of falls amongst the elderly (York Centre for Review and Dissemination 1996). Physical assessment should also investigate organic risks such as poorly controlled blood sugar levels and hypertension which may lead to dizziness and falls. Vision, balance and walking ability should be checked: if the person wears appropriate spectacles and uses walking aids as required this reduces the risk of falls. Health education plays an important part in this strategy and the nurse practitioner is ideally placed to work with elderly patients, particularly women, to reduce the incidence of fractures in osteoporotic bones.

Back pain

If there is evidence of neurological involvement, serious spinal pathology or a suspicion that the cause may be systemic, a medical referral should be made immediately. Simple backache with no obvious physical signs should be managed by advising the use of NSAIDs and heat or cold for pain relief. This regime is more effective than muscle relaxant drugs, which should be avoided in cases of low back pain (Jones 1997). Bed rest should also be avoided if possible and, if really necessary, should only be for a maximum of 3 days as lengthier periods do more harm than good (CSAG 1994). Advise the patient that activity is not harmful and will help to reduce pain, so early activity is encouraged. Discuss key activities such as lifting, sitting, sleeping and walking and offer health education advice. Prolonged absence from work reduces the probability of that person ever returning to work, consequently advise the patient to return to work as soon as possible. Physiotherapy should only be contemplated if this simple advice fails to improve the situation after a week or two.

The back pain school is an innovative approach to chronic back pain that has been pioneered in Sweden and is particularly suitable for nurse practitioner implementation. The idea consists of taking a group of patients and running four teaching sessions, covering the basic anatomy of the spine and associated structures, applied body mechanics and posture, ergonomics and relaxation techniques and exercises (Jenner and Barry 1996). In addition to learning from the nurse practitioner, patients can learn from each other in such a supportive environment.

The long-term problems of individuals with whiplash injury have been referred to on p. 173. Simple analgesics and a soft collar for neck support together with advice about the need for early mobilization will help most of these patients. The minority who suffer long-term problems, like those patients with chronic low back pain, experience significant social disruption and psychological distress. Avoid the temptation to label or stigmatize such individuals and remember the importance of the psychosocial aspects of care, particularly with respect to avoiding isolation and inactivity.

Trauma

The rest of this chapter will focus on minor injuries which you may be involved in managing. It is worth noting some general principles that apply to all injuries, starting with the fact that a minor injury can be painful and therefore by no means minor as far as the patient is concerned.

It is essential always to think beyond the front door of your minor injuries unit or health centre. Consider how, in the light of their injury and your treatment, the patient will manage to get home, how s/he will cope at home and what follow-up arrangements are needed. Discussing these matters with patients before they leave is essential in order to ensure that they will cope and that your treatment will stay in place and be effective, rather than disregarded as soon as the person gets home simply because it is not practical. A further point is to remember that it is not what is taught that counts, but what is learnt. You may feel you have given a comprehensive teaching session about the need to keep fingers mobile, but has the patient *learnt* what you have taught? You should check learning with one or two key questions and have a series of pre-printed advice slips to give to patients to take away and refer to later, as they may well forget what you have taught them. Finally, follow-up arrangements should always be given in writing to patients to be sure they do not make a wasted trip if confused about when they are coming back for a check-up or to see a doctor.

Hand injuries

A key principle in treating hand injuries is to concentrate on mobility rather than immobilization. This is because fingers can become stiff quickly and then require a great deal of physiotherapy to return to normal.

In crush injuries of the fingertip, attention should be paid to healing the wound rather than dealing with any comminuted fracture of the distal phalanx. Little can be done for the bony injury, but preventing infection in the fingertip is essential, hence this priority. A fingertip dressing with silver sulphadiazine cream (Flamazine) and a tubular bandage for the affected finger is recommended.

Undisplaced fractures of a phalanx can best be managed by simple analgesia and strapping the injured finger to its neighbour to act as a splint. Any rings should first be removed as these could act as a constriction around the injured finger if swelling occurs. The strapping must leave the joints free and there should be a piece of gauze between the fingers to avoid potential problems where the two areas of skin would be in prolonged contact. If Elastoplast is to be used as strapping, check first whether the patient is allergic. The patient should be encouraged to keep the finger as mobile as possible and dispense with the strapping when the finger is no longer painful. Mallet fingers should be referred for a medical opinion as if an avulsion fracture is present, an operative reduction and wiring will be needed.

If X-ray reveals that the fracture is displaced or it involves joint surfaces, a medical opinion is needed as manipulation may be necessary. The finger should be gently strapped to its neighbour as support, any rings removed and the hand placed in a high arm sling to reduce swelling as an interim measure while a same-day medical opinion is sought, usually from an A&E department. A simple dislocation of an interphalangeal joint needs reduction as soon as possible and gentle but firm longitudinal traction whilst pressing the base of the displaced phalanx is usually all that is needed. Entonox gas should provide sufficient pain relief for this to be accomplished. A check X-ray will confirm reduction and the patient should then be encouraged to mobilize the finger as much as possible. Whether the nurse practitioner carries out such a procedure is a matter for local determination. Dislocations of the metacarpophalangeal joints are potentially more complex and probably best left for medical management.

Fractures involving the metacarpals, once diagnosed, should be referred to A&E for medical management. If there is likely to be a significant delay before the patient attends A&E, a fracture through the base of the first metacarpal may be best managed by applying a plaster of Paris backslab to immobilize the thumb and wrist. This is particularly important if the fracture involves the first metacarpophalangeal joint (Bennet's fracture). The other likely fracture is of the fifth metacarpal and

temporary immobilization and support with a padded crêpe bandage should be carried out with the metacarpophalangeal joints flexed at 90° and the fingers extended. This position minimizes problems with immobility and may be attained with either a wadge of cotton wool or a rolled bandage applied to the palm and then bandaged in place. In either injury a high arm sling should be applied to reduce swelling and the patient given sufficient NSAID analgesia, such as diclofenac sodium (Voltarol), until an A&E visit.

Fractures involving the carpal bones or distal radius and ulnar should be referred on to the A&E department for management. If there is likely to be a delay in treatment, a plaster of Paris backslab should be applied to immobilize the wrist as this will give considerable pain relief, together with analgesia as described above and a broad arm sling. Patient teaching should emphasize the importance of maintaining finger movement and elevation and watching for any sign of neurovascular compromise. A printed set of plaster instructions explaining these points should be given to the patient. Traditionally, patients with a fracture of the distal radius and ulnar have been starved in case they need manipulation under anaesthesia. This practice is unnecessary where intravenous regional anaesthesia is used (Bier's block) and, as this is the technique of choice, keeping patients nil by mouth should be discontinued (O'Sullivan *et al.* 1996). A national survey by O'Sullivan *et al.* found that in the previous 12 months, no A&E department reported any complications involving the airway – the reason cited for starving – and 42% of departments had abandoned their fasting policy anyway.

Fractures and/or dislocations involving the forearm, elbow, upper arm and shoulder should be referred on immediately to the A&E department. The patient will be greatly helped if every step is taken to immobilize and support the injured limb in the best possible position. Rings and any other constrictions should be removed. A clear account of the injury should be telephoned ahead to the A&E department so that they know what to expect and, if any X-rays have been taken, they should accompany the patient. You will have to make a judgement as to whether an ambulance or private transport is best to transfer the patient. The neurovascular state of the arm should be carefully assessed to ensure there is no nerve or arterial damage and, if this is suspected, the patient's transfer to A&E should then become an emergency undertaken by ambulance. There is a case for a fasting policy where injuries are above the wrist if manipulation or operative surgery will possibly be required, as they are less suitable for the Bier's block technique. This is especially true in the case of children.

Trauma affecting the foot frequently involves heavy objects dropped on to the toes. A simple fracture of a toe can be managed as an undisplaced finger fracture, by strapping to its neighbour. Elevation to reduce swelling and pain is just as important; this involves the patient resting with the foot at least at the same level as the heart. Blunt trauma to the metatarsals which produces bruising but no fracture should also be managed by rest, elevation and analgesics. Recovery will be helped by the application of ice in the initial stages to reduce swelling. If a metatarsal is fractured, a medical referral is needed, although as Crawford Adams and Hamblen (1992) point out, subsequent immobilization in a cast is more for pain relief than to assist fracture healing.

If an ankle injury involves a fracture and/or dislocation, then A&E referral is necessary. Support, immobilization and elevation in the interim are essential to reduce swelling and pain. A plaster of Paris backslab may be needed if there is likely to be a delay in transfer. This can be quickly removed in the A&E department once the patient arrives. An alternative is to use a vacuum splint to immobilize the ankle, providing it is possible to have the splint returned to the minor injuries unit. The nurse practitioner should always check colour, sensation and the presence of a pedal pulse in the foot once immobilization is complete. It may help to mark the exact location of the pulse with a skin marker pen to assist future monitoring.

The large majority of ankle injuries will have no fracture and be diagnosed as a sprain. The traditional treatment involves tubigrip; this approach has recently been questioned. If the rationale is to control swelling and reduce pain, Kennet (1996) argues that tubigrip is of little value, as it fails to exert enough pressure to reduce oedema. A moment's reflection on the shape of the lower leg and the fact that standard tubigrip is all one size reveals part of the problem. If the tubigrip is wide enough to fit over the calf, it will not apply sufficient pressure at the ankle; if it is narrow enough to exert useful pressure at the ankle, it will be too tight over the calf. A graduated compression bandage as used in the management of venous leg ulcers is needed to control ankle oedema effectively, but this would prove much more expensive – possibly prohibitively so given the number of patients with sprained ankles treated every day. Perhaps the only value of tubigrip is psychological rather than physical.

Elevation and ice packs will probably do far more to reduce painful swelling than tubigrip. The use of NSAID analgesia is common in the treatment of sprained ankles but the patient should be made aware of the side-effects such as gastric irritation and hypersensitivity reactions, which are particularly important if the patient is asthmatic. Elevation and ice packs will reduce the need for analgesia. Early mobilization is beneficial for all joints and the ankle is no exception. The patient should therefore be encouraged to begin cautious weight-bearing and mobilization by the following day and the advantages of early mobility should be explained. Crutches should be discouraged as they tend to delay weight-bearing and require careful use if further problems are not to occur. They are also expensive and difficult to recover from the patient. It is possible that some patients may find that the ankle is too painful for weight-bearing even after a day or two. In such cases they should be checked by the local A&E department to ensure that no fracture has been missed and the ankle may require a few days of immobilization in a walking cast before the person can resume normal activity. This may be particularly important for social and economic reasons.

Minor knee injuries where there are no clinical signs of a joint effusion or trauma to a ligament or meniscus may be managed conservatively. Double tubigrip offers support which is probably more psychological than physical and the patient should be advised to rest the knee, take simple analgesics and return if it does not improve, whereupon a medical referral may be made. If the clinical signs suggest a significant injury, then an appropriate medical referral should be made.

A further important strategy in the management of trauma and low back pain is prevention. The nurse practitioner should lose no opportunity to explore the causes of accidents with patients and how they could have been prevented. Many injuries happen at work and could have been prevented by, for example:

- Wearing shoes with reinforced toecaps when working with heavy objects
- Keeping floors clear and dry to avoid trips and slips
- Training in good lifting technique
- Use of lifting aids
- Correct seating and work surface heights
- Good lighting conditions
- Use of protective guards on machinery
- Wearing protective equipment

The waiting room is a good area to convey messages across to patients while they are waiting for treatment, whether by posters, leaflets or even the use of videos and a TV set. Whilst larger companies have occupational health departments, nurse practitioners might usefully target small businesses where this is not the case and organize an accident prevention campaign with the local Chamber of Commerce or branch of the National Farmer's Union/Young Farmers' Club (NFU/YFC). For example, the nurse practitioner could help in the production of much needed literature that is relevant and in language that is easy to understand. S/he could also attend local Chamber of Commerce NFU/YFC meetings to discuss accident prevention and basic first aid.

The use of hip protector pads in the frail elderly can dramatically reduce hip fractures in nursing home environments. One study cited by the York Centre for Review and Dissemination (1996) found a reduction of over 50% in fractures as a result of wearing hip pads. How acceptable they would be to an elderly person living outside a residential home remains to be determined, but they do appear to offer considerable protection against hip fracture which, as we have seen, can carry a mortality rate of 25% in the elderly. The nurse practitioner would be an ideal person to explore their introduction at a local residential home as part of an accident prevention campaign.

Summary

The nurse practitioner has a major part to play in the triage and management of musculoskeletal conditions, whether traumatic or otherwise. The nursing approach to the problem should ensure that treatment takes into account the person's psychosocial well-being as well as the physical disease and/or trauma. Furthermore, the strong health education tradition within nursing means that the nurse practitioner is well-placed to tackle the whole preventive area. This is particularly the case in preventing osteoporosis, which is an issue that is relevant to women of all ages. A community-based accident prevention programme would be another area where s/he could make a significant difference, particularly in high-risk groups such as children (cyclists, roller-bladers), young men (work and sporting accidents) and the elderly (domestic accidents). The nurse practitioner can bring to the field of trauma an extra dimension that has been lacking from traditional A&E medical practice – accident prevention.

References

Akila M., Amos R. (1996) Rheumatism and arthritis: clinical diagnosis. In: Snaith M. (ed.) *ABC of Rheumatology*, London, British Medical Journal.

Bates B. (1995) *A Guide to Physical Examination*, 6th edn., Philadelphia, JB Lippincott.

Bollen S., Scott B. (1996) Rupture of the anterior cruciate ligament – a quiet epidemic? *Injury*, 27(6), pp. 407–409.

British National Formulary (1999) London, British Medical Association/Royal Pharmaceutical Society of Great Britain.

Brown J. (1995) The suspected scaphoid fracture and isotope bone imaging, *Injury*, 26(7), pp. 479–482.

Clinical Standards Advisory Group (1994) *Back Pain*, London, HMSO.

Crawford Adams J., Hamblen D. (1992) *Outline of Fractures*, 10th edn., Edinburgh, Churchill Livingstone.

Dandy D. (1993) *Essential Orthopaedics and Trauma*, 2nd edn., Edinburgh, Churchill Livingstone.

Jenner J., Berry M. (1996) Low back pain. In: Snaith M. (ed.) *ABC of Rheumatology*, London, British Medical Journal.

Jones A. (1997) Primary care management of acute low back pain, *Nurse Practitioner*, 22(7), pp 50–68.

Kennet J. (1996) Tubigrip, ibuprofen and home?, *Accident and Emergency Nursing*, 4, pp. 121–124.

Landy P. (1998) Neurological sequelae of minor head and neck injuries, *Injury*, 29(3), pp. 199–206.

Levi N. (1997) Incidence of Achilles tendon rupture in Copenhagen, *Injury*, 28(4), pp. 311–313.

Mayou R., Bryant B. (1996) Outcome of whiplash neck injury, *Injury*, 27(9), pp. 617–623.

Munro J., Edwards C. (1995) *Macleod's Clinical Examination*, 9th edn., Edinburgh, Churchill Livingstone.

O'Farrel D., Ridha H., Keenan P., McManus F., Stephens M. (1997) An epidemic of roller-blade injuries in children, *Injury*, 28(5), pp. 377–379.

O'Sullivan I., Brooks S., Maryosh J. (1996) Is fasting necessary before prilocaine Brier's block?, *Journal of Accident and Emergency Medicine*, 13, pp. 105–107.

Reid P., Aggarwal A., Browning C., Nicolai P. (1996) The relevance of hearing a crack in ankle injuries, *Journal of Accident and Emergency Medicine*, 13, pp. 278–279.

Ross C. (1997) A comparison of osteoarthritis and rheumatoid arthritis: diagnosis and treatment. *Nurse Practitioner*, 22(9), pp. 20–39.

Salt P., Clancy M. (1997) Implementation of the Ottawa ankle rules by nurses working in an accident and emergency department, *Journal of Accident and Emergency Medicine*, 14, pp. 363–365.

Snaith M. (1996) *ABC of Rheumatology*, London, British Medical Journal.

Spaine L., Bollen S. (1996) The bigger they come: the relationship between body mass index and severity of ankle fractures, *Injury*, 27(10), pp. 687–689.

Spector T. (1996) Epidemiology of rheumatic diseases. In: Snaith M. (ed.) *ABC of Rheumatology*, London, British Medical Journal.

Spicer D., Mullins M., Wexler D. (1996) Roller-blades: should they carry a government health warning?, *Injury*, 27(6), pp. 401–403.

Stiell I., and the Multicenter Ankle Rule Study Group (1995) Multicenter trial to introduce the Ottawa ankle rules for use in radiography in acute ankle injuries, *British Medical Journal*, 311, pp. 594–597.

York Centre for Review and Dissemination (1996) *Effective Health Care; Preventing Falls and Subsequent Injury in Older People*, University of York, NHS Centre for Review and Dissemination.

CHAPTER 13

Basic principles of diagnostic radiography

Scott Bowman and Charles Sloane

Introduction

This chapter will introduce nurse practitioners to the principles of radiography, and then review how accident and emergency (A&E) medical imaging is changing as health-care professional roles are developing. We will then discuss the interpretation of radiographs commonly produced in A&E practice. This is not a definitive text on A&E radiology; many such texts already exist and should be consulted if you want to learn more about this fascinating aspect of A&E work.

Basic principles of radiography

Radiography has traditionally been defined as the production of diagnostic medical images, and radiology as the interpretation of these images. It will be seen later that the boundaries between these two activities are blurring.

The main aim of radiography is to produce medical images which demonstrate the patient's injury with the least possible trauma to the patient. These images are usually produced using X-radiation; in some cases ultrasound and magnetic radiation are used. To demonstrate an abnormality, anatomy must be imaged in at least two planes, ideally 90° apart. Standard projections include anterior–posterior (AP), posterior–anterior (PA) and lateral. Sometimes oblique and angled views are taken. It is important that two views are taken as some abnormalities will not be demonstrated on a single view; even if they are, it will be difficult to estimate displacement.

Medical images produced by X-ray are called radiographs. Radiographs are possible because X-radiation passes through the human body and in so doing is differentially absorbed by various anatomical structures. In general the denser the material the X-radiation is passing through, the more it is absorbed. For example, bone will absorb more radiation than surrounding soft tissue. The radiation that is incident on the patient is a homogenous beam but when it passes out of the other side it has become heterogeneous due to differential absorption. This is shown in Figure 13.1.

The other factor which makes the production of radiographs possible is the fact that X-rays can be detected and recorded. In most cases this is achieved using photographic film and intensifying screens. The intensifying screens convert the X-radiation to light and this in turn exposes the photographic film. The more radiation that passes through the patient the more light is produced and as a result of increased film exposure, the darker the area of the radiograph. This is why on a conventional radiograph soft tissue appears darker than bone, which absorbs more radiation, and hence produces less light in the intensifying screens (Figure 13.2).

In practice, two intensifying screens are used one on either side of the film. Radiographs can also be produced without the use of intensifying screens

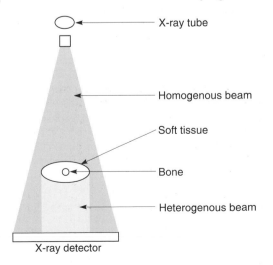

Figure 13.1 X-ray passing through soft tissue and bone

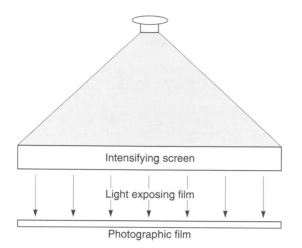

Intensifying screen

Light exposing film

Photographic film

Figure 13.2 How X-rays are detected and recorded

because photographic film is also sensitive to X-radiation, but without intensifying screens up to 1000 times more X-radiation would need to be used.

Some medical imaging departments are changing from a photographic system of recording the image to a electronic one. These systems use solid-state detectors rather than photographic film. The major advantage of this method is that the image data is in digital electronic form and can be manipulated. Image factors such as contrast can be changed after the image is produced without having to subject the patient to another dose of radiation.

Radiation protection

Most images in A&E are produced using X-radiation (X-rays). X-radiation is a form of ionizing radiation. As it passes through the body and is absorbed it produces free radicals in the body's cells. These free radicals are of high energy and can cause cell damage. At very high doses this can kill the cell; at lower doses the cell may become injured. The free radicals can also cause damage to the cells' DNA. This type of damage can cause cancer in the patient or if the cells are reproductive, even in the patient's offspring. Damage to DNA can occur with even the smallest doses of radiation but the higher the dose, the greater the damage. There is no such thing as safe exposure to X-radiation which carries zero risk. Not all cells are equally sensitive to X-radiation. Some cells, such as thyroid and gamete cells, are particularly sensitive and extra care should be taken when considering exposing them to X-radiation. Other cells, such as nerve cells in the spinal cord, are less sensitive but if damaged are incapable of replication, so again extra care is needed. Cells undergoing rapid reproduction tend to be sensitive and it is for this reason that special care is taken when irradiating a fetus or a very young child.

The basic principle of radiation protection is to keep the dose to the patient as low as reasonably practical (ALARP). To ensure the principles of ALARP are followed:

- Only radiographically examine a patient when the benefit from the examination outweighs any risk
- Follow codes of practice in force. Each medical imaging department will have local rules and protocols for radiation protection. There will also be codes of practice to follow in the case of female patients of reproductive capacity
- Where possible, obtain the required information from other sources, including old radiographs, clinical examination and ultrasound examination
- Where practical, use lead protection when radiographically examining patients

All radiographers are well-educated in radiation protection and will be happy to give advice on this subject.

The move towards an imaging team

In many respects nursing has led the way in role development, but other professionals including radiographers are also developing their roles. It is now common to find radiographers undertaking intravenous injection of radiological contrast agents, performing barium enema examinations and, in A&E units, reporting on films. Radiographers qualify with a BSc Radiography degree and many go on to undertake a masters-level qualification in medical image interpretation. It should be remembered that even the most junior radiographer has at least 3 years of experience in viewing radiographs and will have received formal instruction in this task. It is hoped that nurse practitioners will see the radiographer as a valuable resource that they can use to benefit the patient.

With the move towards role development, a new imaging team is developing within A&E which includes nurse practitioners. The changing role of health-care professionals in relation to A&E imaging is shown in Table 13.1.

Interpretation of A&E radiographs

The scope of this chapter does not allow a comprehensive description of all the pathologies one might encounter in the A&E environment. It will give an outline of the steps that must be taken for effective diagnostic decision-making. The further reading section mentioned at the end of this chapter provides a more comprehensive description of

Table 13.1   Changing role of health-care professionals in A&E imaging

Traditional role of the radiographer	New role of the radiographer
The traditional role was to validate requests from medical practitioners to ensure that they are valid for the injury and that the patient is exposed to the minimum amount of radiation. Traditionally, radiographers could not accept requests from nurses Once the radiographer had accepted the request for the examination, s/he had a duty to perform the examination. This duty included a requirement to do no physical harm to the patient, use the least amount of radiation and to offer psychosocial support to the patient through the examination	Like nursing, the degree to which roles have developed varies from one hospital to another. This section outlines the role of radiographers in a hospital where the radiographic role has been most developed The radiographer is still responsible for validating requests for radiographic examinations. Now it is also possible to accept requests from those who are not medically qualified, including nurse practitioners. Those requesting radiographic examinations should indicate the area to be examined, because part of the extended role is to determine exactly what examination to undertake based on the history given and physical examination of the patient. The traditional role of undertaking the radiographic examination remains unchanged Once the image is produced, the radiographer will give some interpretation of the radiograph to the person requesting it. In most hospitals this takes the form of a small red sticker placed on films where the radiographer believes that an abnormality has been demonstrated. Even when only the minimum scheme is in place, radiographers are always happy to discuss the radiographs with those requesting them. In some hospitals radiographers are reporting the radiographs they produce. These radiographers have been on a postgraduate course which allows them to undertake this role. In other hospitals the radiographer reports on the radiograph when it is returned to the medical imaging department. This was traditionally the role of the radiologist
Traditional role of the nurse	**New role of the nurse practitioner**
Traditionally the nurse played no formal role in the imaging of patients in A&E except to accompany seriously ill patients to the imaging department. Informally, nurses often gave advice to medical staff in relation to which radiographic examinations to request and the interpretation on the resulting radiographs	In terms of medical imaging the nurse's role is now greatly expanded. Nurse practitioners now examine the patient and determine if a radiographic examination is required. If this is the case, the nurse indicates the area to be examined and gives a full history to the radiographer. Once the radiograph has been produced the nurse, in consultation with the radiographer, makes an initial interpretation of the radiograph The nurse and radiographer should see the interpretation of the radiograph as a team task. Interprofessional rivalries should not get in the way of making the best possible interpretation of the radiograph for the sake of the patient. If the nurse and radiographer are unsure about the radiograph, then the imaging team should be expanded to include the casualty officer and radiologist
Traditional role of the casualty officer	**New role of the casualty officer**
Traditionally the casualty officer was responsible for determining whether the patient required a radiograph and then requesting such an examination. Once the radiograph had been produced it was the casualty officer's responsibility to interpret the radiograph	The casualty officer is still responsible for requesting radiographic examinations in cases where nurse practitioners are not involved. S/he is also responsible for making the primary interpretation of radiographs; within these bounds s/he will often make this interpretation in consultation with the radiographer and nurse practitioner
Traditional role of the radiologist	**New role of the radiologist**
Traditionally the radiologist gave the definitive interpretation of the radiograph. This was often done after the patient had been treated and left the hospital. In a few cases the radiologist was responsible for giving advice in the use of special imaging techniques such as CT or MRI and the interpretation of some radiographs	In many respects the role of the radiologist has not changed. The main difference is that now s/he shares much of this role with the radiographer and to a certain extent with the nurse practitioner. The radiologist still has an important role to play in terms of giving advice on special imaging techniques and providing reports on difficult cases referred by radiographers and nurse practitioners

common pathologies encountered and pitfalls to be avoided.

An accurate diagnosis can only be made if the correct steps are followed. This starts with the practitioner undertaking a number of vital tasks before the radiographic examination is even requested. Once the radiograph has been obtained the practitioner must possess the skills to examine it. This requires a check of the suitability of the radiograph for diagnosis and an ability to search it in a *systematic* fashion. The process of diagnosis continues when judgements are made regarding any abnormalities present on the radiograph, which means you must be able to recognize the normal appearance of the area under examination. The human body provides many traps for the fledgling diagnostician. A good knowledge of normal anatomy will save time and money and reduce distress caused by unnecessary treatment following a false-positive diagnosis.

Before requesting the radiograph

A comprehensive clinical examination of the patient and a detailed history are the first stages in the process. This information is then relayed to the radiographer undertaking the examination via the clinical indications section of the X-ray request card. The radiographer will then have all the facts needed in order to adapt the radiographic techniques to suit the particular situation. For example, examination of a patient with a badly injured elbow can vary enormously. A procedure designed to demonstrate a supracondylar fracture will be inappropriate if a fractured radial head is suspected. Incorrect technique can easily result in injuries being overlooked. The importance of effective communication between the individual requesting the examination and the radiographer, via the X-ray request form, cannot be overstated.

Examining the radiograph

The first consideration to be made relates to the adequacy of the image and whether or not it fulfils the criteria for diagnosis. This will involve the following stages:

- Check you have the correct radiographs for your patient by referring to the name marker on the image. (It is surprising how often patients' films become mixed up.) The date should also be checked as multiple images of the same body part may exist
- Check the left/right-side marker on the image to ensure that this tallies with the anatomy demonstrated and the site of injury
- Ensure all the region of interest has been included within the image. Ambiguous clinical indications

on the request card may lead to some important anatomy being excluded from the image
- Note if the film density is sufficient to demonstrate all the anatomy to a diagnostic standard within the region of interest

Once you are satisfied the technical factors used to produce the image are adequate you can proceed to search for a pathology. A systematic approach is of vital importance. A surprising number of images contain more than one pathology. The eye will be immediately drawn to the more obvious abnormality. Other less obvious pathologies may therefore be missed as you will be content to have detected the abnormality. If a rigorous and systematic search strategy is employed, the likelihood of missing important injuries will be reduced. Examples of such strategies are given below.

Lateral cervical spine

- Check the alignment of the vertebra. Figure 13.3 shows a number of lines used for this purpose. Trace a line coincident with the anterior and posterior margins of the vertebral bodies (lines A and B). The lines should be smooth and without deviation. Any steps or slippages of greater than a few millimetres could indicate a fracture or dislocation
- Examine the line formed by the facet joints (line C). The inferior articular processes of one vertebra should line up with the superior process of the vertebra below. If it does not, a facetal dislocation may have occurred
- Check the distance between the spinous process (D). If the distance between two spinous processes is significantly greater than the others, ligamentous damage may have occurred
- Trace the outline of each vertebra to look for fractures. Each body should trace a uniform box shape. Look out for wedge or compression fractures
- Examine the soft tissues immediately anterior to the vertebral bodies (E). An abnormal swelling may have been produced by haematoma formation resulting from a fracture. Remember that the prevertebral soft tissues normally widen below C4

The chest radiograph

The chest radiograph is a real challenge, owing to the wide range of pathologies potentially visible. This search strategy represents the simplest method:

- Technical factors: the appearance of the radiograph can vary greatly depending on how the image was obtained. If the examination was performed supine, fluid levels will disappear and the size of the mediastinum will alter. A small

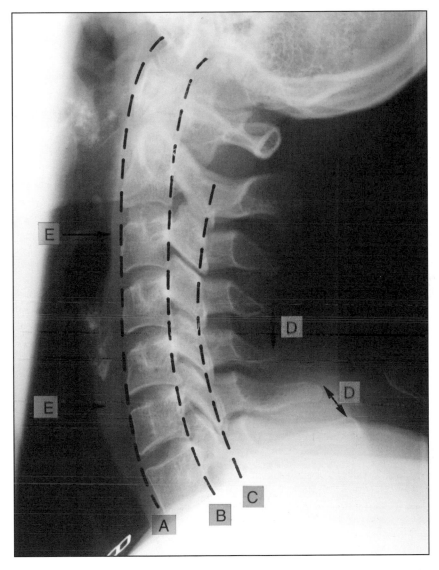

Figure 13.3   Lines used for assessing pathology on lateral cervical spine radiographs

degree of rotation may cause structures which are normally obscured by the heart to become visible. The vena cava is a good example. It will become evident as a line on the right side of the mediastinum if the patient is rotated to the left. The degree of rotation may be assessed by comparing the distance from the medial end of each clavicle to the midline. The phase of respiration will also have a profound effect on normal appearances, especially in the lower regions. The presence of six anterior ribs above the diaphragm indicates that the image was taken on inspiration

- The mediastinum: the diameter of the heart should be less than half the diameter of the chest at the widest point. The outline of the mediastinum should be smooth. A dark line running adjacent to the heart may indicate a pneumomediastinum. The whole mediastinum should be central within the chest, although the heart is situated with two-thirds of its diameter to the right of the midline as you view the image

- The lungs: the lungs should be of equal density. An increase in density, either generally or associated with one of the fissures, is indicative of a pathology such as infection. The blood vessels within the chest should be visible from the lung hilum to the chest wall. Absence of these vessels may indicate a pneumothorax. Pay particular attention to the lung apices if a pneumothorax is suspected

- Diaphragms: these should be smooth with clear costophrenic and cardiophrenic angles. Fluid may collect here as a result of an effusion

- The thoracic skeleton: ribs should be checked for fractures, beginning with the first rib and progressing downward. Start where the rib is joined to the thoracic spine and follow the whole of the rib to its anterior end. Do not forget the clavicles and scapulae
- Other areas: note any artefacts, e.g. buttons. The soft tissues may also demonstrate pathology such as surgical emphysema

Hip radiographs

Shenton's line is defined by the anatomy of the pelvic region and is a useful reference line. It is used as part of a pelvic evaluation routine and to detect femoral neck fractures (Figure 13.4). In the normal hip a line defining the medial border of the femur may be followed continuously round to that defining the upper border of the obturator foramen. If this line cannot be followed, the femoral neck should be scrutinized for a fracture.

The examples above give an idea of the systematic approach used in the evaluation of a radiograph and the processes followed during such evaluations. Each body part requires a different approach. The recommended texts should be referred to for the relevant descriptions.

Recognizing the normal

Before attempting to make diagnoses from radiographs it is imperative to have a good knowledge of bony anatomy and normal radiographic appearances. This should be combined with an understanding of how anatomy can change on the radiograph when the patient is positioned using a non-standard projection. This can radically alter the resultant image and may effect the final diagnosis. There are many variants of normal anatomy which can fool the unwary observer. A few examples are described here; extensive detailed descriptions are given in the recommended texts.

Nutrient arteries

These are channels or pathways that allow the passage of blood vessels into the bone (Figure 13.5). They appear as dark lines within the bone or disruptions visible on its outer margin. They are often confused with fractures but can be quite easily distinguished as they always have smooth edges, whereas fractures will have sharply defined edges. Nutrient arteries are commonly visible within the skull or in long bones.

Accessory bones

Accessory bones are small ossicles that develop close to joints (Figure 13.6). They may be confused with fragments of bone from a fracture. Again they can easily be set apart by their smooth, well-defined edges while bone fragments will have sharp edges. They are often found in the foot, ankle and hand. The os trigonum, found behind the talus, is often mistaken for a fracture.

Epiphyses

The dark lines caused by epiphyses are often mistaken for fractures, especially when they begin to fuse. It is important to be aware where these structures are and note the patient's age when viewing a film. The epiphysis at the base of the metacarpal is frequently mistaken for a fracture. It is quite easy to differentiate as this epiphysis will run in a longitudinal direction whereas a fracture nearly always runs transversely across the bone (see avulsion fractures, below).

Recognizing the abnormal

Having gained an appreciation of normal anatomy and all the variants thereof, the process of diagnosing abnormalities becomes a little easier. For the nurse practitioner working in the A&E department, most pathologies encountered will result from trauma. The remainder of this chapter will focus on the diagnosis of fractures and dislocations; some other acute pathologies will also be mentioned.

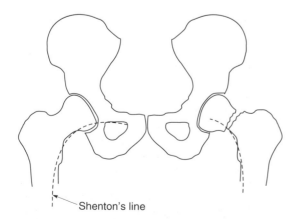

Figure 13.4 Shenton's line can be followed through to the obturator foramen in the right hip. This is not the case in the left hip, which is fractured

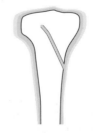

Figure 13.5 The nutrient artery is often mistaken for a fracture. It can be distinguished by its smooth edges

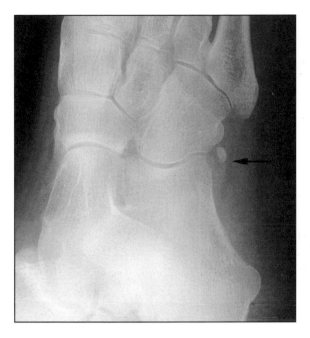

Figure 13.6   Example of an accessory bone in the foot

Recognizing fractures

There is a wide variety of fracture types and each has a characteristic appearance or combination of appearances.

Simple fractures with minimal displacement

The search for a fracture will involve a number of stages. First, the whole of the dense margin on the outside of the bone (the cortex) should be examined for any sharp steps, breaks or disruptions. These can often be subtle and may easily be overlooked. A fracture of the radial head is a good example of a commonly occurring fracture that will only manifest itself with a cortical abnormality. Figure 13.7 shows an example of a torus fracture in a child; this occurs when a longitudinal force is applied to an immature bone. The relatively soft bones of children often do not completely fracture but will bend or partially break, rather like bending a cardboard tube. The only evidence of damage to the tube may be a ridge in the cardboard. Similarly, the torus fracture will often appear as a slight buckle or raising of the outer bone cortex. Tibial plateau fractures may only be evident as a small defect in the cortex or a small flake of bone raised above the surrounding cortex.

The hunt for a fracture will continue with an examination of the intricate honeycomb pattern that constitutes the centre of a bone (the trabeculae). This should be scrutinized since disruptions in the continuity of the trabecular pattern or areas of increased film density (radiolucency) would be indicative of a fracture. In the case of a radiolucency the X-rays are able to pass through the space within the bone caused by a slight displacement of the fracture. They are then free to pass through to the film, thus causing an increase in blackening compared to the surrounding bone. When a fracture occurs, bone fragments may be forced together and could overlap. This will provide an additional barrier to the X-rays. Thus fewer will reach the film compared to those from areas immediately adjacent to the fracture. A lighter area defined by sharp edges will then be observable within the normal trabecular pattern. Good examples of these appearances may be found as a result of an impacted fracture of the hip or a depressed skull fracture (Figure 13.8).

Compression and comminuted fractures

An injury that results in a compressive force being applied to a bone may result in a comminuted fracture in which the bone is shattered into a number of pieces. Many of these fractures will be easily identified but some are less obvious.

A compressive force applied to the top of the head may cause a total disruption of C1. This is referred to as a Jefferson fracture and can be identified by the increased distance between the odontoid peg and the lateral masses of C1. The articular surfaces between C1 and C2 will not be in alignment (Figure 13.9). Compression fractures are common elsewhere within the spine. A hyperflexion injury may result in the collapse of the anterior portion of the vertebral body, causing the characteristic wedge deformity (Figure 13.10). This may be dramatic or subtle and

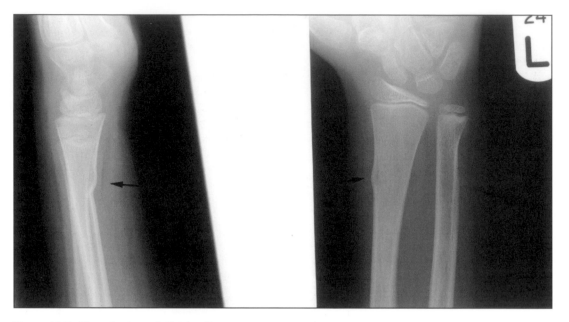

Figure 13.7   Torus fracture of distal radius

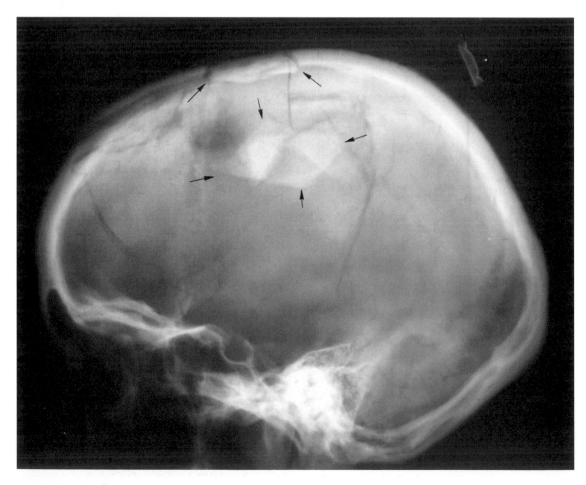

Figure 13.8   Multiple skull fractures. Arrows indicate depressed fractures

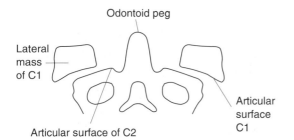

Line drawing of 'open mouth' projection of C1/2

Figure 13.9 Jefferson fracture of C1. Note how the lateral masses of C1 have been displaced outwards and the articular surfaces are no longer in alignment

hardly visible. The shape of each vertebral body should therefore be carefully examined and compared to its neighbours.

Avulsion fractures

An avulsion fracture results from a force being transmitted along a tendon or ligament, resulting in a piece of bone being pulled off at its attachment. This often occurs at the greater tuberosity of the humerus where the tendons of the supraspinatus, infraspinatus and teres minor muscles are attached (Figure 13.11). The base of the fifth metatarsal is also prone to avulsion fractures. The peroneus brevis tendon will be responsible for a transverse fracture

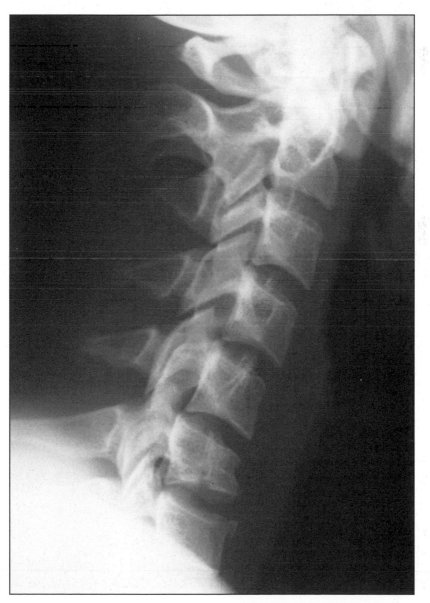

Figure 13.10   Wedge fracture of C6 with a 'teardrop fracture' to the body of C7

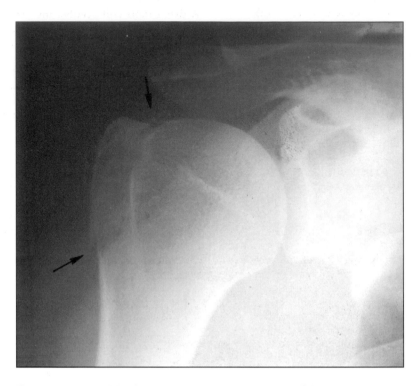

Figure 13.11   Avulsion fracture at the greater tuberosity of the humerus

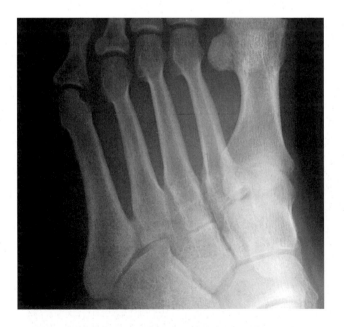

Figure 13.12   Avulsion fracture to base of fifth metatarsal

across the base of the metatarsal following an inversion injury to the ankle (Figure 13.12).

Epiphyseal injuries

A range of injuries may occur at any growth plate. These may be quite subtle and only involve the smallest displacement of the epiphysis, or could involve fractures with epiphyseal separation. If the injury involves an impaction of the epiphysis there may be no separation, which makes diagnosis difficult. Figure 13.13 shows slippage of the upper femoral epiphysis. This is often encountered in overweight boys and may not be evident on an AP hip projection. A second 'frog-leg' lateral will be required in such cases.

Contrecoup fractures

These injuries occur where the force causing a fracture in a bony ring is transmitted to the other side of the ring, causing another fracture. It is rather like trying to break a biscuit with a hole in the middle. You will have difficulty in causing a break in one place only; you always end up with two or more breaks. Common sites for these fractures include the skull, mandible and the tibia and fibula. An injury to the medial malleolus of the ankle may be accompanied by fracture at the upper end of the fibula just below the knee. This is often overlooked both clinically and radiographically.

Dislocations

A dislocation will involve the articular surface in one component of a joint being completely separated from the other articular component. They are most often encountered in the shoulder, although other sites such as the hip or interphalangeal joints are not uncommon. An anterior dislocation of the glenohumeral joint will involve a considerable amount of forward and inferior displacement of the humerus. Posterior dislocations are quite rare but difficult to diagnose. The degree of displacement is much less and will take place in a posterior direction. An AP shoulder radiograph may not appear significantly abnormal due to the direction of the displacement. A second projection of the shoulder is always required if an obvious anterior dislocation is not evident. The acromioclavicular joint is also prone to dislocations or subluxation (partial dislocations) and should merit special attention when assessing the shoulder radiograph.

Other pathologies

Soft-tissue injuries and evidence of bleeding are sometimes evident on radiographs. A classic example is the elbow effusion (Figure 13.14). A build-up of fluid in the elbow joint capsule following an injury will cause the fat pads in the capsule wall to be displaced outwards. These can be identified as two sail-like radiolucent areas found anteriorly and

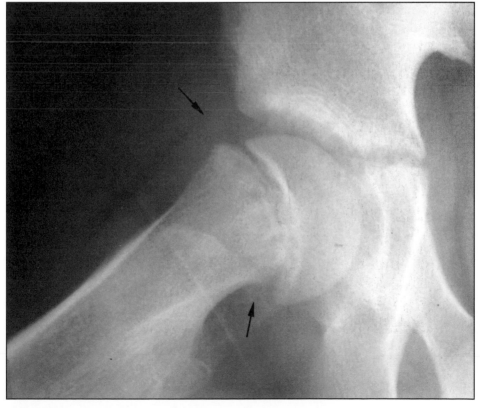

Figure 13.13   Slipped femoral epiphysis

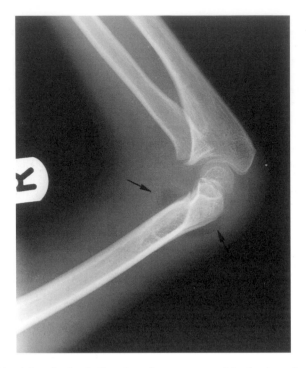

Figure 13.14   Joint effusion in the elbow from supracondylar fracture. Arrows indicate raised fat pads

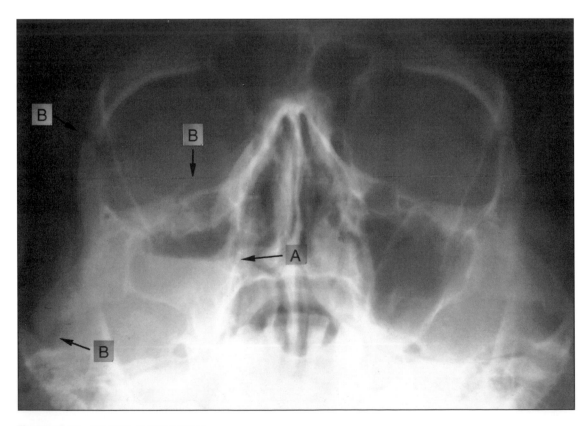

Figure 13.15   Fracture of facial bones

posteriorly to the joint. If the fat pad sign is noted then careful analysis of the joint should follow, as a fracture is likely to be present.

Bleeding may also occur in the maxillary sinuses following a fracture to the facial bones (Figure 13.15). As before, a careful inspection of the bones should follow; sinusitis may also result in a fluid build-up within the sinuses.

Infection in a bone or joint may be difficult to identify. The joint space may become slightly wider as a result of fluid build-up in the joint. The bone periosteum may lift slightly or the sharp cortical outline of the bone may become indistinct when infection is present. Chronic bone infection will result in the gradual destruction of bone.

Summary

The key to successful diagnosis from radiographs is to ensure you are equipped with a good knowledge of normal anatomy and to adopt a thorough and systematic approach when viewing the image. Abnormalities have characteristic patterns of appearance with which you will become familiar over time. A few have been mentioned above but you should use the recommended texts and as well as your colleagues in the A&E and radiology departments as valuable learning resources.

References

Keates T. (1996) *An Atlas of Normal Roentgen Variants that may Simulate Disease*, St Louis, Mosby.

Moller T., Reif E., Stark P. (1992) *Pocket Atlas of Radiographic Anatomy*, New York: Thieme.

Nicholson D.A., Driscoll P.A. (eds.) *ABC of Emergency Radiology* (1995) London, *British Medical Journal* Cambridge, BMJ Publishing Group.

Raby N., Berman L., de Lacey F. *Accident & Emergency Reporting (1995) A Survival Guide*, London, WB Saunders.

CHAPTER 14

The assessment of child health: setting the context

Fiona Smart

Children are users of health-care services. Before birth and throughout childhood and adolescence, children make contact with health-care professionals for numerous reasons. Operating in diverse roles in various settings, nurse practitioners are involved in meeting the health needs of children. This chapter centres on the process underpinning health-care interventions, that of child health assessment. It will argue that the process needs to be framed by a knowledge base which extends beyond an understanding of the child as a biological entity vulnerable to the experience of ill heath and disease because of developmental immaturity. It will show that such a within-individual, biologically based, disease-oriented biomedical frame of reference is inherently limited (Moon and Gillespie 1995). Instead, the chapter will provide evidence that children's experiences of health and illness are rooted in unstable social worlds which need to be understood by nurse practitioners if they are to assess child health. Immature as they may be from a biological perspective, not all children have the same chances of health. This chapter will not dispute the place for the systematic assessment of bodily systems, but will argue that such skills need to be grounded in a knowledge base which extends beyond the fact of biological immaturity and cognizant of the impact of the social world on child health.

Written primarily for the nurse practitioner, this chapter sets out to challenge the reader and to provoke debate. It does not seek to prescribe, but rather to heighten understanding. Ultimately it aims to influence the process of child health assessment and to enhance children's experiences of care within adult-constructed health-care systems. To achieve this goal, theoretical perspectives and research findings will be drawn on. However, readers are asked to remain focused on their own practice and the every day reality of working with children to assess and meet their health needs. It will be argued that it is in the world of the every day that differences can be made and that caring practices can advance.

The exploration of caring practices as extended to and experienced by children begins in a world seemingly divorced from their everyday lives – international law, as embodied in the United Nations (UN) Convention on the Rights of the Child (1989, cited by Leenders 1996). Having examined both its potential and inherent limitations, this chapter moves to unmask the myth of the medical model which portrays health and illness as biologically based facts and immutable truths (Moon and Gillespie 1995). Statistics show otherwise; the picture of child heath will be shown to be unstable. Having explored these data and exposed the reality of difference, the chapter centres on children themselves, developing in terms of their understanding of the world and their ways of relating to it. If children sometimes seem a mystery to health-care professionals, then just what the world of health care seems to them can only be surmised. This chapter will draw together these three interrelated themes – the law, health/illness statistics and the child as a developing individual – and propose that they form a framework within which the assessment of child health should take place. It will be argued that to do otherwise threatens to silence children's voices, ignore their lives and set aside their needs as developing individuals. The assessment of child health should extend beyond the body and the world of medicine and needs to begin with children themselves, drawing the family unit into the process with the intention of developing relationships from which all gain and grow.

A concern for children?

It is curious to think that our professed concern for children and their health is of recent origin. As Kurtz and Tomlinson (1994) remind us, the middle of the 19th century in this country saw children living in desperate circumstances, suffering severe ill health and premature death. One in three children failed to reach adulthood (Kurtz and Tomlinson 1994). Dickensian fiction mirrored a reality experienced by large numbers of children. Survival was the primary issue and was important in that it enabled children to contribute to the family income. Children's health was of concern only if they could not meet this expectation. Kurtz and Tomlinson (1994) speak of widespread indifference to the fragility of childhood.

Superficially, at least, much seems to have changed since Dickensian times. In the UK we have child-focused laws, child education programmes and child health services (Leenders 1996). It seems that children are no longer viewed in terms of their earning capacity. Conversely, some might see them as the ultimate consumer good – the accessory which cannot be done without. And yet our beliefs and values are ambivalent and contradictory; so too are our laws and the policies which drive service provision (Mayall 1994; Payne 1995). For example, we speak of protecting children, but condone potentially damaging child-rearing practices that allow children to be hit by adults, although similar chastisements carried out on adults might be deemed assaults (Newell 1989; Lansdown 1994). We talk of children's best interests, yet use the principle to justify the actions of adults and to overrule the wishes and feelings of children (Lansdown 1994). We set store by educational opportunity, but fail to appreciate the negative aspects of schooling – the boredom, the noise and the enforced social interaction with peers and teachers from whom children cannot escape without sanction (Mayall 1994). We speak of prioritizing child health, yet seem to tolerate inequality of opportunity to enjoy this phenomenon. Poverty ensures that health eludes some children and damages future generations (Spencer 1995; Dennehy et al. 1997). So, whilst much has changed in a short period of time, childhood remains challenging for children in the UK. What of the world beyond?

White (1991) writes that worldwide 30 million children live on the streets; 80 million undertake work detrimental to their development; 7 million live in refugee camps and 200 000 children under 15 years of age are part of the armed forces. Looking at these figures, it is possible to conclude that, whilst childhood in the UK may not be easy, it is nothing like as difficult as that faced by others. None the less, children in the UK do face difficulties and their health is challenged, some more than others. Inequality of opportunity is a fact that must be understood by concerned parties, including nurse practitioners who have a role in assessing and meeting the health needs of children.

Concern for children and their health and well-being should extend beyond the boundaries of health care. Argued by Paton and Cockburn (1995) to be society's canaries, vulnerable to the full blast of societal ills, all children, whether in developing or developed countries, whatever the lives lived, need to have first call on adult concerns and should be able to depend upon that commitment (Black 1996). It was this spirit that drove the formulation of the UN Convention on the Rights of the Child (1989).

The UN Convention on the Rights of the Child (1989)

The UN Convention recognizes the vulnerability of children and sets out their rights to special consideration under three headings (Fatchett 1995; Leenders 1996).

1 Provision: the right to possess, receive or to have access to certain things or services:

- a name
- a nationality
- health care
- education
- rest and play
- care for the disabled and parentless children

2 Protection: the right to be shielded from harmful acts and practices:

- separation from parents
- commercial or sexual exploitation
- physical and mental abuse
- engagement in warfare

3 Participation: the right to be heard on decisions affecting his or her life; the right to increasing opportunity to take part in the activities of society, as preparation for adulthood.

It is possible to question the relevance of at least some of these rights to nurse practitioners operating in the UK. The UK is not at war; children are given names; laws protect children from exploitation. The Dickensian era has passed and the Children Act (1989) promotes and safeguards the welfare of children (Leenders 1996), or at least it purports to do so, although only for children in England and Wales (Scotland and Northern Ireland make separate provision for children) and only in relation to matters coming to court which concern children's upbringing (Lansdown 1994). Contrary to popular belief, the Children Act (1989) is limited in its jurisdiction (Lansdown 1994). It does not have power in tribunals hearing immigration and nationality appeals, nor in educational tribunals addressing issues concerned with school choice, special needs and school exclusion (Lansdown 1994). In the arena of health care, there is no obligation to listen to children, nor to take account of their views. The goals of efficiency and economy can hold sway over children's best interests (Lansdown 1994).

Those in health care who look to the Gillick judgement (1986) instead of the Children Act (1989) find that subsequent case law has exposed the fragility of children's rights to dissent (Alderson and Montgomery 1996). However, McCall Smith (1992) seems to approve this challenge to the Gillick judgement's fundamental principle that children of sufficient understanding and intelligence should be enabled to make their choice, arguing that the ability to consent and dissent require different degrees of capacity.

Given the Children Act's (1989) limited frame of reference and the fragility of the Gillick principle, the UN Convention on the Rights of the Child (1989) seems increasingly significant to those working with and for children. Constituting international law, the Convention brings together 54 articles concerning civil, economic, social and cultural rights (Hill and Tisdall 1997). All signatories to the Convention, whether rich or poor, are expected to work to achieve these standards (Fatchett 1995). Signatories must report on progress towards implementation of the articles – a requirement which has applied to the UK since 1991 when government ministers signed up to the Convention (Lansdown 1994).

Hill and Tisdall (1997) note the particular significance of three articles.

- All rights guaranteed by the Convention must be available to all children without discrimination of any kind (article 2)
- The best interests of the child must be a primary consideration of all actions concerning children (article 3)
- Children's views must be considered and taken into account in all matters affecting them, subject to the children's age and maturity (article 12)

The potential for conflict in aiming to uphold both articles 3 and 12 is worthy of consideration. Whilst article 12, echoing the Gillick principle, gives children a voice, article 3 focuses on children's best interests. In theory it is possible to see that adults' roles in acting for children in their best interests should diminish as children become more capable of acting for themselves (Charles-Edwards 1991). However, this leaves open to dispute situations where children make competent decisions that they argue to be in their best interests, but with which adults disagree. Experience suggests that adults support children's rights to choose when the decisions concur with their own opinions. Therein lies the rub. Children's rights to a voice and to choose may only be partial and depend on children seeing situations in the same way as adults do. Moreover, in a country where the history of hearing children's voices is short and

inconsistent (Mayall 1994) and where there is much emphasis on protecting children, perhaps the fact that children's rights to autonomy do not always hold sway should not be too surprising. The UN Convention may well be international law, but its enactment cannot be divorced from the sociocultural context. As contended earlier, beliefs and values concerning children in the UK are ambivalent and contradictory; thus, achieving a balance between articles 3 and 12 proves challenging and is likely to remain so.

Heath-care professionals know of the tension arising from attempts to confer children's rights to autonomy whilst ensuring the protection of current and future interests. Practice is replete with instances that typify the challenges faced. Situations vary, as do issues raised, but certainly the tightrope of everyday health care practice is testing, especially given that it is not possible to construct prescriptions for action. However, informed by statute and case law, the UN Convention is a framework within which health care professionals must operate. Documents such as that published by the British Association for Community Child Health (1995) help translate its ideals into practice and in so doing focus emphasis on children's health rights, as set out in article 24 of the UN Convention.

Meeting the health needs of children

The recognition that children have health needs requiring specific provision is significant, given that some might argue that children's needs are no more and no less than those adults. However, neither the International Council of Nurses (ICN 1997) nor Price (1994) would hold with this view. And yet, focusing on young people, the ICN (1996) cites evidence of unmet need. It identified 'complex' and 'cold', non 'youth-friendly' health care systems staffed by professionals viewed as 'negative' and 'judgemental' in their approach. Although it is unclear as to the source of this material, and thus the extent to which criticisms can be levied at UK health care provision, the ICN's (1996) analysis offers food for thought and challenges nurse practitioners, amongst others, to look at the services they provide, how they are offered and the extent to which they disable or support children and young people in the process of assessing their health needs and subsequent health-care provision. If due weight is to be given to article 12 of the UN Convention, such a critique of services should be informed by children themselves. Their understanding of what enables and what constrains the assessment of health needs and the provision of 'child and young-friendly' health services may differ from adult perspectives. Such evaluation of heath-care provision is beginning. Examples of good practice are emerging which challenge Mayall's (1994) assertion that the UK is locked in a culture that does not attend to children (Dennehy *et al.* 1997). The Northumberland Young People's Health Project (1997) is one initiative that is illustrative of others. Significantly, it demonstrates a change of emphasis in that, in addition to young people working with each other, they work with adults, not vice versa, to address issues of concern. The venture is collaborative, but it is driven by young people.

Leaving aside the question as to how commonplace or exceptional such initiatives are, it seems opportune to consider how far health-care professionals are themselves enabled to offer services grounded in the recognition of children's needs, cognizant of their rights. If Mayall (1994) is right in her portrayal of a culture which does not attend to children, it may be that, despite the best intentions, health-care professionals are as disabled in their attempt to offer health-care services that facilitate the assessment and meeting of children's needs as children are when they come into contact with them. Understanding the law – international, statute and case – and its potential and limitations, subscribing to a belief in children's rights and appreciating differences in needs between children and adults does not of itself change practice. The gap between theory and practice has been much explored and the chasm exposed (Rolfe 1996). However, as Rolfe suggests, it may be that the gap could be minimized by a reorientation wherein, instead of theory and research being seen as the starting place for development, practice takes the lead role, informed as appropriate by theory and research. Child-sensitive health-care services have emerged from practice (Dennehy *et al.* 1997) and suggest the need to understand better what supports and what constrains such innovation.

Frameworks for assessing child health

Attention to children's health needs and their assessment raises important questions as to which models might be used to frame the process. Having acknowledged the long-standing and continuing dominance of the medical model, Fatchett (1995) writes of a competing social model of health which is further explored by Moon and Gillespie (1995). The limitations of the medical model are exposed by mortality and morbidity statistics which demonstrate that child health is challenged less by biological immaturity than social circumstance. Whilst children as a group are healthier than, for example, their historical counterparts, not all children

are equally likely to enjoy health. Children live dissimilar lives, even in the UK. Childhood is an unstable phenomenon; the experience of it varies (Alderson and Montgomery 1996; Scatton 1997). Some children face inequality of opportunity in terms of their experience of health because of, for example, where they live, their cultural group or their gender (Spencer 1995; Dennehy *et al.* 1997). Some have an increased risk of premature death; some will live with continuing illness (Dennehy *et al.* 1997). Consequently, despite its continuing dominance (Fatchett 1995), the appropriateness of the medical model as a framework for assessing child health is suspect. In its quest to diagnose ill health in the individual, it allows significant factors such as social structuring and organization to be ignored (Moon and Gillespie 1995). Moreover, its focus is disease, not health. Assessment of child health and meeting of child health needs must extend beyond a bodily system-based approach and locate child health in a sociocultural context within which it is understood that the experience of childhood is not uniform and that there is inequity in terms of health chances and access to health services. Failure to draw on a social model of health risks locating health-care practices in knowledge which is at best partial. At worst, they might be described as deluded.

A picture of health?

Having spoken of inequality of opportunity and access, this section sets out to capture the picture of child health, recognizing that it is dynamic. Statistics date with speed. None the less, the data now available illuminate the fact that some children's experiences of health are different to others' and that these differences cannot be explained simply by reference to biological immaturity or lifestyle behaviours, either of families or of children themselves. Health is a complex phenomenon that defies simplistic accounts as to its roots, processes and outcomes. It is argued that the assessment and provision of child health needs must be grounded in data that recognize difference and do not assume a homogeneity of experience.

Given the focus on health it is curious to note that its measures are frequently assessed via mortality and morbidity statistics. This section continues this tradition. It also acknowledges a bias to UK data.

Causes of death

The previously made claim that children's health is improving is borne out by mortality data, especially those focused on infants. Botting and Crawley (1995) cite data that show a 50% fall in stillbirth and infant mortality rates from 1971 until 1991 for both sexes, with the greatest falls recorded for stillbirth (63%) and neonatal (62%) deaths. During the same period the postneonatal death rate fell by 49% (Botting and Crawley 1995). Given that some, including Botting (1997) and Moon and Gillespie (1995), have argued that a nation's health can be assessed by its infant mortality statistics, it might be concluded that child health, as measured via infant mortality statistics, is improving in the UK. Yet this analysis is flawed because the data mask differences.

Throughout the first year and continuing through life, males have a higher mortality rate than females (Botting and Crawley 1995). Likewise, the data conceal another fact. Despite falling death rates in the first year of life, social class differentials persist (Botting 1997). From 1993 to 1995 the infant mortality rate (IMR) for births classified in social class V was 70% higher than that of social class I (Botting 1997). Whilst Botting (1997) concedes that infant mortality differentials by social class have narrowed, she identifies a slightly widening gap in those for childhood mortality.

Focusing on those childhood mortality rates, Botting (1997) cites falling rates for males aged 1–15 years from 37/100 000 in 1979 to 21/100 000 in 1995. For females aged 1–15 years the fall was smaller – 26/100 000 in 1979 to 17/100 000 in 1995. From the 1981 census, Botting (1997) reports that mortality increased from social classes I and II through to V, with the gradient most marked at ages 1–4 where children in social class V had death rates three times higher than those in social class I. This trend persisted in the 1991 census. In each age group the mortality rates for children in social class V were noticeably higher than those for other classes (Botting 1997). Despite the fact that social class membership as decided by occupational group is a less than ideal measure of health, it acts as an indicator and shows that health, disease and death are not matters of fortune (Moon and Gillespie 1995). The social positioning of adults has an impact on children, with evidence demonstrating that ascription to social class V is associated with an increased risk of premature death in childhood. It is important to reflect on just how health services might respond to such data, as well as on the risk of stereotyping and labelling individuals on the basis of social class. Assumption-based practice seems wholly inappropriate and yet health-care professionals, including nurse practitioners, need to appreciate the association between social class and experience of health, disease and death. Data relating to accidental death illustrate the point. Moreover they highlight the need for health-care professionals to consider the social worlds within which children live and the increasing risk of danger faced by children whose families belong to social classes IV and V.

The Health of the Nation (Department of Health 1992) target was set to reduce accidental deaths among children under 15 years by at least 33% between 1995 and 2005. This has already been met (Botting 1997). This said, there is a differential in terms of the rate of accidental deaths between the social classes. Between 1981 and 1991 the rates fell by 21% for social class IV and by 2% for social class V, in comparison with 32% and 37% for social classes I and II respectively (Botting 1997). More specific data concern death by fire and flames. Statistics show an increase for children in social classes IV and V between 1981 and 1991, with residential fires the primary cause of death (Botting 1997).

The risk of morbidity

Turning to morbidity statistics, the mainstay of health status measurement, the social gradient is similar to that noted for child mortality (Spencer 1995). Children in less favoured socioeconomic circumstances experience greater levels of morbidity (Spencer 1995). This said, Spencer (1995) acknowledges a paucity of data relating to specific diseases or medically defined conditions. Thus, the picture of child health as constructed by morbidity data is incomplete. Nevertheless, the statistics make challenging reading. Particular attention is drawn here to two areas of morbidity – respiratory illness, the most common health problem for children aged 0–15 years (Botting and Crawley 1995) and mental illness, argued by some to be the new epidemic (for example, see Shooter 1997). This is not to say that other aspects of child ill health are unimportant.

Data drawn from the General Household Survey (GHS) identify respiratory illness as the major health problem affecting children aged 0–15 years (Botting and Crawley 1995). Although seemingly small in percentage terms at 7%, Botting and Crawley (1995) write that respiratory conditions account for over 50% of children's consultations with GPs – a fact that would seem to underline its significance to nurse practitioners operating in primary care settings, especially given known seasonal variations and the increased pressure for consultations at certain times. Similarly, the demand for beds at particular times of the year is understood by hospital-based practitioners. However, not all children are equally likely to have a respiratory illness, especially one that is acute in type. To illustrate this point, Spencer (1995) cites a case-control study of hospital admissions for clinically suspected bronchiolitis during an outbreak in Sheffield in the winter of 1989–1990. It confirmed the association between acute respiratory infections and urban living, overcrowding and poor housing conditions.

Reading (1997) explores the relationship between

infection, social deprivation and child health further. He focuses on the 1.5 million dwellings (7.6%) found to be unfit in the English House Condition Survey (1991). Poorer families tend to live in the private rented sector and local-authority housing – the two types of tenure with the worst conditions; 30% of private rented homes were deemed unfit (Reading 1997). The most common reason for unfitness was lack of food preparation facilities (Reading 1997, citing the Department of the Environment 1993). Thus some children are more at risk not only of acute respiratory infections, but also of gastrointestinal ones (Reading 1997). Poor housing has been implicated in the incidence of less clearly defined respiratory problems too. Children in social classes IV and V are more likely to have a cough, a symptom linked with cold and damp housing, especially where fungal mould is a problem (Dennehy *et al.* 1997). Night coughing disturbs sleep of the child and of the family and may impact on family functioning within and without the home. The effects on schooling and the capacity to learn are important to consider and should not be left out of any analysis of educational failure.

Whilst care must be taken not to conflate social class ascription and financial resources (Moon and Gillespie 1995), children of families in social classes IV and V and, indeed, those falling into the unclassified group are more likely to experience poverty than those in social classes I and II (Spencer 1995). Much debated and sometimes ignored as a factor, data indicate that poverty is associated with the re-emergence of old diseases, namely tuberculosis, and with the incidence of the new, specifically HIV and AIDS (Reading 1997). However, citing Mann (1992, 1995), Reading argues that the AIDS pandemic is not simply related to poverty, but also to the failure to ensure human rights. Thus it affects the disenfranchised, discriminated against and stigmatized and includes children in its number, either directly or indirectly. The extent to which article 2 of the UN Convention on the Rights of the Child (1989) is being achieved in respect of equality of access to health care provision (article 24) is questionable. This said, it remains a goal to be strived for by both governments and individual practitioners.

The link between poverty, deprivation and ill health is less clear in respect of asthma, a chronic respiratory problem with acute exacerbations (Spencer 1995). In fact, Spencer notes that, although a few studies suggest an increased risk of asthma associated with lower socioeconomic status allergic conditions generally show a reverse class gradient in children and young adults. However, of interest is the increased risk of hospital admission for asthma for children from areas with high poverty levels (Spencer 1995). Possible explanations for such a referral pattern are interesting to consider, although it may result simply from the fact that asthma seems more severe in children from poorer social circumstances (Spencer 1995, citing Starfield and Budetti 1985; Wise and Meyers 1988; Wissow *et al.* 1988; Schwartz *et al.* 1990) and that they therefore need admission to hospital. However, alternative explanations are possible. Whatever the reasoning, families may face increased financial costs because of their child's admission to hospital. Transport costs may be an issue, as may the outlay needed to eat and drink away from home (Callery 1997).

Reading's (1997) critique of social disadvantage and child health offers a means to understand the causes of mortality and morbidity extending beyond the usual reference to lifestyle behaviours and structural inequalities. Reading (1997) looks at infection as both an aspect of poor health and as an explanatory factor for health inequalities. Centring on respiratory illness, he cites the Office of Population Censuses and Surveys (1988) which identified the death rate for pneumonia and bronchitis in social classes I and II as 13.3/million, while in social class V and 'unoccupied' it was 34.5/million. This analysis suggests that we have not learned the lessons of Dickensian times when infection was both a killer and a constraint on child health. All too often, Reading (1997) argues, either lifestyle behaviours or structural factors or both are used inappropriately to explain ill health. Those concerned about child health should not overlook the obvious. The prevalence of infection is associated with social class.

If infection was the scourge of the past, and is a factor even now, then today's pandemic would seem to be mental ill health and distress. Whilst Dennehy *et al.* (1997) note difficulties in establishing the extent of the problem, Shooter (1997) estimates that about 2 million children in the UK under 18 years of age (equivalent to 1 : 5) have problems sufficient to interfere with normal enjoyment of childhood and adolescence. Carlisle (1997) elaborates the picture, estimating that:

- 10% of all children suffer severe emotional and behavioural problems. Of these children:
- 50% have disruptive behaviour problems such as conduct disorder and hyperactivity
- 40% have emotional difficulties such as depression, disabling anxiety, eating disorders or psychosomatic illness
- 10% have a learning disability such as autism

These estimates mask difference. Not all children are equally likely to experience mental health problems – once again, social class and its association with poverty cannot be ignored, nor can gender (Dennehy *et al.* 1997). Their explorations of depression, schizophrenia, suicide, parasuicide and eating disorders prove illuminating in respect of both variables and draw into view a third, that of ethnicity. Dennehy *et al.* (1997) challenge the capacity of a health service dominated by white middle-class professionals to meet the mental health needs of individuals from minority ethnic groups. However this assumes that children with mental health problems access health-care professionals. Hill and Tisdall (1997) write that this is not necessarily so. They go on to claim that children who present with mental health problems may be assessed differently depending on the professional they come into contact with. Consequently, the interventions planned to meet their needs may differ and might not be appropriate. Hill and Tisdall (1997) note that GPs tend to medicalize mental health problems and to seek psychiatric diagnoses and treatment. Given Shooter's (1997) claim that only about half of the 2 million under-18-year-olds experiencing mental health problems will have a recognized psychiatric illness, the potential for inappropriate intervention becomes apparent. Equally possible is the potential for psychiatric illness to be missed by professionals who look to other causes of mental health problems. Mental health and ill health are complex phenomena; an assessment framework which situates health in sociocultural settings but recognizes the possibility of psychiatric illness would seem to be essential.

This leads thinking on to the much prized goal of interagency collaboration (Naidoo and Wills 1994; Wass 1994) – a laudable aim, ultimately limited in its application by history, tradition and the multiple and competing perspectives held by practitioners from different professional groups (Delaney 1996). The likely losers in this scenario are children. Perhaps it is that training opportunities across professional boundaries might enhance understanding not only of children's mental health and the factors which threaten it, but of roles and the potential for collaborative action. The government white paper, the *New NHS: Modern and Dependable* (1997) published in 1997, also opens up opportunities (Crail 1997). It looks to GPs and community nurses commissioning services for local communities and advocates working closely with social services (Crail 1997). However, the need to draw other agencies such as housing, leisure, education and indeed preschool care into the commissioning process is imperative, given the potential of each to impact on child health. So too would it seem vital to involve communities, families and children themselves in the process. Heath extends beyond the domain of GP practices, health centres and hospitals. GPs and community nurses cannot speak for children and develop health services for them without reference to their social worlds and to the voices of children themselves.

Understandings of health

Whether spurred on by the Gillick judgement (1986, cited by Lansdown 1994), the spirit of the Children Act (1989), the UN Convention (1989) or other factors, evidence suggests that children are becoming involved in health-care decision-making (Alderson and Montgomery 1996). However, the extent to which they are equally involved in the underpinning process of assessing their own health is open to debate. Research findings accumulated over the past 20 years suggest that children have knowledge of health and of their bodies and could play an active role in the process. Interestingly, one of the most recent analyses of the literature portrays children as cognizant of behaviourist health-promoting messages which link diet and lifestyle; nevertheless they seem capable of resisting them, much as adults do (Hill and Tisdall 1997). Children report a discrepancy between what they know about health and what they do in practice (Hill and Tisdall 1997). Even with healthier choices available to them, children may not take them. Research carried out by Prout (1996) identified trading arrangements for the contents of packed lunches. Factors other than knowledge affect choice. This is exemplified by smoking behaviours. Whilst the risks of cigarette smoking seem widely known (Oakley *et al.* 1995), about 1 in 5 children in their mid-teens smoke (Power 1995). Such information perhaps fuels the fires of those wishing to limit children's rights to choose, in order to protect future interests.

Significantly, while Hill and Tisdall (1997) argue that children have knowledge of how to keep healthy, it seems that they do not incorporate structural explanations into their accounts. They appear unaware that some of them face an increased risk of illness and disease. Health beliefs and behaviours are complex and warrant careful attention, beyond the remit of this chapter.

Knowledge of illness and of health care encounters

The body of knowledge accumulating in respect of children's understandings of illness is fascinating and has been enhanced in recent years by exposure of the limitations of stage theories in explaining developments in children's understanding over time (for example, see Yoos 1994). Yet the domination of Piagetian theory seems to persist and with it the belief that, regardless of previous experience the younger children are, the less likely they will be to understand illness causation and subsequent treatments. The consequence of this belief persisting is that children may not be informed because 'they are too young to understand'. Without information, children's capacity to be involved in their own health care becomes constrained. The only voice children may have is one of protest and non-co-operation. The end-result may be frustrated health-care professionals, dissatisfied families and mistrusting children. This would not seem to be the ideal recipe for engaging children in a health-care system which assesses and meets their needs, both now and in later life.

Although Piagetian theory remains powerful, alternatives exist. For example, the work of Lev Vygotsky suggests that children have the capacity to understand complex ideas if enabled to do so by more knowledgeable others (Berk 1994). Of equal potential value to the nurse practitioner is the work of Nelson (1986, cited by Eiser 1989) who speaks of children's abilities to formulate scripts. Eiser (1989) recognized the potential of scripts both in terms of understanding children's responses in health-care settings and as a means of explaining health and illness to them. Eiser (1989: 97) defines scripts as: 'Schemata for episodes extended in time that contain representations of events that go to make up such an episode and the order in which such events typically occur'

Scripts generate expectations about what will happen. Eiser (1989) cites research conducted by Nelson and Gruendel (1986) that identified the capacities of children as young as 3 years of age to develop scripts for routine everyday events. Eiser (1989) took the concept of scripts into the world of health care and investigated children's knowledge of everyday medical events. The study involved 5-year-olds ($n = 20$) and 8-year-olds ($n = 20$). Children in both groups gave well-ordered descriptions of a visit to the doctor, although the older ones tended to include a larger number of specific acts. Rather than explain the age-related difference in terms of maturation, Eiser (1989) identified the significance of experience in allowing scripts to develop.

This study raises a number of points pertinent to the nurse practitioner. For example, what events contribute to the formation of scripts? Does experience have to be direct or might it be vicarious? What of faulty scripts and the possibility of their being refashioned to an accurate understanding? How do children manage situations when the anticipated does not happen – for example, when the child expects to see the doctor or a nurse, but instead meets a nurse practitioner? Can children be prepared for events by helping them to develop scripts? How might nurse practitioners work together with families to this end? Certainly, the extent to which the newness of situations, the unanticipated, can be addressed via preparation is worthy of consideration and points to the possibility of parents and nurse practitioners forming alliances

to build and enhance children's scripts concerning health-care encounters.

The concept of scripts as identified by Nelson (1986) and pursued by Eiser (1989) alerts professionals to the fact that children's ideas about events may differ from those of adults. Cognitively children are developing over time; less experience may result in their having a smaller pool of previous knowledge on which to draw, which may lead to them seem lacking in understanding and more open to the possibility of surprise and fear in new situations (Yoos 1994). However, this may not be true of all children. Moreover, because they are individuals, children cope differently with new situations; some seem to be more vulnerable while others are more resilient (Pellegrini 1990).

Beyond cognition

Whatever the nature of children's scripts, their responses to health-care encounters and their capacity to be active in the process by which their health is assessed will be affected by what they know and understand. However, given that children are not simply thinking beings, their interpretations of and responses to situations will also be influenced by their feelings. Just as cognition develops over time, so too do the emotions. In describing such change, Berk (1994) seems to suggest that in terms of emotional expressiveness what children become with age is ever more in control of their emotions. Instead of the display of feelings developing over time, they come to conform with sociocultural and gendered expectations. Emotional display becomes dampened by what is required; such regulation is seen as an indicator of maturity (Berk 1994).

Given that mature emotional displays are gendered (Berk 1994), questions are raised as to the roles played by health-care professionals in regulating the emotions of male children in health-care interactions. It may be that 'big boys don't cry' is a maxim which operates in practice from early years. Quite what the consequences of this might be are unknown. Evidence suggests that in later years it is difficult to diagnose and treat depression in young men because of their tendency to conceal their feelings in displays of bad behaviour (Dennehy et al. 1997). Citing Agnew (1996), Dennehy et al. (1997) claim an underdiagnosis of about 65% and make links to worrying statistics concerning the increasing suicide rate for young men. Perhaps less dramatic, but equally important are consultation patterns for adult males (GHS 1995, cited in Rowlands et al. 1997) and their decreased likelihood of taking up preventive health care opportunities (Jones 1994). Whilst other explanations for such health behaviours are possible, the effects of early expectations made of boys by health-care professionals, perhaps even in collaboration with the children's parents, cannot be ruled out and require consideration.

Whilst children have to learn to control their emotions in order to fit in with expectations of them, Berk (1994) writes of their capacity to understand the emotions of others from birth onwards. They sense the feelings of others from birth and are able to detect the meaning of others' emotional signals from 7 months of age (Berk 1994). Parents are able to tell of times when their own feelings seemed to be communicated to their children; indeed this phenomenon has been sufficiently recognized to be labelled as emotional contagion (Muller *et al.* 1986). Informal discussions with health-care practitioners support the conclusion that children are equally responsive to the emotions of others. Anxious, busy ward nurses find that babies will not feed; infants seem to sense the practitioner about to give an immunization for the first time. If nothing else, such behaviours illustrate that children, even young babies, are not passive recipients of caring practices, but rather are active within the process, capable of reading situations and responding to them. Even without words, young children can make themselves understood. Whether practitioners listen and understand is another matter.

One particular feature of young children's emotional understanding is their use of social referencing to feed them information. Children under 1 year of age can be seen assessing situations via the responses of others (Berk 1994). The same phenomenon can be evidenced in the behaviour of older children too. This knowledge is significant to nurse practitioners because it makes clear the fact that when working with children there is more than one person to be concerned about. An anxious or fearful child may have an anxious or fearful parent. The needs of both demand attention.

Working with families for children

Much has been written about the bedrock on which child health care should be founded, namely family-centred partnerships established between health-care professionals and parents (for example, see Casey 1993). Only some of the literature, including that of Darbyshire (1994), has acknowledged the challenges that its attempted implementation brings to the world of health care. It is argued that more debate is needed in respect of what amounts to a prescription for action, particularly given the dearth of material exploring what it is that families and their children want in respect of models for practice.

Yet it would seem that whatever their roles and areas of operation, nurse practitioners need to work with families for children. Children's lives are interwoven with those of their families (Casey 1993; Whyte 1996); the former cannot be understood in isolation from the latter. Given the explorations of this chapter thus far, it is clear that an assessment of child health divorced from an understanding of the family and its social circumstances would be incomplete. Yet discussions with nurse practitioners reveal an inherent tension embedded in relationships between health-care professionals and families, especially parents. In a range of settings and in diverse roles, nurse practitioners speak of common experiences and shared difficulties. For example, they talk of:

- Believing that the presence of parents is not always beneficial to children
- Parents' tendencies to speak for their children and so affect the assessment of health and meeting of needs
- Difficulties in understanding parental behaviours

It seems that, despite believing they should be working with families for children, nurse practitioners struggle to do so. The time would seem ripe for a more thorough examination of the relationship between parents and nurse practitioners viewed from both perspectives. A phenomenological study might allow understanding to develop as to what constrains and what enhances caring practices as experienced by one and given by the other. Undoubtedly there is a need to understand parents' perceptions of the emerging role of the nurse practitioner in the UK and to uncover their beliefs about what makes a difference to them. On the basis of such knowledge, the world of everyday practice might develop.

Meanwhile the need to work with families for children remains and searches for guidance. Rushton (1994), writing of critical care settings, draws on a framework originally offered by Shelton *et al.* (1987). Its key elements are outlined below:

- Recognition that the family is the constant in the child's life while the service systems and personnel within those systems fluctuate
- Facilitation of parent/professional collaboration at all levels of health care
- Sharing of unbiased and complete information with parents about their child's care on an ongoing basis in an appropriate and supportive manner
- Implementation of appropriate policies and programmes that are comprehensive and provide emotional and financial support to meet the needs of families
- Recognition of family strengths and individuality and respect for different methods of coping
- Understanding and incorporating the developmental and emotional needs of infants, children and adolescents and their families into health-care delivery systems

- Encouragement and facilitation of parent-to-parent support
- Assurance that the design of health-care delivery systems is flexible, accessible and responsive to family needs.

It is accepted that some elements of Shelton *et al*'s (1987) framework as adapted by Rushton (1994) may be more relevant to some nurse practitioners than others, depending on their role and area of work. Equally it is clear that as a framework it is less than perfect. Certainly, it would benefit from attention to the need for professionals to understand beliefs held by parents that might impact on their behaviour, since anecdotal evidence suggests this to be an area of conflict in practice. Carter-Jessop and Yoos (1994) maintain that working to understand parental beliefs offers a way forward in the development of relationship, opening lines of communication and even perhaps enabling professionals to learn from parents. However, imperfect as it is and in the absence of a more complete understanding as to what works and what does not work in practice, the adaptation of Shelton *et al*'s (1987) framework offers a starting place for nurse practitioners. Moreover it could serve to guide parents as they attempt to make sense of a system which may seem foreign and within which they are trying to act for and with their children.

On this note it seems that the explorations of the chapter have almost turned full circle. The UN Convention (1989) embodies the ideal of balancing two principles – protecting children and their best interests (article 3) and enabling them to have a voice and to choose to the limits of their decision-making capacity (article 12). Parents carry a heavy responsibility as they work both to protect children and to facilitate their developing autonomy. Health-care workers are similarly charged and, as with parents, may find their roles complicated by their own beliefs and values concerning children. There is the potential for conflict between parents and professionals as they take on their responsibilities to children, equally there is space for collaboration. Perhaps the greatest challenge for the nurse practitioner lies in negotiating steps towards the latter.

Towards the assessment of child health

From the outset this chapter did not purport to be a recipe book – a 'how to' on the assessment of child health. Had it pursued a biomedical model it might have done so. However we began by arguing, and have illustrated, that child health is a complex phenomenon, rooted in diverse social worlds, variously experienced, affected not only by beliefs, values and the law, but by children themselves, developing as individuals and learning to make sense of their worlds. Child health is not simply a matter of understanding biological immaturity and of knowing how to assess bodily systems. Its assessment requires practitioners to go beyond the borders of the medical model and into the world wherein child health is nested. Doing so will allow practitioners to identify not only the factors that sustain and those that close down children's opportunities to enjoy health, but to look for ways of preventing disease and promoting health in collaboration with communities, families and children themselves (Billingham 1995; Scriven and Orme 1996). Such is the principle underpinning the concept of Health Action Zones (Crail 1997) and, before that, the Health Cities initiative (Wass 1994). And yet the extent to which such a social health role is congruent with that which has emerged for nurse practitioners is debatable. Even although a circumscribed approach to the assessment of child health that begins and ends with the individual threatens to be partial in the data it collects, to the nurse practitioner operating within the still-dominant paradigm of biomedicine (Moon and Gillespie 1995) and looking to identify undifferentiated, undiagnosed health problems (South Thames Regional Health Authority 1994) it may seem more congruent. Indeed, the very idea of assessing child *health* may seem foreign to those practising within a biomedical paradigm. However, care needs to be taken in pursuing this argument further. The diversity of roles undertaken by nurse practitioners in a range of settings and the fact that the full extent of what nurse practitioners do is as yet unknown (Reveley 1997) means that generalizations should not be made. This said, as long as the dominance of biomedicine endures (Moon and Gillespie 1995), it may be that nurse practitioners, who are knowledgeable of the impact of the social world on child health, are challenged as they work to assess it and meet needs. It will be for each nurse practitioner to negotiate what is undoubtedly a difficult path between two very different fields of understanding. Moreover it will be important to the continuing development of the nurse practitioner role that knowledge of practice which treads the path between biomedical and social understandings of factors impacting on child health is made public.

This chapter closes by drawing together the themes explored and arguing that together they promise to inform the process of working with children and their families in order to assess child health and meet needs. Although challenging to implement, the UN Convention (1989) offers direction to practitioners working with and for children. Yet in emphasizing the centrality of children's rights, it leaves aside issues concerning how children might be enabled to exercise their rights responsibly. Just as children, and indeed adults, must learn that rights are not absolutes, so too understanding needs to grow in respect of the fact that rights should be exercised with care and concern for others. Nurse practitioners have a role in facilitating such a process. So too do they have a role in taking into account the reality of difference in children's everyday lives – difference which impacts on health and can disadvantage some more than others. However, the challenge within this understanding is not to blame those experiencing health inequalities, as all too often has seemed to have happened (Naidoo and Wills 1994). Social organization and structuring support inequality of opportunity in all aspects of people's lives. Nurse practitioners are left to reflect on how they might use their voices to children's and families' advantages given the reality of disadvantage. And finally, as developing individuals learning to make sense of their worlds and working out their responses to it, children are active participants in all interactions. Yet adult power can operate to silence voices and shape behaviours – those of children and adults too. Nurse practitioners must look to develop caring practices that embrace children and families so that each gains and grows from the experience. Collaborating with families in the development of services is one way forward, needs-led health care will not emerge from the minds of providers without reference to users.

In conclusion, there is much scope for the nurse practitioner working with children and their families and there is room to advance sensitive caring practices. Restricting the nurse practitioner role to one that is framed by the biomedical paradigm appears to represent a loss of opportunity. Moreover, harnessing an exciting, and as yet unbounded role, to a biomedical model which should whither away (Moon and Gillespie 1995) would seem to threaten its existence. Children and their families can benefit from the emerging role of the nurse practitioner, but only if it responds to their needs and reaches beyond the constraints of the medical world into the reality of their everyday worlds wherein health is rooted and is lived.

References

Alderson P., Montgomery J. (1996) *Health Care Choices: Making Decisions with Children*, London, Institute for Public Policy Research.

Berk L. (1994) *Child Development*, Boston, Allyn and Bacon.

Billingham K. (1995) *Child Health Surveillance*. In: Fatchett A. (ed.) *Childhood to Adolescence: Caring for Health*, London, Baillière Tindall.

Black M. (1996) *Children First: The Story of UNICEF, Past and Present*, New York, Oxford University Press.

Botting B. (1997) Mortality in Childhood. In: Drever F., Whitehead M. (eds.) *Health Inequalities*, London, Stationery Office.

Botting, B., Crawley R. (1995) Trends and patterns in childhood mortality and morbidity. In: Botting B. (ed.) *The Health of our children*, London, OPCS/HMSO.

British Association for Community Child Health (1995) *Child Health Rights*, London, British Paediatric Association.

Bukatko D., Daehler M.W. (1995) *Child Development: A Thematic Approach*, Boston, Houghton and Mifflin.

Callery P. (1997) Paying to participate: financial, social and personal costs to parents of involvement in their child's care in hospital, *Journal of Advanced Nursing*, **25**, pp. 746–752.

Carlisle D. (1997) Disturbed young minds, *Health Visitor*, **70**(3), pp. 95–96.

Carter-Jessop L., Yoos L. (1994) Parental thinking: assessment and applications in nursing, *Maternal-Child Nursing Journal*, **22**(2), pp. 49–55, 64.

Casey A. (1993) Development and use of the partnership model of nursing care. In: Glasper, E., Tucker A. (eds.) *Advances in Child Health Nursing*, London, Scutari.

Charles-Edwards I. (1991) Who decides?, *Paediatric Nursing*, December 6–8.

Crail M. (1997) Modern Times?, *Health Service Journal*, December 11, **107**(5583), pp. 10–11.

Darbyshire P. (1994) *Living with a Sick Child in Hospital: The Experiences of Parents and Children*, London, Chapman & Hall.

Delaney F. (1996) Theoretical issues in intersectoral collaboration. In: Scriven A., Orme J. (eds.) *Health Promotion: Professional Perspectives*, Basingstoke, Macmillan Press.

Dennehy A., Smith L., Harker P. (1997) *Not to be Ignored: Young People, Poverty and Health*, London, Child Poverty Action Group.

Department of Health (1992) *The Health of the Nation*, London, HMSO.

Department of Health (1997) *The New NHS: Modern Dependable*, London, HMSO.

Eiser C. (1989) Children's concepts of illness: towards an alternative to the "stage" approach, *Psychology and Health*, **3**, pp. 93–101.

Fatchett A. (1995) *Childhood to Adolescence: Caring for Health*, London, Baillière Tindall.

Hill M. Tisdall K. (1997) *Children and Society*, Harlow, Addison Wesley Longman.

Jones L. (1994) *The Social Context of Health and Health Work*, Basingstoke, Macmillan Press.

Kurtz Z., Tomlinson J. (1994) How do we value our children today? As reflected by children's health, health care and health policy. In: Gott M., Moloney, B. (eds.) *Child Health: A Reader*, Oxford, Radcliffe Medical Press.

International Council of Nurses (1996) *Healthy Young People – A Brighter Tomorrow*, Geneva, ICN.

Lansdown G. (1994) Children's Rights. In: Mayall B. (ed.) *Children's Childhoods Observed and Experienced*, London, Falmer Press.

Leenders F. (1996) An overview of policies guiding health care for children, *Nursing Standard*, **10**(28), pp. 33–38.

Mayall B. (1994) *Children's Childhoods Observed and Experienced*, London, Falmer Press.

McCall Smith A. (1992) Consent to treatment in childhood, *Archives of Diseases in Childhood*, **67**(10), pp. 1247–1248.

Moon G. Gillespie R. (1995) *Society and Health: An Introduction to Social Science for Health Professionals*, London, Routledge.

Muller D., Harris P.J., Wattley L. (1986) *Nursing Children: Psychology, Research and Practice*, London, Harper and Row.

Naidoo J., Wills J. (1994) *Health Promotion: Foundation for Practice*, London, Baillière Tindall.

Nelson B. (1986). In: Eiser C. Children's Concepts of Illness: Towards an Alternative to the Stage Approach, *Psychology and Health*, **3.**

Newell P. (1989) *Children are People too: The Case against Physical Punishment*, London, Bedford Square Press.

Northumberland Young People's Health Project (1997) *Ford Castle – The Weekend: Some Young People under 18 Talking about 'Health'*, Ashington, Northumberland Young People's Health Project.

Oakley A., Bendelow G., Barnes J., Buchanan M., Husain N. (1995) Health and cancer prevention: knowledge and beliefs of children and young people, *British Medical Journal*, **310,** pp. 1029–1033.

Paton J.Y., Cockburn F. (1995) Core knowledge, skills and attitudes in child health for undergraduates, *Archives of Disease in Childhood*, **73,** pp. 263–265.

Payne M. (1995) Children's rights and children's needs, *Health Visitor*, **68**(10), pp. 412–414.

Pellegrini D. (1990) Psychosocial risk and protective factors in childhood, *Developmental and Behavioral Pediatrics*, **11**(4), pp. 201–209.

Power C. (1995) In: Botting B. (ed.) *The Health of Our Children*, London, OPCS/HMSO.

Price S. (1994) The special needs of children, *Journal of Advanced Nursing*, **20**(2), pp. 227–232.

Prout A. (1996) *Families, Cultural Bias and Health Promotion*, London, Health Education Authority.

Reading R. (1997) Social disadvantage and infection in childhood, *Sociology of Health and Illness*, **19**(4), pp. 395–414.

Reveley S. (1997) *Introducing the Nurse Practitioner into General Medical Practice: The Maryport Experience*, Lancaster, University College of St Martin.

Rolfe G. (1996) *Closing the Theory–Practice GAP: A New Paradigm for Nursing*, Oxford, Butterworth-Heinemann.

Rowlands O., Singleton N., Maher J., Higgin V. (1997) *Living in Britain*, London, Stationery Office.

Rushton C.H. (1994) Strategies for family centred care in the critical care setting. In: Gott M, Maloney B. (eds.) *Child Health: A Reader*, Oxford, Radcliffe Medical Press.

Scatton P. (1997) *'Childhood' in 'Crisis'*, London, UCL Press Ltd.

Scriven A., Orme, J. (1996) *Health Promotion: Professional Perspectives*, Basingstoke, Macmillan Press.

Shooter M. (1997) Halting the downward spiral, *Health Visitor*, **70**(3), pp. 97–98.

South Thames Regional Health Authority (1994) *Nurse Practitioner: A New Insight into Primary Care*, South Thames Regional Health Authority.

Spencer N. (1995) *Poverty and Child Health*, Oxford, Radcliffe Medical Press.

United Nations (1989) *United Nations Convention on the Rights of the Child*, Geneva, United Nations.

Wass A. (1994) *Promoting Health: The Primary Health Care Approach*, Sydney, Harcourt Brace.

White C. (1991) Child health in the 1990s. *British Medical Journal*, **302,** pp. 7.

Whyte D. (1996) *Explorations in Family Nursing*, London, Routledge.

Yoos H.L. (1994) Children's illness concepts: old and new paradigms. *Pediatric Nursing*, **20**(2), pp. 134–138, 145.

CHAPTER 15

Promoting health

Alison Crumbie

Introduction

The promotion of health falls firmly into the remit of nursing. That is not to say that health promotion is an exclusively nurse-led activity; rather, that it lies at the very heart of nursing. The practice of nurse practitioners encompasses the principles of health promotion; indeed, every consultation can be seen as a health-promoting opportunity. Amelia Mangay Maglacas (1991) states that the role of the nurse practitioner is to carry out a wide range of health-care services, including nursing, medical care, preventive care and health promotion. Theo Schofield (1991) lists one of the attributes of nurse practitioners as the ability to focus on health promotion and whole-person care and Barbara Stilwell (1991) records that nurse practitioner consultations include health teaching and exploration of clients' attitudes to follow-up and treatment. Clearly much of the work of the nurse practitioner is involved in the promotion of health and well-being.

There is much debate about the definition of health promotion and health education. Downie *et al.* (1996) offer a comprehensive overview of the two defini-tions. They state that health education is 'communica-tion activity aimed at enhancing positive health and preventing or diminishing ill health in individuals and groups through influencing the beliefs, attitudes and behaviour of those with power and of the community at large'. Health promotion is defined as 'efforts to enhance positive health and reduce the risk of ill health through the overlapping spheres of health education, prevention and health protec-tion'. Clearly, nurse practitioners have a role to play at a variety of levels of health promotion, however, during individual consultations, the activity of nursing intervention will tend to be focused upon health *education* at an individual level. The purpose of this chapter is to examine a variety of approaches to promoting the health of clients in the practice setting.

Health

In a survey of 9000 adults in England, Scotland and Wales Cox *et al.* (1987) discovered that 30% of the respondents defined health as 'not ill' or 'no disease'. Whilst it is important to remain cognizant of the perspectives of the general population, many authors have defined health as a concept which incorporates a sense of well-being and is not merely the absence of disease. The World Health Organization (WHO) in 1948 defined health as 'a state of complete physical, mental and social well-being' and in 1984 a WHO working group on health promotion defined health as:

> the extent to which an individual or group is able, on the one hand to realise aspirations and satisfy needs and on the other hand to change or cope with the environment. Health is therefore seen as a resource for everyday life, not the objective of living: it is a positive concept emphasising social and personal resources as well as physical capabilities.

The ability to adapt to a changing environment underpins Ewles and Simnett's statement that health is to do with the ability to adapt to constantly changing demands, expectations and stimuli (Ewles and Simnett 1995).

David Seedhouse (1986) in his exploration of the concept of health states that a single uncontroversial definition of health is not waiting to be discovered. What is required is a theory of health which incorporates the multitude of possible definitions and provides us with a meaningful resource to guide our practice. In an attempt to clarify the fuzzy limits of health, Seedhouse uses an analogy which helps to clarify the objective of health-promoting inter-ventions:

> The key is that work for health is work on building a solid stage, and keeping that stage in good condition. The roles that people perform and how they choose to perform these roles upon that stage is up to the individuals provided that the platform is sound.

Seedhouse suggests that the most important issue is that we work to clarify the priorities of other people without imposing our own. We need to ask ourselves questions such as: 'Does this person want what I regard as health?' 'How can I find out what this person wants?' 'What am I trying to do when I work towards health promotion with this client?' In this way we avoid imposing our own values and beliefs on other people. A common understanding between the patient and the nurse practitioner can lead to clarification of the goals for health-promoting interventions.

Factors affecting health

It is clear that ill health does not happen by chance. There are many factors which affect a person's health status. Naidoo and Wills (1994) list the main influences upon health as genetic, biological, lifestyle, environmental and social factors. The nation's health promotion activity can therefore be focused on any or all of these factors. Genetic factors used to be considered as the one area health-care professionals could do nothing about; however, research into the human genome is creating possibilities for health promotion even at a genetic level and society will have to address the implications and the ethics of such activity. It is important to remain aware of the multiplicity of factors affecting an individual's health and therefore to consider the range of influences upon the person including family, employment, learned behaviour, health beliefs, politics, housing and available health services.

Health promotion

It is clear that there are a variety of definitions of health and that each client will bring his or her own definition to the consultation. Working towards an understanding of the meaning of health for the individual will help the nurse practitioner to determine the goals of nursing interventions. If we consider that health is something greater than the absence of disease, the concept of health promotion becomes an area of activity with limitless boundaries. If a client is unable to administer preventive steroid inhalers for uncontrolled asthma because s/he is unable to pay for the prescription, the focus of health promotion could be seen to be working towards an improvement in that patient's financial security. If a child attends a casualty department with injuries sustained in a car accident where she was not wearing her seat belt, the focus of health promotion could be aimed at changing the laws of our country to ensure that no child ever travels in the back of a car without a seat belt. Clearly there are several levels of health promotion activity.

WHO has defined health promotion as 'the process of enabling people to increase control over and to improve their health' (WHO 1986). Implicit in this statement is the need to address not only individual-specific needs but also environmental influences upon a person's health status. Health promotion according to the WHO definition is an *action*, and it includes activity at an individual level as well as at a national level. Health promotion is defined by Tones (1993) as the product of healthy public policy and health education, with the major function of health education being empowerment.

Implementing health promotion in practice

Health promotion in acute settings

Traditionally the focus of health promotion has been seen as an activity which occurs in primary care. Nurse practitioners can also be located in hospital settings where time and resources are frequently cited as reasons for not putting health promotion into practice (Wilson-Barnett and Latter 1993). The health promotion message is just as important in acute care as it is in primary care. Indeed, the patient may be having a life-changing experience during the hospital stay or in the A&E department and the nurse practitioner should be prepared to offer the health promotion message at the appropriate moment for the patient.

Latter (1993) found that nurses in acute-care settings tended to follow the traditional medical approach to health promotion. The activity of the nurses was focused on disease processes and tended to ignore the social aspects of health. Jones (1993) analysed transcripts of taped conversations between nurses and patients and found that there seemed to be little spontaneous health education in the acute-care setting. Jones points to the need for improvement in communication skills for nurses and that nurses themselves need to feel empowered before they are able to empower others. Wilson-Barnett and Latter (1993) came to a similar conclusion; their findings suggest that the organization of the acute-care setting should offer continuity, autonomy and responsibility and should maximize empowerment for nurses. The nurses' level of knowledge was an essential component in the process of health promotion.

Nurse practitioners educated to an advanced level will clearly address many of the difficulties outlined in the research above. Nurse practitioners have a level of autonomy and responsibility beyond the level of the ward-based nurses addressed in Wilson-Barnett and Latter's research and consequently should experience a greater level of empowerment. As Jones (1993) points out, to empower others it is essential for the nurse to feel empowered. Nurse practitioners should therefore work towards an organizational structure which supports not only themselves but also their nurse colleagues and other members of the health-care team.

Health promotion in primary care

In 1978 the WHO held an international conference which resulted in the Alma Ata declaration exhorting governments to strengthen primary health care (WHO 1978). There are a variety of definitions of primary health care; most agree that it represents the first contact for community-based health care, provides open access to generalist services and takes a patient-centred, holistic approach (Coulter 1996). Nurse practitioners in primary health care consult with people who have undifferentiated undiagnosed problems. The nurse practitioner's role is to assess, diagnose, treat and discharge or refer. The nurse practitioner consultation therefore may be the patient's only interaction with the health service. It is essential then that every opportunity is taken to reinforce health promotion messages and to work towards the self-empowerment of each individual who chooses to consult with the nurse practitioner.

Primary care in the UK is dominated by general practice. Orme and Wright (1996) point out that this could potentially lead to a medical model of health promotion in the primary health-care setting. The introduction of the 1990 GP contract led to a system of remuneration for the number of health promotion clinic sessions held in the GP surgery. This approach emphasized a task-oriented style and fits neatly with the medical approach to health promotion. A diabetic clinic would be held for people with diabetes, an asthmatic clinic for people with asthma and a weight reduction or lifestyle clinic for people who need to reduce weight. This type of clinic does not provide the foundation for a holistic approach to health care and health promotion.

There is incredible potential for the practice of health promotion in each nurse practitioner consultation. If a nurse practitioner views the individual client as a presenting problem then health promotion will be conducted in the traditional medical approach which tends to address the problem in isolation from the multitude of influencing forces upon the individual. Viewed from the perspective of the individual's health beliefs and lifestyle and as a product of genetic factors, family influences and the society in which he or she lives, the nurse practitioner will gain an understanding of the person which will help to direct the focus of health-promoting activities.

Approaches to health education

In order to work with individuals who have a wide variety of definitions of health and have numerous influences upon their health status, it is necessary to consider the variety of approaches to health promotion. Katz and Peberdy (1997) outline five approaches to health promotion: medical, behavioural, educational, client-centred and social change. Naidoo and Wills (1994) also outline five approaches; however, they refer to the client-centred approach as empowerment – a concept seen as central to the activity of health promotion by Tones (1993).

Medical approach

The medical approach to health promotion uses scientific methods to address the problems of disease and ill health. Preventive measures include immunizations and screening to allow for prevention and the early detection of medically defined illnesses. This approach relies heavily upon a national infrastructure to deliver the service and on individual compliance. The medical approach to health promotion will evaluate the level of success by the incidence and prevalence of disease.

Behavioural approach

The behavioural approach seeks to encourage individuals to adopt healthy behaviours. The individual should then be at a decreased risk of developing diseases which are associated with high-risk behaviours such as smoking, consumption of alcohol, excessive consumption of fatty foods or, in some cases, sexual intercourse with no barrier protection. Health education is often focused on behaviour change and relies heavily upon the individual's willingness to adopt a healthier lifestyle. The result of the behaviour change approach should be that the individual no longer indulges in high-risk activities and ultimately that the potential diseases associated with those activities do not develop.

Educational approach

The educational approach aims to provide individuals with the knowledge and understanding necessary to make an informed choice about their health. This approach does not set out to persuade an individual to change in a certain direction; rather, the aim is to provide the individual with the information necessary to make an appropriate decision. Clearly an individual may choose not to make any lifestyle changes having understood the information provided and weighed up the pros and cons of change. This result is acceptable within the educational model as it respects the individual's right of free choice and the health educator has fulfilled his or her responsibility of providing the necessary educational content to ensure that the individual can make an informed choice.

Client-centred approach

The client-centred approach helps the client to identify concerns and priorities. The role of the health educator is to provide the client with the necessary tools and skills to set the agenda and to act upon the identified concerns. This approach sets the client firmly at the centre of the activity; the client is an equal partner in the health education process and the health promoter simply addresses the areas of concern to the client. Tones (1993) points out that it is beneficial for individuals to believe that they have some control over their lives. This sense of control can be seen as self-empowerment. Tones states that there are four factors which are central to the dynamics of self-empowerment: the environment, level of individual competency, sense of belief in control and emotional state. An individual who is empowered will be able to challenge the world and the social reality of life. The role of the health promoter is to help the individual identify areas of concern and to provide the necessary tools for the individual to make change.

Social change

Social change is directed at the environment within which a person lives. Political action is focused upon changing the social, physical or economic environment and thereby making it possible, or more likely, for individuals to make healthy lifestyle choices. An example of this top-down approach might be an organization choosing to make its premises a non-smoking area or the government introducing a greater level of taxation on cigarettes. As smoking becomes increasingly socially unacceptable, it could be suggested that individuals will be more likely to make the decision to stop smoking.

Nurse practitioners working in both primary care and hospital settings have an important role in women's health. Preconceptual care is an area of practice which clearly involves a number of health education messages. It is possible to consider preconceptual care by linking it to each of the five different health education approaches listed above. The medical approach would be to consider the administration of folic acid to prevent the development of neural tube defects in the infant before commencing with the pregnancy. The educational approach would involve making sure that the woman and her partner were fully aware of all the information available for people considering pregnancy. They could then make their own informed choices about lifestyle change and the adoption of healthy lifestyle behaviours based on the knowledge they have gained from the nurse practitioner. The behavioural approach would address high-risk behaviours and aim to change those behaviours. The client-centred or self-empowerment approach would aim to identify the agenda of the woman and her partner, recognizing the importance of their own values and ideas around pregnancy. The social approach would consider community and societal influences upon the couple. Health promotion might address issues around societal expectations of smoking in pregnancy or the demands upon a woman to drink alcohol when in fact she is trying to abstain.

The approach to health promotion adopted by the nurse practitioner will be determined by the needs of the individual or, in other situations, the client group. A variety of approaches can be utilized to address any one particular issue and in some situations several approaches will be necessary to produce the desired outcome. Nurse practitioners will be involved in each approach to a varying degree. In addition to considering the variety of approaches available, it is also worth considering models of health promotion to help analyse clinical practice and evaluate outcomes.

Models of health promotion

A model of health promotion helps to provide a framework to analyse and guide practice (Figure 15.1). There are many models of health promotion

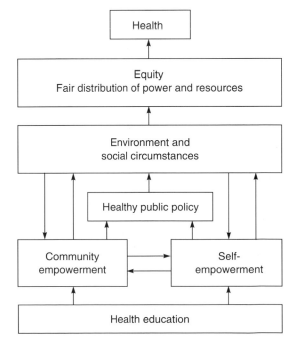

Figure 15.1 Empowerment model of health promotion

Source: Adapted from Tones (1996)

and an individual practitioner may find one model suits the style of activity with certain clients or client groups more than another. Tones (1996) has developed a model of empowerment and health promotion which brings together health education, self- and community empowerment, healthy public policy, environment and social circumstances and equity. Each of these concepts underpin the individual's ability to achieve health.

Beattie (1991) suggests that there are four strategies for health promotion: individual persuasion, legislative action, personal counselling and community development (Figure 15.2). The strategy employed can therefore be authoritative or based on negotiation and may be an individual activity or the focus of collective activity.

Mode of intervention

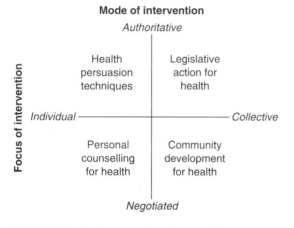

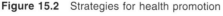

Figure 15.2 Strategies for health promotion

Source: Adapted from Beattie (1991)

It is clear from each of these models that the activity of health education forms only one part of a health promotion strategy. If nurse practitioners are to be successful in working towards acceptable levels of health for each individual it is essential to consider the variety of levels of activity required to achieve the goal of optimum well-being. Most frequently nurse practitioners will be focusing nursing interventions on health education, self-empowerment, personal counselling and health persuasion and will less frequently be involved in the creation of legislation or public health policy. The following are examples of models which can be applied to practice and can be utilized within each nurse practitioner consultation.

The health belief model

The health belief model (Becker 1984) focuses on the role of health beliefs in determining an individual's actions. The health belief model is based on the assumption that each person will consider the costs and benefits of a particular behaviour and engage in health actions accordingly. In order to engage in behaviour which will prevent illness and/ or promote health and well-being, the individual must believe that:

- he or she is susceptible to the disease
- the disease is serious
- the preventive behaviour or activity will be beneficial
- the benefits of the behaviour or action will outweigh the costs.

An additional influence on the individual's behaviour is the presence of cues. A cue is a reminder to engage in a certain behaviour.

Originally this model was developed to predict preventive behaviours but it has also been used to predict the behaviour of both chronically and acutely ill patients (Bennett and Hodgson 1992). The success of the implementation of this model can be measured by assessing the number of preventive actions undertaken by the individual and by determining the strength with which the individual holds the four key beliefs (Tones and Tilford 1994).

Nurse practitioners regularly consult with patients who are overtly weighing up the pros and cons of a particular action or behaviour. The health belief model can help to refine the approach taken in the consultation and assist the nurse practitioner in understanding why some individuals may choose not to adopt a behaviour which may prevent illness or promote their general well-being. For example, consider a man who presents to the A&E department with an acute myocardial infarction. At this stage he will have a clear understanding that he is susceptible to heart disease; he will be experiencing the pain of infarction which emphasizes the seriousness of the problem; he will be aware that his smoking habits could be linked to his present problem and during the acute phase he could well be weighing up the advantages and disadvantages of smoking cessation. As the patient recovers from the acute phase of the illness the trigger of the pain will subside. As the memory of the crushing chest pain fades, his perception of the seriousness of his illness may also change. He may no longer believe that he is susceptible to heart disease and as time passes he may decide that his illness is not too serious. He may tell himself that the smoking probably was not linked to the infarction as he has an aunt who is in her 80s and who has smoked all her life, and after a few days at home that irresistible urge to smoke overcomes his temporarily changed beliefs during his time in hospital.

The nurse practitioner could utilize the framework of the health belief model to enhance the possibility of the patient in the above scenario engaging in health-promoting activities. The patient could be encouraged to join a cardiac rehabilitation programme which would continue to educate him about his susceptibility to the disease, the seriousness of the illness and the benefits of changing his behaviour. The patient's family could be involved in providing cues such as congratulating the patient on the number of days without smoking or working together on exercise and healthy eating. The nurse practitioner might also explain to the patient the need to monitor lipid levels, blood pressure and weight and may also explain that he should receive an annual influenza vaccination. Each of these activities would emphasize the seriousness of the disease and, according to the health belief model, this will have an influence on the patient's behaviour.

Theory of reasoned action

Ajzen and Fishbein's (1980) theory of reasoned action is another model which can help the nurse practitioner to understand the behaviour of patients and the reasons why some choose to adopt healthy lifestyle actions and others do not (Figure 15.3). Ajzen and Fishbein (1980) argue that behaviour is influenced by an individual's attitudes towards a certain behaviour and also by subjective norms. An individual's attitude is comprised of a belief and the strength of feeling towards this belief. For example, an individual may think that excessive alcohol consumption causes liver damage but it doesn't happen often. In this example the individual holds the belief but the strength of that belief is weak. Subjective norms are the individual's perceptions of what others might think of their behaviour. If the individual's peer group believe that smoking marijuana helps to reduce stress and helps everyone have a good time the subjective norms of the group will influence the individual's lifestyle choices. The individual's attitude and the individual's subjective norms form the two major influences creating an *intention* to behave in a certain manner. The intention is closely linked to the behaviour itself, although people do not always behave consistently with their intentions.

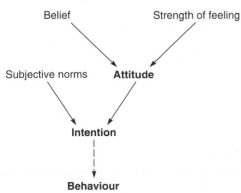

Figure 15.3 Theory of reasoned action

Ajzen and Fishbein separated beliefs from attitude and emphasized the importance of significant others in influencing health behaviour (Tones and Tilford 1994). This is a particularly useful model in helping to understand the behaviours of people who choose to engage in risky actions even when they have all the information and a full understanding of the implications of their behaviour. Young people who have type one diabetes are often labelled as non-compliant when they choose to stop their insulin injections and to go out on the town with their friends. In this example the overwhelming pressure of subjective norms outweighs the attitude toward the behaviour and, even though the intention might be to maintain the blood glucose levels, the behaviour is an overindulgence in alcohol and results in an admission to the A&E unit with health-care professionals and parents left scratching their heads in wonderment at the futility of the behaviour.

The theory of reasoned action can be used by nurse practitioners to consider the possible outside influences which have an impact on the patient's behaviour. It may be that a woman has the belief that smoking is harmful. She may have a fairly weak strength of feeling about the harm of smoking and therefore when she is socializing with her friends who smoke regularly she will indulge in smoking behaviour. If the theory of reasoned action is applied to this situation, the patient might be advised to find an alternative to the social circle who provide the subjective norms and clearly affect her intentions. The nurse might provide literature for the patient in an attempt to enhance the strength of feeling related to the harmful effects of smoking behaviour. The theory of reasoned action provides a framework for nurse practitioners to engage in more effective health education with clients.

Helping people change

It is clearly of great concern to any health-care professional involved in health promotion that if changes are made towards a healthier lifestyle, those changes should be permanent. Prochaska and DiClemente (1984) developed a stages model of behaviour acquisition which outlines the stages involved in changing behaviour (Figure 15.4).

In the precontemplation stage the individual has not yet become aware of the need to change. The health professional has a role here in bringing healthy lifestyle issues to the attention of the individual so that the contemplation stage can begin. Heron's (1990) six-category intervention analysis model can be utilized by the nurse practitioner to plan an intervention which aims to highlight healthy lifestyle issues to the individual. The nurse practitioner could

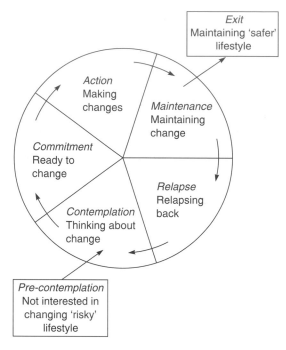

Figure 15.4 Stages model of behaviour acquisition

Source: Adapted from Ewles and Simnett (1995)

plan to engage in an informative intervention or could choose to be confronting, depending upon the needs of the client. Heron's six-category intervention analysis model is discussed in more detail on p. 256.

After precontemplation, the individual moves on to contemplation. In this stage the individual is aware of the benefits of change but may be thinking about the change and awaiting further information. S/he then becomes ready to change and may require some extra support at this stage to move on to make the change. It is possible for an individual to take weeks or even years over any stage and s/he may move back and forth between stages until ready to move on. After making the change the individual may relapse and then return to the precontemplation stage. If relapse does not occur the individual has maintained the healthy lifestyle and the new behaviour is sustained. The important message for health-care professionals is that relapse may be part of the cycle and is not necessarily a sign of failure.

The stages model of health promotion, which has been widely used in primary health care, is particularly relevant in the management and support of people who are overweight and attempting to change their dietary habits. In the precontemplation stage individuals have not become aware that their weight is a potential risk to health; indeed they may even see their size as healthy. Discussing a weight-reducing diet at this stage would be a waste of time for both patient and nurse practitioner as the patient

is not interested in making a change and has no awareness of the need to change. Patients may move into the contemplation stage for a variety of reasons, including objective changes in their own health such as the development of hypertension or diabetes mellitus or health problems in their friends and family. In the contemplation stage the patient has entered the cycle and has enough motivation to consider seriously changing dietary or exercise habits. During the contemplation stage the nurse practitioner could provide the patient with dietary information to help in the decision-making process. If the patient continues to progress through the stages, the next stage is a commitment to change. At this stage the patient requires support and encouragement and may benefit from regular meetings, either with a group of other patients who have made the same decision or on an individual basis with the nurse practitioner. The patient's subsequent actions should be supported by clear goals and a realistic plan. Rewards help to promote the patient's actions at this stage; obvious rewards in the case of diabetes mellitus are the fact that the patient begins to feel better as the blood glucose is reduced.

Maintaining a reduction in weight can cause a great deal of anxiety and patients have to adopt coping strategies to deal with the change in their dietary habits. It is not uncommon for relapse to occur and for a previously highly motivated patient to begin to put on weight after several weeks or months of weight reduction. It is essential that the patient is made aware that this is simply one of the stages in the cycle of change and that it is common to go through several revolutions of the cycle before adopting a permanent change to lifestyle behaviours. (Indeed, Ewles and Simnett (1995) point out that on an average successful former smokers take three revolutions of change before they finally stop smoking.) At the exit stage the patient undertaking weight reduction will have made permanent alterations to dietary habits and exercise routines and will be able to maintain an acceptable body mass index without the anxiety of relapse and the struggle to maintain the behaviour changes.

The stages model of health promotion can help the nurse practitioner to support and understand the patient through the change process. The problem arises when the patient is in the precontemplative stage, is unaware of the risky behaviour and is not motivated to do anything about it. Naidoo and Wills (1994) point out that there are several prerequisites to change which are worth considering when faced with a patient who refuses or is unable to change. It is important that the change is self-initiated. Telling patients that their behaviour is a risk to their health and that they must stop smoking will probably result in an angry, highly demotivated patient. It is also important that the risky behaviour becomes salient. A patient who shares a house with four student friends, all of whom smoke, will reappraise her smoking behaviour when she moves into a new house with her non-smoking partner. The smoking activity which was previously automatic and habitual has become problematic as she is now more aware of her habit; this leads to a reappraisal of her behaviour and a greater chance of moving into the contemplative stage. If the behaviour is a coping mechanism for the patient it will be extremely difficult to change. In this case the patient needs to consider alternative coping strategies. It is not always easy to find alternatives to smoking; however, some people find that chewing gum at times when they would have smoked or engaging in diversions such as exercise or other activities can help.

Naidoo and Wills (1994) point out that there is a limit to an individual's ability to change. Lifestyle change is stressful and if life is problematic and uncertain then the capacity to cope with change is limited. Social support is essential to reinforce the need for behaviour change and to maintain the change. Nurse practitioners need to consider all the prerequisites for change and to ensure that the patient has adequate support. Only then can success be achieved in the form of reduction of risky lifestyle behaviours and the promotion of health.

Evaluation

Nurse practitioners who engage in health promotion activities either as individual practitioners or as a member of a health care team must be aware that evaluation of their practice is essential. Evaluation helps to demonstrate whether a particular programme has achieved its stated aims. It is often extremely difficult to determine whether the number of clients who received advice about exercise and coronary heart disease actually remained free of heart disease. There are so many other potential factors to consider that absolute proof is often elusive. Attempts must be made to develop overall aims and objectives of a particular health-promoting activity and then to measure outcomes against measurable objectives. For example, a practice might decide that the primary health care team will target the prevention of heart disease as a specific programme of activity. The aims and objectives of the programme might be developed by the team before a plan of activity is developed.

Aim
- To reduce the incidence of coronary heart disease in the practice population

Objectives
- To enhance awareness of the risk factors for heart disease
- To reduce the number of people who smoke in the practice population
- To reduce the number of people with a body mass index over 25

Measures
- The incidence of heart disease in the practice will be monitored and reduced
- Patients will be able to describe what the risk factors for heart disease are when asked
- Numbers of people who smoke in the practice can be recorded and reduced
- Numbers of people with a body mass index over 25 can be recorded and reduced

It is clear that it may take a decade of sustained health promotion to produce any recordable results relating to the aim of the programme; however, other objectives such as number of people with a body mass index over 25 in the practice population can easily be recorded and the number before the programme was initiated can be compared with the number of people after 12 months of targeted health promotion. Evaluation of health promotion programmes is a complex process, yet without evidence it is difficult to be sure of the value of activities carried out in practice.

This chapter has provided an overview of the meaning of health and illness, health promotion and health education. Several approaches to health education and models of health promotion have been presented to provide a framework to help guide activity in practice. Whilst it is clear that health promotion is a multidisciplinary, multilevel activity many clients require continued individualized support to work towards a healthy lifestyle. Nurse practitioners working in both the primary health care and hospital setting are ideally placed to offer that support.

References

Ajzen I., Fishbein M. (1980) *Understanding Attitudes and Predicting Behaviour*, Englewood Cliffs, New Jersey, Prentice-Hall.

Beattie A. (1991) Knowledge and control in health promotion: a test case for social policy and social theory. In: Gabe J., Calnan M., Bury M. (eds.) *The Sociology of the Health Service*, London, Routledge.

Becker M.H. (ed.) (1984) *The Health Belief Model and Personal Behaviour*, New Jersey, Charles B. Sack Thorofare.

Bennett P., Hodgson R. (1992) Psychology and health promotion. In: Bunton R., Macdonald G. (eds.) *Health Promotion Disciplines and Diversity*, London, Routledge.

Coulter A. (1996) Why should health services be primary care-led?, *Journal of Health Service Research Policy*, **1**(2), pp. 122–124.

Cox B.D. *et al.* (1987) The health and lifestyle survey: preliminary report. The health promotion trust. Cited in: Katz J., Peberdy A. (1997) *Promoting Health Knowledge and Practice*, Hampshire, The Open University/Macmillan.

Downie R.S. Tannahill C., Tannahill A. (1996) *Health Promotion Models and Values*, 2nd edn., Oxford, Oxford University Press.

Ewles L., Simnett I. (1995) *Promoting Health*, 3rd edn. London, Scutari.

Heron J. (1990) *Helping the Client*, London, Sage Publications.

Jones K. (1993) Opportunities for health education: an analysis of nurse–client interactions in acute areas. In: Wilson-Barnett J., Macleod J. (1993) *Research in Health Promotion and Nursing*, London, Macmillan.

Katz J., Peberdy A. (1997) *Promoting Health Knowledge and Practice*, Hampshire, The Open University/Macmillan.

Latter S. (1993) Health education and health promotion in acute settings: nurses' perceptions and practice. In: Wilson-Barnett J., Macleod J. (eds.) *Research in Health Promotion and Nursing*, London, Macmillan.

Mangay Maglacas A. (1991) A global perspective. In: Salvage J. (ed.) *Nurse Practitioners Working for Change in Primary Health Care Nursing*, London, Kings Fund.

Naidoo J., Wills J. (1994) *Health Promotion. Foundations for Practice*, London, Baillière Tindall.

Orme J., Wright C. (1996) Health promotion in primary health care. In: Scriven A., Orme J. (eds.) *Health Promotion Professional Perspectives*, London, Macmillan.

Prochaska J.O., DiClemente C. (1984) *The Transtheoretical Approach: Crossing Traditional Foundations of Change*, Illinois, Harnewood.

Schofield T. (1991) Commentary. In: Salvage J. (ed.) *Nurse Practitioners Working for Change in Primary Health Care Nursing*, London, Kings Fund.

Scriven A., Orme J. (1996) *Health Promotion Professional Perspectives*, London, Macmillan.

Seedhouse D. (1986) *Health The Foundations for Achievement*, Chichester, John Wiley.

Stilwell B. (1991) An ideal consultation. In: Salvage J. (ed.) *Nurse Practitioners Working for Change in Primary Health Care Nursing*, London, Kings Fund.

Tones K. (1993) The theory of health promotion: implications for nursing. In: Wilson-Barnett J., Macleod Clark J. (eds.) *Research in Health Promotion and Nursing*, London. Macmillan.

Tones K. (1996) The anatomy and ideology of health promotion: empowerment in context. In: Scriven A., Orme J. (eds.) *Health Promotion Professional Perspectives*, London, Macmillan.

Tones K., Tilford S. (1994) *Health Education Effectiveness, Efficiency and Equity*, 2nd edn., London, Chapman & Hall.

Wilson-Barnett J., Latter S. (1993) Factors influencing nurses' health education and health promotion practice in acute ward areas. In: Wilson-Barnett J., Macleod J. (eds.) *Research in Health Promotion and Nursing*, London, Macmillan.

World Health Organization (1948) Preamble of the constitution of the World Health Organization, WHO. Cited in: Katz J., Peberdy A. (1997) *Promoting Health Knowledge and Practice*, Basingstoke, Macmillan.

World Health Organization (1978) Alma Ata declaration, WHO. Cited in: Katz J., Peberdy A. (eds.) *Promoting Health Knowledge and Practice*, Basingstoke, Macmillan.

World Health Organization (1984) Report of the working group on concepts and principles of health promotion, Copenhagen, WHO. Cited in: Katz J., Peberdy A. (1997) *Promoting Health Knowledge and Practice*, Basingstoke, Macmillan.

World Health Organization (1986) Ottawa charter for health promotion, Geneva, WHO. Cited in: Katz J., Peberdy A. (1997) *Promoting Health Knowledge and Practice*, Basingstoke, Macmillan.

CHAPTER 16

Assessment and management of the patient with chronic health problems

Alison Crumbie

Introduction

Whether based in a hospital or a primary health-care setting, nurse practitioners will be constantly interacting with people who live with chronic conditions. Longevity and the impact of medical progress and social reform upon people who previously might have died from their disorder or would have faced a life in institutionalized care have resulted in chronicity becoming an ordinary feature of family life (Cole and Reiss 1993). Some nurse practitioners may be responsible for managing people who are chronically ill whilst others whose work is focused on the patient with acute problems will have to consider the effect of the chronic condition on the presenting condition.

The aim of this chapter is to consider the meaning of chronicity and its impact upon the care of people who consult with nurse practitioners. The physical examination and history-taking of people who live with diabetes mellitus and those who live with chronic pain will be outlined as an example of the way in which a chronic condition might influence the nurse practitioner's assessment technique and management plan.

Chronic conditions

People who live with a chronic condition live with a permanent alteration in their way of existing in the world. Most people live with rather than die from a chronic condition (Verbrugge and Jette 1994). There are a variety of definitions of chronicity. Lyons

et al. (1995) state that a chronic illness is not a singular event; rather it signifies a set of complex processes that develop and endure over time. Cameron and Gregor (1987) argue that chronic illness is a lived experience which involves a permanent deviation from the norm caused by unalterable pathological changes. Bleeker and Mulderij (1992) speak of the body losing its silence and Morse *et al.* (1994) describe a body in dis-ease. Clearly chronicity involves a heightened awareness of the physical self which permeates the whole being.

Physical implications

Kelly and Field (1996) point out that chronic illness results in the physical reality of 'bad' bodies. The body changes in chronic illness and can be seen as letting the person down. This has been reinforced in medical sociology by Parsons (1951) who viewed the sick role as a form of deviance. According to Parsons a person who takes on the sick role should legitimize the role by seeking advice from doctors or healers and must do everything possible to get well. This is often not possible for someone who has a chronic illness. S/he is often not able to get well and, indeed, in some forms of chronic illness the person's well-being gradually deteriorates over time. When western medicine does not provide the answers or a cure for people who live with chronic illness, they may be more likely to seek the views of complementary therapists or healers. Society may be even less sympathetic to their condition as they may be seen as seeking less legitimate forms of care. In this way someone who lives with a chronic condition may be seen as deviant and this has an effect which permeates beyond the physical manifestations of the disease process.

Self-concept and personal relationships

The patient who lives with a chronic problem experiences a change in self-concept associated with the physical changes which occur in the body. Jerret (1994) states that a chronic condition results in a reappraisal of functioning and health while Price (1996) makes an interesting connection between the patient's case notes and the experience of chronic illness. He states that 'as the case notes get fatter so does the catalogue of experiences and with each successive passing year the redefinitions of what happiness and hope means'. The changes in self-concept, reappraisal of life and redefinitions of hope and happiness clearly impact upon the person's relationship with family, friends, health-care professionals and the world. Lyons *et al.* (1995) state that health challenges can threaten the stability of close relationships. Roles and responsibilities alter and changes in autonomy can cause additional stressors within the relationship. Lyons describes illness as removing the window dressing of everyday life, leading to the exposure of elements in a relationship which are of central importance. This can ultimately strengthen and improve a relationship or the subsequent emotional distress may compromise the links between individuals.

Relationships are under threat from chronic conditions. However, a relationship can also be a source of strength and support for the person who has the chronic condition and can be an additional beneficial tool in the nurse practitioner's interventions aimed at promoting coping strategies. While there is no comprehensive model detailing strategies for relationship-focused coping, Lyons *et al.* (1995) suggest that the re-evaluation of self and relationships, the containment of the impact of illness on relationships, network modelling, relationship adaptation, relationship reciprocity and communal coping provide a viable framework for relationship coping.

Spirituality

Having considered the physical effects of chronic illness, the social impact and the effect it might have upon family relationships, the nurse practitioner might also consider the spirituality of the person who lives with a chronic condition. In Heriot's discussion about spirituality and ageing (1992), she states that 'Even though physical functions decline with ageing, the spiritual dimension of life does not succumb to the ageing process even in the presence of debilitating physical and mental illness'. This statement has interesting connotations for people who live with a chronic condition. In the presence of debilitating illness a person can still achieve a sense of wellness. Pilch (1988) states that wellness spirituality is 'a way of living, a lifestyle that views and lives life as purposeful and pleasurable, that seeks out life sustaining and life enriching options to be chosen freely at every opportunity and that sinks its roots deeply into spiritual values or specific religious beliefs'. The nurse practitioner therefore should not only consider the physical manifestations of the chronic illness but should also focus attention on the individual's sense of meaning and purpose in life. By focusing upon spiritual well-being a person can feel well even in the presence of disability and ill health.

Assessment of people who live with chronic conditions

Chronicity then has an enduring quality; it permeates a person's whole being and affects relationships. Chronic illness is a condition with which a person has to learn to live; it represents a permanent alteration and affects the physical, mental, social and spiritual well-being of the person. Examples of chronic conditions are asthma, epilepsy, cardiovascular disease, arthritis, diabetes mellitus, psoriasis, cancer, multiple sclerosis, Parkinson's disease, AIDS/HIV, thyroid disease, chronic back pain, a bipolar disorder of mental health and stroke, to name but a few. It is clear from this list of conditions that the impact of the illness will vary enormously according to the perceived level of intrusion of the illness into the person's life. A person with type I diabetes constantly has to inject with insulin – indeed, life depends upon it – and the individual's sense of self will become intricately tied into the routines associated with the management of blood glucose levels. A person who has lived with diabetes for many years, however, finds the management of the condition less intrusive than a person with acne who may be acutely aware that the condition is obvious to the world.

The care of people who have a chronic condition represents an exciting challenge for nursing. Not only do they require medical interventions to improve their physical functioning, they also require the skills of nursing to be sensitive to their needs, offer appropriate levels of assistance, include the person as a partner in care and provide a flexibility that acknowledges the individuality of each person who presents with the condition. McBride (1993) states that the care of people who have a chronic condition is central to the mission of nursing and Funk *et al.* (1993) describe it as being at the heart of nursing. Nolan and Nolan (1995) state that the medical model is appropriate when cure is the aim and so often in the management of chronic conditions cure is not the aim. Nurse practitioners have the skills and a variety of models of care which can be utilized to address the various levels of need for people who live with chronic conditions.

Kelly and Field (1996) state that the management of physical problems in chronic illness is at the epicentre of the coping experience. Social coping, family relationships and spiritual well-being all depend on ability to cope with the physical body. Conversely, it could be argued that spiritual well-being can have a positive impact on the individual's ability to cope with the physical manifestations of the disease process. Indeed, Leetun (1996) points out that no amount of body healing will work if the spirit is not also healed. In a study of women with advanced breast cancer Doris Coward found that self-transcendence directly affected emotional well-being and that emotional well-being led to a reduction in illness distress (Coward 1991). The following framework for assessing people who live with chronic conditions will take a holistic approach considering physical well-being, social coping, family relationships and spiritual health, recognizing the impact of each upon the other.

History-taking for people who live with a chronic condition

History-taking has been addressed in Chapter 2. History-taking in people who live with a chronic condition should follow the same structured format as for any person in the health-care setting. It is vitally important that the nurse practitioner creates the space for individuals to tell their story. People who live with chronic conditions will have had many interactions with people in the health service and are often more expert in the assessment and management of their condition than the myriad of health-care professionals with whom they interact.

Chief complaint

The nurse practitioner must consider if the chief complaint is associated with the underlying condition and if not, what its impact might be upon the chronic condition. It is important to ensure that an awareness of the chief complaint does not cloud the judgement in making a clinical assessment. It is equally important that the nurse practitioner does not forget to consider the possible impact of the condition upon the chief complaint. This becomes particularly complex in the management of people who have more than one chronic condition, such as people who have diabetes mellitus and coronary heart disease or people who have hypertension and chronic obstructive airways disease.

In answer to the question 'what brought you here?' the patient may immediately identify the chronic condition as the source of the presenting problem when it may not necessarily be so. The patient may not have made the connection between the chief complaint and the chronic condition. For example, a patient who presents with a sore throat and who has hypothyroidism may have a throat infection or may be experiencing a sore throat due to the presence of a goitre. The nurse practitioner must be alert for all possibilities and therefore a structured and thorough history-taking approach is essential in making an accurate diagnosis.

Present problem

A detailed analysis of the presenting problem will begin to help differentiate between the chronic condition and the presenting problem or may link them together. Exploring issues around current health status and health status before the presenting problem became an issue will provide clear clues about the impact of the chronic condition on the presenting problem and/or the impact of the presenting problem on the chronic condition. The PQRST framework (p. 16) is a useful tool for this purpose.

Palliation

It is important to explore with the patient what interventions have been tried to improve the condition, what medications have been used and what impact they have had. People who live with chronic conditions may have tried altering their own medications before seeking help, for example, just taking a few extra thyroxine tablets to help arrest weight increase or increasing antihypertensive agents if the person experiences headaches. Patients have their own rational decision-making process for trying such interventions and the nurse practitioner must be alert to this to ensure that alterations in medications are properly evaluated.

Provocation

Exploring the issues of provoking factors with the individual can help the nurse practitioner identify links between the problem and the chronic condition. Individuals may have their own ideas about the cause of the problem and this should be explored with them to give them a clear message that the nurse practitioner values their input to the assessment process.

Quality or quantity

Asking patients to describe the problem in their own words will help the nurse practitioner to assess patients' level of concern. This is particularly important in people who live with chronic conditions as the patient can often learn to live with extraordinary levels of discomfort. The onset of symptoms may be gradual and insidious and it is therefore essential to carry out an accurate assessment.

Region or radiation

Asking the patient to locate the source of discomfort and what region of the body it radiates to is particularly helpful in differentiating between sources of pain. This is an important aspect of the assessment in people who suffer from a skin disorder. The nurse practitioner should consider the whole body and ask appropriate questions to determine if the patient is experiencing symptoms in areas beyond the immediately obvious.

Severity scale

An accurate assessment of the type and level of severity of the presenting problem is essential in obtaining a clear picture of the progression or regression of problems for people who have chronic illnesses. This is particularly important in the management of chronic pain and an assessment tool should be utilized to help provide a subjective and objective measurement of the level of discomfort.

Timing

Exploration of the timing of the presenting problem is valuable in the assessment of any problem for a person who has a chronic condition. Timing can relate to time of year. This is particularly important in the assessment of people who have allergic conditions. Timing in the week can help make links between environmental triggers in asthma, for example, or occupational hazards leading to repetitive strain injuries. Timing in the day will be particularly valuable when considering the impact of medications upon the presenting problem. For example, night-time restlessness or diaphoresis in people with type I diabetes mellitus may lead the nurse practitioner to consider the timing and dosage of insulin injections.

Past medical history

This is of particular importance in the assessment of people who have a chronic condition. The patient may have experienced the presenting problem before and may have a clear idea of how to treat it. Exploring the patient's past medical history will help to piece together the complex picture of his or her current health status. Past illnesses, immunizations, allergies, surgery, medications and mental health status all contribute towards the patient's ability to cope with the presenting complaint and will also have an impact upon his or her perception of the complaint.

Family history

In taking a history from someone with a chronic condition it is important to enquire about other family members and their health status. A person who has been diagnosed with ischaemic heart disease may have a high level of anxiety if other family members have experienced debilitating illness associated with heart disease and may logically assume that the same will happen to them. However, a person who has been diagnosed with diabetes mellitus may have family members who have had no ill effects from their diabetes and have continued to eat whatever they like. Clearly this will have an effect upon the patient's perception of their problem and this issue should be explored in order to address any anxieties or concerns.

Personal and social history

The patient's culture, financial situation, personal values and beliefs, occupation, home environment, religion, spiritual beliefs, general life satisfaction and support networks are all important to help determine the impact of the complaint upon the well-being of the individual. Spirituality is a particularly important aspect of the personal assessment as it assists the nurse practitioner in determining the level of personal distress an individual may be experiencing.

Leetun (1996) suggests that an assessment of wellness spirituality can be carried out by utilizing a wellness spirituality protocol. The protocol includes an assessment of clinical presentation and an evaluation of self-actualization activities, connectedness activities, healing and new life activities and religious or humanistic activities. A person who lives with a chronic condition should be assessed for spiritual well-being as many of the problems which may emerge in an assessment of personal and social history could be addressed by creating a treatment plan which is focused on reducing the spiritual distress of the individual. For example, a patient may state that s/he feels out of touch with the world and that the chronic condition has resulted in a withdrawal from society. The nurse practitioner may be able to suggest support groups or voluntary organizations to improve connectedness. A person who states that finances are the main concern could be offered benefits counselling from the appropriate source. A tool such as the wellness spirituality protocol can be utilized at an appropriate moment or the nurse practitioner can use it as a mental framework throughout the history-taking process.

Review of systems

A review of the systems will be guided by the presenting complaint and/or the chronic condition.

Chronic conditions tend to affect several body systems and, in some cases, all body systems. The review of systems is particularly appropriate in this situation. Of particular importance is an assessment of mental health. The nurse practitioner should ask about mood changes, sleep disturbances, depression and ability to concentrate. Living with a chronic condition, particularly chronic pain, can lead to alterations in mental health status. Callaghan and Williams (1994) state that living with a chronic illness affects the psychosocial aspects of a person's life. Psychosocial effects include anxiety, feelings of fear, uncertainty and decreased self-esteem. Any of these outcomes will adversely affect other treatment plans and therefore taking a focused history from a person who lives with a chronic condition will not be complete without a full review of systems.

Sexual history

A sexual history is an important consideration in many nurse practitioner consultations. In the management of people with chronic conditions it is particularly important. Many chronic conditions adversely affect a person's ability to achieve an optimum level of sexual health. The nurse practitioner should be sensitive to this issue and create a safe and open therapeutic environment so that the patient feels able to discuss such sensitive issues. The question: 'in what way has your condition affected your sexual relationships?' is open and may pave the way for a discussion around sexual health and sexuality. This is clearly an important consideration in consultations with men who live with diabetes mellitus as erectile dysfunction is a common complication. The same is true for people who live with skin disorders as their bodily appearance can be a source of great damage to their self-esteem and identity and hence their sexual health.

Treatment issues for people who live with a chronic condition

The treatment regimes for people who live with a chronic condition will vary according to the condition and also according to the individual concerned. Issues common to all people living with a chronic condition are the feeling of uncertainty, loss of control over their body, negative self-concept, concern with the management of treatment regimes and alterations in the balance of family relationships. Callaghan and Williams (1994) suggest that people adopt a variety of coping strategies for living with diabetes. However, in an effort to make their lives as normal as possible, some people attempt to limit the effect of the condition on their lives by not attending for hospital appointments, not taking their medications or choosing not to monitor their condition.

Wichowski and Kubsch (1997) report that non-compliance is a major concern in the management of people with chronic conditions; Kyngas *et al.* (1998) quote a series of studies which estimate that approximately 50% of young diabetic people do not comply with treatment regimes.

Compliance

Compliance is often defined as the extent to which a patient follows medical advice. Hentinen (1988) views compliance as an active responsible process of care in which the person works to maintain his or her health in close collaboration with health-care professionals. In a review of the literature Yoos (1981) identified six classes of variables associated with compliance to treatment regimes: sociodemographics, the nature of the disease, the patient's beliefs and values, the nature of the treatment regime, factors associated with the organization and delivery of care and the quality of the care-giver–patient interaction. Nurse practitioners can acknowledge the first three and positively impact the latter three.

More recently, an editorial in the *British Medical Journal* (1997) stated that the concept of concordance, which suggests a frank exchange of information, negotiation and a spirit of co-operation, probably more accurately reflects the desired approach in prescribing treatment regimens for patients. Collaboration and partnership are important considerations in the treatment of people who have chronic conditions. The individual has to live with the condition and therefore must be allowed to own the management plan and to feel that there is some control over treatment. When making decisions about the treatment regime and being involved in the organization of services, nurse practitioners as leaders and clinicians can help people become involved with the treatment regime of their choice.

Diabetes mellitus as an example of a chronic condition

Potential changes in the history and physical examination

Diabetes mellitus is a chronic condition because it represents a permanent alteration in an individual's life. The nurse practitioner should be alert to potential changes in all body systems and therefore the physical examination and history taking should be particularly focused on the following.

History-taking and symptoms

Polyuria, polydipsia, weight loss, blurred vision, fatigue and weakness are all symptoms of diabetes mellitus. It is likely that this information will be elicited in the history-taking process and will guide the nurse practitioner to carry out the appropriate clinical investigations if the person has never been diagnosed or consider blood glucose control if the person has already been diagnosed with diabetes. The history should also focus on the symptoms of the potential complications of diabetes such as intermittent claudication, chest pain, breathlessness, changes in vision, erectile dysfunction, loss of sensation and pain in the peripheries, gastrointestinal disturbances and dizziness.

Cardiovascular system

Hypertension and cardiovascular disease occur with greater frequency in people with diabetes than in the general population. In young patients (under the age of 45) the increased risk of dying from a heart attack in men is five times more likely in those with diabetes than in the general population and 11.5 times more likely in women (Mackinnon 1993). When assessing the cardiovascular system of a person with diabetes the nurse practitioner should carry out the usual assessment as outlined in Chapter 7 but should also consider the high incidence of cardiovascular disease and the possibility of silent myocardial infarction in people with diabetes.

Neurological examination

Diabetes leads to neurological dysfunction in both peripheral and autonomic systems. The mechanism by which this occurs is poorly understood. An assessment of the neurological system could result in discovering autonomic dysfunction including problems with heart rate control, postural hypotension, pupillomotor function, gastrointestinal motility and genitourinary function. Symptoms include dizziness on standing, nocturnal diarrhoea, vomiting, constipation, abnormal sweating, bladder and erectile dysfunction.

Erectile dysfunction is thought to have a prevalence of 30–50% in the male diabetic population and may not necessarily be caused by the neurological complications of diabetes (Tiley 1997). Other possible causes include venous, arterial and psychological causes. Medications such as digoxin, beta-blockers, thiazide diuretics and tricyclic antidepressants can all have an effect on the ability to maintain an erection. A focused and thorough history will help determine possible causes and hence the most appropriate management plan.

Foot examination

A thorough examination of the foot is essential in the assessment of people with diabetes. The importance of foot care cannot be overemphasized and the nurse practitioner should take every opportunity to reinforce this message with the patient. The examination of the foot incorporates an assessment of peripheral vascular sufficiency, macrovascular sufficiency, peripheral neuropathy and autonomic neuropathy.

The foot should be inspected for distribution of hair, colour, calluses, corns, ulcers and dry skin. Skin temperature should be assessed; it will be found to be unusually warm for the neuropathic foot and cold for the ischaemic foot. Palpate the dorsalis pedis and posterior tibial pulses. If the pulse is full and bounding this may be a sign of a neuropathic foot. If it is diminished or absent this may be a sign of an ischaemic foot. Absence of dorsalis pedis can be a normal variant in the general population and therefore this finding should be considered alongside the inspection and the rest of the foot examination.

Neurological examination should be carried out from toe to mid-calf. Test for motor strength and compare sides. Light touch can be assessed using a fine microfilament. The skin is touched lightly over a wide area of the feet and lower legs covering dermatomes S1 and L5 (Figure 16.2). Areas of decreased sensation should be mapped out in detail to determine the boundaries and the extent of the deficit.

Vibration sense is checked using a low-pitched tuning fork of 128 or 256 Hz. Vibration sense is often the first sensation to be lost in peripheral neuropathy. The tuning fork is placed on the interphalangeal joint of the patient's finger, then over the interphalangeal joint of the big toe (Figure 16.1). The patient should be able to report a vibrating sensation. If this is impaired the nurse practitioner should proceed to other bony prominences such as the metatarso-phalangeal joint. Differential diagnoses of alcoholism, vitamin B_{12} deficiency and tertiary syphilis should be considered if there is an impairment in vibration sensation.

Position sense is assessed by grasping the patient's big toe by its sides and then moving it up towards the patient and then downwards away from the

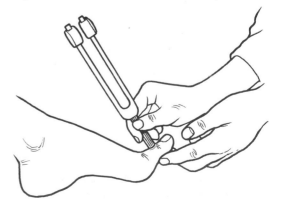

Figure 16.1   Vibration testing

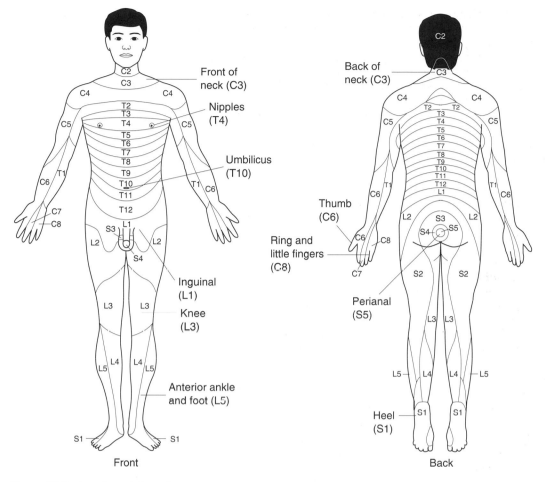

Figure 16.2   Location of dermatomes

patient. With the patient's eyes closed s/he should be able to report if the toe has been moved upwards or downwards. If this is impaired, move proximally to test the ankle joint. Assessment of the ankle reflex concludes the neurological assessment of the foot (Bates 1995).

Eye examination

Diabetic eye disease is the main cause of blindness during adult working life. The eye examination has been covered in detail in Chapter 6. In assessing a person who has diabetes the nurse practitioner should be alert to the possibility of refractive changes, diabetic retinopathy, cataract, rubeosis of the iris, glaucoma and squints or double vision, all of which occur with greater frequency in the person with diabetes mellitus (Figure 16.3).

Skin

The skin of the foot should be inspected for signs of ulceration, dry skin and potential sources of infection. In addition to changes in the feet there is an incidence of necrobiosis lipoidica in diabetes. This appears as symmetrical plaques on the anterior aspect of the lower legs with an atrophic yellow appearance. The plaques are waxy to the touch and are considered to be a skin manifestation of diabetes mellitus (Epstein *et al.* 1997).

Renal system

Chronic renal failure has been found to be 25.2 per 1000 population in a study of South Asian diabetic people living in Leicester compared to 0.3 per 1000 in the general population (Gujral *et al.* 1997).

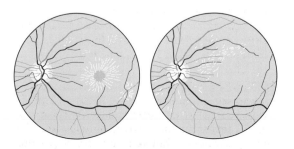

Figure 16.3   Examples of diabetic retinopathy

Diabetic renal disease develops through five stages:

- Stage 1: no detectable abnormality
- Stage 2: detectable microalbuminuria
- Stage 3: proteinuria
- Stage 4: chronic renal failure
- Stage 5: end-stage renal failure

Physical examination in the early stages of renal disease will show no abnormality and therefore screening for microalbuminuria at annual review can help in the detection of early disease when there is still a possibility of reversing the damage. Serum creatinine is another indicator of renal disease and this should be checked annually. In the later stages of renal disease complications such as retinopathy, foot ulcers, angina and intermittent claudication are common, detectable in physical examination and may have a link to renal disease.

Assessment and treatment options for people who live with chronic pain

Pain, either acute or chronic, is the commonest reason why people seek advice from health-care professionals (Tollison 1989). Pain is an extremely individual yet common experience that seems to knit the fabric of humanity together (Jaros 1991). Nurse practitioners regularly consult with people who are in pain. The acute pain of minor illness and injury can be managed with an adequate understanding of methods of analgesic relief and patient education. Chronic pain provides more of a challenge to health-care professionals as it is difficult to define and there is a great deal of disagreement between health-care professionals about its management. The pain can occur anywhere in the body and the causes may be known or unknown. McCaffery *et al.* (1994) developed a working definition of chronic non-malignant pain which can assist nurse practitioners in providing a framework for understanding. These authors define chronic non-malignant pain as:

> pain that has lasted three months or longer, is ongoing on a daily basis or recurs on a regular basis, is due to non life threatening causes, has not responded to currently available treatment methods and may continue for the remainder of the patient's life.

A distinction must be drawn here between chronic non-malignant pain and the pain of cancer. Examples of chronic non-malignant pain are low back pain, osteoarthritis, peripheral neuropathy, headaches, rheumatoid arthritis, irritable bowel syndrome, vascular insufficiency and postherpetic neuralgia. Pain which is associated with cancer has a different dynamic. The US Department of Health and Human Services developed comprehensive clinical practice guidelines for the management of cancer pain in 1994 which address the complex issues related to the treatment of people with cancer (Agency for Health Care Policy and Research (AHCPR) 1994). The guidelines state that pain can be managed effectively in 90% of all people with cancer. Ongoing assessment is essential as the patient's needs will change over time. Cancer pain is associated with considerable fear and anxiety about the meaning of the pain and this can only heighten the patient's perception of the painful stimuli. The management of the pain of cancer is a specialized area of practice. Most nurse practitioners will have the support of a wide range of other health-care professionals in dealing with people who have cancer pain. The following section will focus on people who have chronic non-malignant pain; the assessment tools and many of the underlying pain management principles can also be related to people who have cancer.

One of the main principles of the management of chronic pain is that the person who has the pain is the only authority on the existence and nature of the pain since the pain can only be felt by the person experiencing it (McCaffery *et al.* 1994). It is essential that all nurse practitioners respect the patient's perspective on the existence of the pain and that every effort is made to work with the patient to reduce the hurt and suffering. McCaffery *et al.* (1994) list seven important attitudes which should be communicated by the nurse to the patient and family. These include:

- I care
- I believe you
- I respect the way you are reacting to the pain
- I want to explore with you what you think will help relieve your pain
- I want to discuss with you what your pain means to you
- I am willing to stay with you even if I fail to help control your pain
- If you cannot relate to me I will try to find someone else for you

If the nurse practitioner maintains an open and accepting attitude to the patient's report of pain and is guided in assessment and management by the principles outlined above, the patient will feel that every effort is being made to relieve the discomfort and that alone can help reduce the burden of anxiety and fear experienced by people who suffer from chronic pain.

Theories of chronic pain

Severn (1998) describes four theories of chronic pain; the gate control theory, central sensitization, the neuromatrix theory of pain and the biopsychosocial model. Melzack and Wall originally proposed the gate control theory in 1965. Melzack and Wall's theory states that the fast conducting fibres conveying touch sensation are capable of inhibiting the discharge of spinal interneurones which respond to painful sensation. Opening the gate results in pain and closing the gate produces a decrease in the intensity of the pain and can even alleviate the pain. This theory provides the rationale for the use of transcutaneous electrical nerve stimulation (TENS) and the observation that 'rubbing makes the pain feel better'.

Central sensitization is a theory which refers to the progressive sensitivity of the central nervous system to painful stimuli. The dorsal horn becomes sensitized and this can last a long time after the original painful stimulus stops. Postherpatic neuralgia is an example of central sensitization which may even become irreversible.

The neuromatrix theory of pain relates to the idea of pain having its origin within a specific but diffusely organized set of neurones within the brain. This theory can be linked to people who have a spinal cord injury and yet are able to continue to report pain in a specific area when in fact the neural pathways to that area are no longer intact (Severn 1998).

The biopsychosocial model views pain as a disease in its own right, regardless of the cause of the pain. People who live with chronic pain often develop the complications of progressive disability, dependence upon others, depression and a gradual reduction in physical fitness. Treatments for this group of people are often focused upon the complications of the chronic pain disease rather than the subjective symptoms of the pain.

Assessment

A thorough assessment is an integral component of nurse practitioner practice. This is particularly important in the management of people who are experiencing chronic pain. A thorough assessment provides a baseline measurement of the patient's pain and an objective basis for the evaluation of treatment regimes. An accurate assessment of pain relies on the effective use of communication skills to explore the PQRST of the pain sensation, as outlined earlier in this chapter.

- P : what *provokes* the pain and what *palliates* the pain?
- Q: a description of the *quality* of the pain using terms initiated by the patient, such as burning or stabbing
- R: *radiation* of the pain to discover which parts of the body are included

- S: *severity* of the pain, for example using a visual analogue scale
- T: the *timing* of the pain

In addition to PQRST the patient should be observed for non-verbal expressions of pain and should be asked to report any associated symptoms such as nausea or syncope. This is an absolute minimum in pain assessment. In an ongoing complex pain management situation a more thorough pain assessment tool may be used so that a record can be developed of the patient's experience of pain.

There are a variety of visual analogue scales for use in practice. A numeric scale consists of a straight line with the numbers 0–10 placed from left to right representing the extreme limits of the pain experience. Zero represents no pain and 10 represents the worst possible pain. There are variations of this scale, including some which start at 1 instead of 0 and it is important that there is consistency between members of the health-care team to ensure that assessments can be compared over time. It is also possible to use a verbal rating scale, asking the patient to state whether the pain is absent, mild, moderate, severe, very severe or excruciating (Thomas 1997). Pictorial analogues can be used for children, with smiling, frowning and crying faces, and culturally sensitive analogues can be used with pictures of the faces of children from a variety of cultures; examples of these can be found in Thomas (1997). The important point is that the scale to which the patient is most able to relate should be used rather than the one which is convenient for the health-care professional.

In addition to the visual analogue scales an assessment tool such as the one developed by McCaffery *et al.* (1994) can be used to guide a thorough and comprehensive assessment of the patient's pain (Figure 16.4).

An assessment tool is particularly useful if treatment regimes have failed, treatments are being initiated or changed, the treatment includes high-dose opioids or if the patient is displaying complex symptoms in several body systems. The assessment of the patient is essential to guide treatment and to evaluate progress in relieving the patient's suffering.

Treatment

The treatment of chronic pain can once again be guided by a series of underlying principles which have been developed by McCaffery *et al.* (1994). These principles include:

- Be open-minded about what may control the pain
- Include what the patient believes will be effective
- Consider whether the patient is able or willing to be active or passive in the implementation of pain control measures

INITIAL PAIN ASSESSMENT TOOL

Date _____

Patient's name _____   Age _____   Ward _____

Diagnosis _____   Doctor _____

Nurse _____

1   LOCATION: Patient or nurse mark drawing:

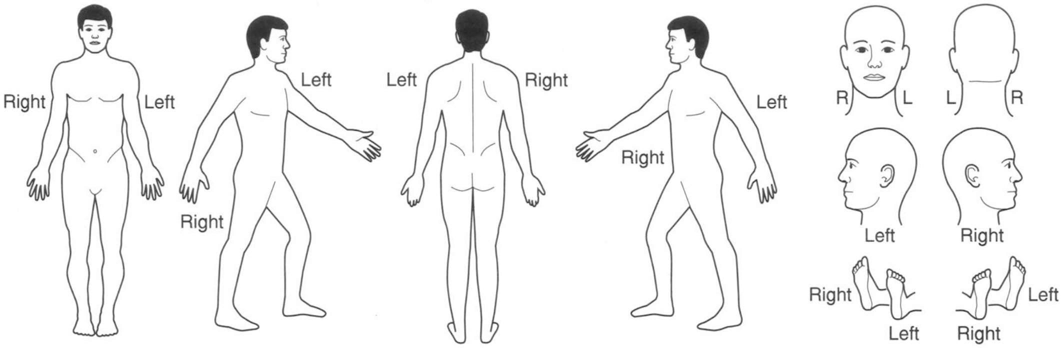

2   INTENSITY: Patient rates the pain. Scale used: _____

Present: _____

Worse pain gets: _____

Best pain gets: _____

Acceptable level of pain: _____

3   QUALITY: (use patient's own words, e.g. prick, ache, burn, throb, pull, sharp) _____

_____

4   ONSET, DURATION VARIATIONS, RHYTHMS: _____

_____

5   MANNER OF EXPRESSING PAIN: _____

_____

_____

6   WHAT RELIEVES THE PAIN? _____

_____

_____

7   WHAT CAUSES OR INCREASES THE PAIN? _____

_____

_____

8   EFFECTS OF PAIN: (Note decreased function, decreased quality of life.)

Accompanying symptoms (e.g. nausea) _____

Sleep _____

Appetite _____

Physical activity _____

Relationship with others (e.g. irritability) _____

Emotions (e.g. anger, suicidal, crying) _____

Concentration _____

Other _____

9   OTHER COMMENTS: _____

_____

10 PLAN: _____

_____

Figure 16.4   Pain assessment tool

Source: Adapted from McCaffery *et al.* (1994)

- Be proactive and use pain control measures before the pain becomes severe
- Use a variety of methods of pain control
- Monitor the patient's response and modify pain control methods accordingly
- If the pain control measure is ineffective the first time it is used, try to encourage the patient to try it at least once or twice more before abandoning it
- Keep trying
- Do no harm

The treatment options for the management of chronic non-malignant pain are many and varied. Whatever treatment plan is agreed with the patient, it is essential that the efficacy of the treatment is reassessed and modified if necessary. It is common to use a variety of approaches, including pharmacological and non-invasive methods. In pharmacological approaches analgesia should be offered on a regular basis rather than as required; this helps to prevent the return of the pain and will provide a more satisfactory level of consistent pain relief. The *British National Formulary* (1999) provides a thorough overview of analgesic medications and antidepressants which are sometimes required to manage the complications of pain. Patients who suffer from chronic pain will sometimes have acute exacerbations of their pain or may experience other causes for acute pain. Acute pain episodes must be treated effectively and reassessments will be necessary so that the patient can return to the baseline treatment as soon as the acute episode is over.

Non-pharmacological approaches include physiotherapy, heat, cold, massage, relaxation, distraction and interventions such as the TENS machine. The choice of treatment plan should be based on the patient's style and the level of active involvement required by the patient and his or her significant others. It is essential to be alert to the risk of suicide in the patient with chronic pain and make appropriate referrals if necessary.

People who live with chronic pain and those who live with diabetes mellitus are examples of the challenges of living with a chronic condition. Nurse practitioners have the skills to carry out comprehensive history-taking, physical examination and to communicate therapeutically to arrive at a diagnosis and plan a treatment regime in partnership with the patient. These are the skills which are at the core of the role of the nurse practitioner. Utilizing these skills effectively will enhance the health and well-being of people who live with chronic conditions.

References

Agency for Health Care Policy and Research (1994) *Management of Cancer Pain*, Rockville, MD, United States Department of Health and Human Services.

Bates B. (1995) *A Guide to Physical Examination and History Taking*, 6th edn., Philadelphia, JB Lippincott.

Bleeker H., Mulderij K. (1992) The experience of motor disability, *Phenomenology and Pedagogy*, 10, pp. 1–18. Cited in: Price B. (1996) Illness careers: the chronic illness experience, *Journal of Advanced Nursing*, 24, pp. 275–279.

British Medical Journal (1997) Editorial: Compliance becomes concordance, *British Medical Journal*, 314, pp. 691–692.

British National Formulary (1999) London, British Medical Association/Royal Pharmaceutical Society of Great Britain.

Callaghan D., Williams A. (1994) Living with diabetes: issues for nursing practice, *Journal of Advanced Nursing*, 20, pp. 132–139.

Cameron K., Gregor F. (1987) Chronic illness and compliance, *Journal of Advanced Nursing*, 12, pp. 671–676.

Cole R.E., Reiss D. (eds) (1993) *How do Families cope with Chronic Illness?*, Hove, Lawrence Erlbaum.

Coward D.D. (1991) Self-transcendence and emotional well being in women with advanced breast cancer, *Oncology Nursing Forum*, 18(5), pp. 857–863.

Epstein O., Perkin G.D., deBono D.P., Cookson J. (1997) *Clinical Examination*, 2nd edn., London, Mosby.

Funk S.G., Tornquist E.M., Champagne M.T., Wiese R.A. (eds.) (1993) *Key Aspects of Caring for the Chronically Ill. Hospital and Home*, New York, Springer.

Gujral J.S., Burden A.C., Iqbal J., Raymond N.T., Botha J.L. (1997) The prevalence of chronic renal failure in non-diabetic white Caucasians and south Asians, *Practical Diabetes International*, 14(3), pp. 71–74.

Hentinen M. (1988) Hoitoon sitoutuminen hoitotyon nakokulmasta *Sairaanhoitaja*, 4, pp. 5–7. Cited in: Kyngas H., Hentinen M., Barlow J.H. (1998) Adolescents' perceptions of physicians, nurses, parents and friends: help or hindrance in compliance with diabetes self-care?, *Journal of Advanced Nursing*, 27, pp. 760–769.

Heriot C.S. (1992) Spirituality and ageing. *Holistic Nursing Practice*, 7(1), pp. 22–31.

Jaros J.A. (1991) The concept of pain, *Critical Care Nursing Clinics of North America*, 3(1), pp. 1–10.

Jerret M. (1994) Parent's experience of coming to know the care of a chronically ill child, *Journal of Advanced Nursing*, 19, pp. 1050–1056.

Kelly M.P., Field D. (1996) Medical sociology, chronic illness and the body, *Sociology of Health and Illness*, 18, pp. 241–257.

Kyngas H., Hentinen M., Barlow J.H. (1998) Adolescents' perceptions of physicians, nurses, parents and friends: help or hindrance in compliance with diabetes self-care? *Journal of Advanced Nursing*, 27, pp. 760–769.

Leetun M.C. (1996) Wellness spirituality in the older adult *Nurse Practitioner*, 21(8), pp. 60–70.

Lyons R.F., Sullivan M.J.L., Ritvo P.G., Coyne J.C. (1995) *Relationships in Chronic Illness and Disability*, California, Sage.

Mackinnon M. (1993) *Providing Diabetes Care in General Practice*, London, Class Publishing.

McBride A.B. (1993) Managing chronicity: the heart of nursing care. In: Funk S.G., Tornquist E.M., Champagne M.T., Wiese R.A. (eds) (1993) *Key Aspects of Caring for the Chronically Ill. Hospital and Home*, New York, Springer.

McCaffery M., Beebe A., Latham J. (eds.) (1994) *Pain Clinical Manual for Nursing Practice,* London, Mosby.

Melzack R., Wall P.D. (1965) Pain mechanisms: a new theory, *Science,* **150**, pp. 971–979. Cited in: McCaffery M., Beebe A., Latham (ed) (1994) *Pain Clinical Manual for Nursing Practice,* London, Mosby.

Morse J., Borttorff J., Hutchinson S. (1994) The phenomenology of comfort, *Journal of Advanced Nursing,* **20**, pp. 189–195.

Nolan M., Nolan J. (1995) Responding to the challenge of chronic illness, *British Journal of Nursing,* **4**(3), pp. 145–147.

Parsons T. (1951) *The Social System,* London, Routledge and Kegan Paul.

Pilch J. (1988) Wellness: wellness spirituality, *Health Values,* **12**(3), pp. 28–31.

Price B. (1996) Illness careers: the chronic illness experience, *Journal of Advanced Nursing,* **24**, pp. 275–279.

Severn A. (1998) What is chronic pain and how should it be managed?, *Lancaster and Westmorland Medical Journal,* **3**, pp. 42–43.

Thomas V.N. (ed.) (1997) *Pain: Its Nature and Management,* London, Baillière Tindall.

Tiley S. (1997) Impotence: what is it?, *Diabetic Nursing,* **25**, pp. 5–7.

Tollison C. (ed.) (1989) *Handbook of Chronic Pain Management,* Baltimore, Williams & Wilkins. Cited in: Cupples S. (1992) Pain as a hurtful experience, *Nursing Forum,* **27**(1), pp. 5–11.

Verbrugge L.M., Jette A.M. (1994) The disablement process, *Social Science and Medicine,* **38**(1), pp. 1–14.

Wichowski H.C., Kubsch S.M. (1997) The relationship of self perception of illness and compliance with health care regimes, *Journal of Advanced Nursing,* **25**(3), pp. 548–553.

Yoos L. (1981) Compliance: philosophical and ethical complications. The nurse practitioner, *American Journal of Primary Health Care*, **6**(4), pp. 27–34.

CHAPTER 17

The patient as partner in care

Alison Crumbie

Introduction

As the boundaries between medicine and nursing become increasingly blurred, nurse practitioners must not lose sight of one of the main advantages of the delivery of health services by a nurse – the ability to work with the patient as partner. Brearley (1990) states that patient participation is seen as a positive part of the nurse's role whereas participation can be construed as a potential threat to the autonomy of medicine.

> 'If they ask me what's wrong with them, I say to them, that's my business. Do as I tell you and take your medicine and you'll get better': Dr John Pickles at the turn of the century (Livesey 1986 p. 8).

Few patients today would accept such an approach from any health-care professional. As nurse practitioners take on many of the tasks of medicine, however, there is a risk that patients will perceive the nurse in a different way and may be less willing to enter into a partnership. It is essential therefore to consider why we want to encourage partnerships with patients and how we might go about enhancing such a relationship. This chapter aims to explore the nature of partnerships with patients from an ethical, sociological, psychological and political perspective. Models of nursing and the skills that can be used to enhance partnerships with patients will be explored with a particular focus on the consultation process.

Partnerships

Participation means getting involved or being allowed to become involved in a decision-making process of the delivery of a service or the evaluation of a service or even simply to become one of a number of people consulted on an issue or matter (Brownlea 1987).

A partnership is a relationship between parties working towards a joint venture. At its most basic level, this partnership is between the nurse and an individual patient during the consultation process. The relationship is commonly more complex than this and can include any or all of the following: the patient's family, other groups of patients, the local community and the population of the nation. Similarly, the nurse practitioner can be influenced by other members of the health-care team, the organization within which s/he works, the local health authority, the NHS and even the government (Figure 17.1).

The one-to-one relationship is the most frequently occurring partnership in the everyday practice of nurse practitioners and therefore this chapter will focus most attention at this level. Brearley (1990) states that individual patient participation can be viewed as a continuum with complete passivity at one end and complete activity at the other. The completely passive patient is moribund on arrival in the A&E department or an unconscious patient

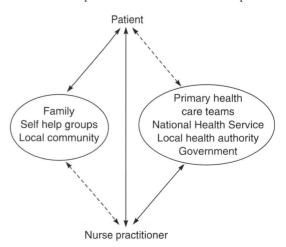

Figure 17.1 The links in partnerships

on a ward. This patient requires health-care providers to make all the decisions and actively to carry out all aspects of care. The completely active patient cares for his or her own health-care needs without any input from the health-care professional.

Brearley goes on to state that the activity of the health-care professional is inversely proportional to the activity of the patient. As the patient becomes more active, the health-care provider can become less active. The level of activity of the patient depends on the nature of the problem and also on the willingness of the health-care professional to allow the patient to be an active participant in the process. There is inequality in the relationship between the patient and the health-care professional as the power lies with the clinician and this clearly influences the nature of the partnership. It could be suggested that in order to enhance a patient's level of activity the nurse practitioner needs to increase his or her level of activity to form a dynamic active relationship with the patient (Figure 17.2). If the health-care professional remains passive, the two parties could slip into the traditional roles of submissive patient and dominant physician or nurse.

Toop (1998) describes three models which have been used to describe the types of relationship between clinicians and patients originally developed by Szasz and Hollender over 20 years ago (Szasz and Hollender 1976). The activity–passivity approach outlined above is based on a parent–infant model; the guidance–co-operation model is based on a parent–child approach and the mutual participation approach is based on adult–adult interaction. Toop (1998) states that none of these models is claimed to be better than the other as any of the three approaches may be appropriate in certain situations. Mutual participation (the basis of patient-centred care) has been gaining popularity over recent years.

In primary health care the relationship between the nurse practitioner and the patient often develops over a period of time. The US Institute of Medicine (Donaldson *et al.* 1994) have recognized this enduring relationship and developed the concept of sustained partnerships. Leopold *et al.* (1996) have developed

a model of sustained partnership and state that the defining features include the following:

* Focus on the whole person
* Clinician's knowledge of the person
* Caring and empathic approach
* The patient has trust in the clinician
* The care offered to the patient must be appropriately adapted to the patient's goals
* The patient participates in the decision-making process

Health-care professionals have tended to discourage patients from taking sole responsibility for their health and well-being for a variety of reasons. In the past many ailments were treated without referral to the health services and the individual would rely upon acquired knowledge, the family or other members of the community to manage the problems of ill health. Downie *et al.* (1997) point out that sleeplessness is an example of a problem which used to be treated by individuals as it was seen as a normal condition which could be managed effectively at home. Grief or anxiety are further examples of normal experiences which would have been managed quite effectively by visiting a member of the clergy or a supportive friend or neighbour. We now turn to the health services for all our problems and we expect an expert and a cure. This has been encouraged by people in the health service who warn against delays in diagnosis and the possible lethal consequences of missing those early warning signs in meningitis, malignancies or heart disease, for example. As a result the public have lost confidence in their ability to diagnose and treat minor conditions (Downie *et al.* 1997) and consequently the expectation is that the health service is responsible for curing all the problems facing each individual and the broader community. Other risks associated with patients playing an active role in their health care include the possibility of misusing treatments, exposure to the ill effects of self-medication and diagnosis without expert advice. It is difficult for nurses to accept any level of risk when dealing with an individual's health. Nurses who work as nurse practitioners, however, have to accept uncertainty and risk management as part of everyday practice. The advantages of patient participation therefore must outweigh the disadvantages if it is to be encouraged.

Tudor Hart (1988) points out that the active, intelligent contribution of the patient to the diagnostic process becomes obvious when one considers the difficulty faced by clinicians when a patient is unable to communicate due to cultural or language barriers. When the patient is unable to provide a history for the nurse, the diagnosis relies upon other methods of detection such as the physical examination or other investigations. Tudor Hart

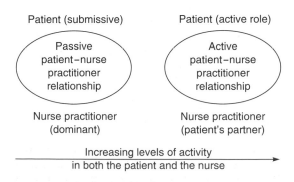

Patient (submissive)	Patient (active role)
Passive patient–nurse practitioner relationship	Active patient–nurse practitioner relationship
Nurse practitioner (dominant)	Nurse practitioner (patient's partner)

Increasing levels of activity in both the patient and the nurse

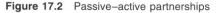

Figure 17.2 Passive–active partnerships

states that, in 80 newly referred medical outpatients, the final diagnosis could be reached after reading the GP's letter of referral and taking a history in 82% of patients, a further 7% could be diagnosed after physical examination and 9% after technical examinations. This emphasizes the importance of patient participation in the diagnostic process. Livesey (1986) adds that participating patients will save time in the long run as their greater level of knowledge will enhance satisfaction and reduce the number of return visits in the search for reassurance and understanding.

The accuracy of diagnosis associated with patient participation can also have advantages at a community level. According to Brearley (1990), the advantages of patient participation include not only increased patient responsibility and commitment to health and health-promoting behaviours and activities but also the contribution to the health system of new community-based resources. Consumer demand can lead to the development of new health services and improved integration of existing health services combined with better utilization of those services. Patient participation can therefore have a positive effect at both individual and community level.

Clearly partnerships with patients are complex relationships which may or may not involve a wider community. Waterworth and Luker (1990) raised the point that some patients may not wish to be involved in the decision-making process about their health care. Their research found that some patients comply with active involvement as it is a means of 'toeing the line'. Collaboration can be seen as a duty rather than a desirable approach to care and Waterworth and Luker question whether the encouragement of active involvement respects the rights of human beings.

Nurse practitioners therefore must consider the issue of partnerships whilst remaining mindful of the individuality of each patient. Taking the risk of encouraging the patient to play an active role in health care could potentially enhance patient satisfaction. In order to implement the concept of partnership in your practice you need a clear understanding of the principles which underpin your actions. The principles which govern the nurse practitioner's practice can be examined from ethical, sociological, psychological and political perspectives.

The ethical perspective

The involvement of the patient with the health-care process involves a number of complex ethical decisions. The issues of autonomy, paternalism, beneficence and non-maleficence and justice are worth considering, as each can help to inform decisions about the level of passivity or activity a patient should have in the health-care relationship.

Autonomy

Autonomy refers to individuals' capacity to choose freely for themselves and to direct their own life. Autonomy in its pure form is not attainable and therefore should not be thought of as an absolute; rather it is something which can be gained to a greater or lesser degree. Respecting autonomy involves respecting another person's rights as a human being. The rights relating to health-care include the right to information, the right to privacy and confidentiality and the right to appropriate care and treatment (Naidoo and Wills 1994). If the nurse practitioner utilizes the ethical principle of autonomy to consider the patient as a partner then each patient has a right to information relating to his or her diagnosis and treatment and this information should be provided for the patient in an appropriate and understandable way.

Paternalism

Paternalism refers to an action taken by one person in the best interests of another without the latter's consent (Childress 1979). Thomasma (1983) distinguishes between strong and weak paternalism. Weak paternalism is an action taken in the absence of consent when a person does not have the ability to give consent. Strong paternalism is a decision which has been taken against the wishes of another. The provision of health-care has tended to be based on a paternalistic framework. For example, health-care professionals who made decisions for the patient because they thought that they knew what was best were behaving in a paternalistic manner. Paternalism does not respect the rights of the human being and results in the patient taking a passive role in health care.

Beneficence and non-maleficence

Beneficence and non-maleficence relate to promoting good and doing no harm. Patients should be informed that the course of action aims to promote their well-being and do them no harm in the process. A patient who is participating in the process of health care therefore needs to be fully informed of the consequences of treatment decisions. Possible harmful side-effects should be discussed so that a decision can be made about the advantages and disadvantages of a particular treatment. Livesey (1986) states that where there is some debate about treatment plans, a patient who is fully informed about the pros and cons of the treatment is most likely to choose not to proceed with the prescription. This saves health service resources and saves the patient from possible iatrogenic effects of a medication, which may not have been necessary.

Justice

Justice refers to the fair distribution of scarce resources, respect for individual and group rights and following morally acceptable laws (Naidoo and Wills 1994). This is a particularly important concept when the nurse practitioner considers the patient's voice in the planning and evaluation of health-care services. Patients' views can be sought by forming patient advisory groups. Pritchard and Pritchard (1994) state that one of the major benefits of patient advisory groups is that the patient becomes a member of the health-care team at an organizational level. It is hoped that the patient's voice will help to inform decisions about health-care services and to provide a more equitable and fair system for all patients in the community. Patient participation in advisory groups does not necessarily guarantee a fair system; however, it is one method of enhancing the possibility of justice.

The issues considered above help nurse practitioners to include patients in the decision-making process by respecting each individual as a human being and providing full and appropriate information to ensure that they are fully informed. Ethical principles dictate that patients should be treated as active partners in their care and that the nurse practitioner has a duty to engage the patient in this way.

The sociological perspective

A sociological perspective on the issue of patients as partners considers the issue of the roles people play in society. Strong (1979) explored the ceremonial order of the clinic by analyzing over 1000 observations of the parents of children who were consulting with doctors. Strong found that even though there were a whole variety of circumstances for the meetings the ceremonial order of the occasion was the same. He argued that medical consultations have a distinct social form and pointed out that the imbalance of power within this bureaucratic format was most striking. Parents might be partners but it was certainly not an equal partnership. The parents were cast in a role that was subordinate to the doctor. The doctors had more rights than the parents and largely controlled the sequence of events. For example, it was acceptable for the doctor to leave the room without explanation and to turn and speak with students or nurses during the consultation but it would not have been acceptable if the parents had engaged in such behaviour.

A further exploration of the roles people play during the consultation process can be informed by Talcot Parson's concept of the sick role (Parsons 1951). Parsons viewed health and illness as being intimately involved with the social system. Illness is seen as sociologically deviant behaviour – a negative and undesirable state. The effective performance of social roles is diminished by ill health. Once a person is in a state of ill health s/he is obliged to reverse this situation as it is a state of being which threatens the normal equilibrium of society. This leads us to the four fundamental responsibilities and obligations of a person who is an occupant of the sick role: the person becomes exempt from normal responsibility, is not responsible for his or her own condition, is obliged to get well and must seek competent help. The sick role then requires sanctioning from other members of society; it places clinicians in a powerful position and patients in a dependent position. If we consider the patient as a partner in care, Parson's sick role certainly requires that the patient actively seeks competent help and should get well and therefore should play an active role in the health-care process; however, medical dominance is present in the power to legitimize the illness by providing a label or diagnosis for the patient.

Both Strong (1979) and Parsons (1951) outlined roles that health-care professionals and patients play in the health-care setting. It is useful for nurse practitioners to be aware of the social meaning of the roles we adapt in each consultation with a patient. If we adopt the trappings of the medical profession with consulting-room desks, large chairs, white coats, stethoscopes and prescription pads, we too may exhibit the power which was uncovered in the study by Strong. We should then question the value of this power, the lack of equality in our relationship with our patients and the effect it might have on the outcome of our interventions. If we analyse our consultations from the perspective of the sick role, it could be perceived that once again the relationship between the nurse practitioner and the patient is unequal. It would be possible to address some of the inequality by utilizing the patient's need to actively seek help and to get well and engage them in the diagnosis and treatment planning process.

The psychological perspective

The contention that an increase in patient participation in health care will prove beneficial to patients has been supported by psychological theory, albeit with some reservations (Brearley 1990). A variety of personal characteristics, including hardiness, learned helplessness, self-efficacy and locus of control can be examined within a psychological framework and linked to the patient's willingness or ability to participate in health care.

Hardiness

Kobasa *et al.* (1981) described hardiness as a group of characteristics that function as a resistance to stressful life events, including commitment, control and challenge. Commitment is the tendency to be actively involved in whatever you are doing, control is the tendency to feel and act as though you have influence over your life and challenge is the belief that change rather than stability is normal in life. Lee (1983) conducted a review of the literature relating to hardiness and found that endurance, strength, boldness and power to control were all related to hardiness. People who have a high level of hardiness have been found to engage in good self-care behaviours (Payne and Walker 1996). This has strong implications for nurses who wish to engage patients as partners in their care. If the nurse practitioner can recognize hardiness in a patient then it might be possible to anticipate their reaction to the illness experience. A hardy person may need to take more control over the course of his or her treatment once in the health-care system and therefore be more participatory. If nurse practitioners can recognize hardiness and utilize this quality in individual patients then it may be possible to judge more accurately those patients who may respond to being offered the opportunity to take a more active role in self-management.

Learned helplessness

Learned helplessness means learning that one's own actions have no influence upon outcomes (Seligman 1975). Seligman demonstrated the concept of learned helplessness in the laboratory by administering a series of minor electric shocks to two dogs. One dog was provided with the means to stop the shock and the other was not. When the dogs were transferred to another setting the dog that had learned to stop the shocks soon learnt to jump over a small barrier to escape whereas the second dog made no attempt to move, failed to recognize the escape routes and appeared very miserable. The difference in the behaviour of the two dogs was attributed to the learned behaviour in the first situation. Payne and Walker (1996) relate these findings to human depression, suggesting that it is necessary to help depressed people relearn that they are capable of doing something positive to gain control over their lives.

People who have experienced a lack of control over their surroundings have fewer personal resources to allow them to become partners in health care. Learned helplessness can result in a person who has poor motivation, an emotional deficit and a cognitive deficit, rather like the second dog in Seligman's experiments. It is not sufficient simply to tell a person that s/he can regain control. The nurse practitioner should focus on assisting the person to identify his or her personal skills, which can be utilized to help them act in a positive way to influence their lives.

Self-efficacy

Self-efficacy is a sense of self-competence or self-mastery, which leads to a sense of self-esteem or self-worth (Payne and Walker 1996). This sense of self is derived from beliefs about oneself which are generated from life experiences and feedback from others, from successes and failures in life and from humiliations (Burns 1980). This collection of experiences results in the construction of a self-picture and the person behaves according to this picture, which in turn generates feedback from others. This is a vicious cycle and results in a person believing and therefore behaving in a certain manner and this in turn is reinforced by others. Self-esteem is a value judgement based on the sense of self. Self-efficacy is the conviction that it is possible to carry out a behaviour to achieve a desired outcome. People avoid activities that they believe are beyond their capabilities and will engage in behaviours that they judge they are able to perform (Payne and Walker 1996). Nurse practitioners can use these principles to influence a person's behaviour. By providing information and education for a patient the person can begin to believe that he or she does have the ability to achieve whatever the behaviour is that is expected of him. By making the activity seem achievable to the client and by understanding the client's sense of self-efficacy, the nurse practitioner can tailor health-care advice and information to the client's needs to optimize the self-care behaviour.

Locus of control

Learned helplessness, hardiness and self-efficacy all involve the issue of personal control. A person's locus of control is the degree to which the person believes that the events which happen to him or her occur as a result of his or her own behaviour or as a result of luck or fate (Strickland 1978). It has been found that people who have an internal locus of control are more likely to engage in screening and other health-care behaviours as they feel that this behaviour might in some way make a difference (Payne and Walker 1996). People who have an external locus of control have a sense that they are controlled by external forces and therefore there is little point in carrying out any health-care behaviour as it will not have any impact on the outcome of events. It has been suggested that a person's locus of control is generated from past experiences (Brearley 1990) and therefore it may change with current and future experiences (Payne and Walker 1996).

Nurse practitioners can intervene on a variety of levels to enhance a person's self-esteem, self-efficacy, internal locus of control, motivation, active problem-solving, level of success and achievement and overall confidence and optimism. Payne and Walker (1996) links each of these concepts and suggests a variety of therapeutic interventions to improve a patient's level of control over his or her problem situation (Figure 17.3).

A desire for control over health care is aimed at coping (Brearley 1990). Nurse practitioners can help patients to gain a sense of control over their situation by providing information, educating patients about their rights and recognizing the fallibility of health-care professionals.

Political context

The current political climate in the UK has helped to enhance awareness of patients' rights and the value of engaging patients as partners in care. The health service has not always been so attuned to the views of patients and in 1974 community health councils were set up throughout England and Wales (there are similar bodies in Scotland and Northern Ireland) in response to evidence that the NHS was not sufficiently patient-centred (Tschudin 1995). Community health councils represent the patient's

voice in the health service and they have rights to visit health-care premises, to inspect them and to make reports on their findings. The services of the community health council are available to patients who wish to make comments about health services or those who wish to complain. The Association for Community Health Councils in England and Wales (ACHCEW) published its own *Patient's Charter* in 1986 (ACHCEW 1986) outlining a list of 17 rights for all who may need to access health services. This list included such issues as the right to be fully informed, the right to refuse treatment, the right to be treated with respect at all times and the right for a second opinion. The National Consumer Council issued a similar document in 1983 which outlines the patient's rights in relation to choice and consent, information, the rights of children and the right to complain. These documents set the stage for *Working for Patients* (Department of Health 1989) and *The Patient's Charter* (Department of Health 1991). *Working for Patients* outlines several key government proposals, including the patient's right to information, explanation and rapid notification of results, which clearly emphasizes the value of the provision of information for patients. If the patient had been considered equal in his or her relationship with the health service, however, the document might have been more appropriately titled *Working **with** Patients*.

The *Patient's Charter* was said to be 'a big disappointment' by ACHCEW, 'rather flabby' by

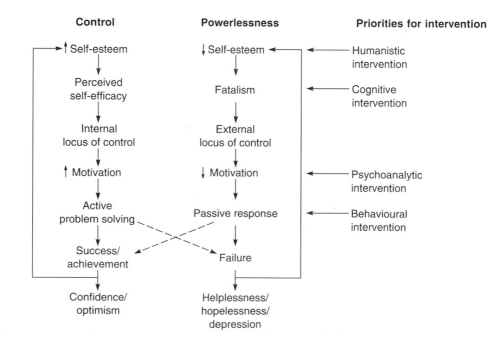

Figure 17.3 Hypothetical model of the dynamic relationships between control related concepts and outcomes

Source: Adapted from Payne and Walker (1997)

the Patient's Association and 'something of a middle class charter' by the Director of the King's Fund Centre (Stocking 1991). The charge that the *Patient's Charter* did not represent the rights of people who are in ethnic minorities or people who are homeless, for example, was countered by others who felt that it was a step in the right direction (Millar 1991). Many of the rights identified in the *Patient's Charter* are a repeat of previous rights for all citizens in relation to the health care service, however, the *Patient's Charter* re-emphasized these established rights, introduced new rights and promoted the public's awareness of them. In 1993 the National Consumer Council found that 64% of the respondents to a MORI survey had heard of the *Patient's Charter*.

The white paper *The New NHS: Modern, Dependable* was published in 1997 and recognizes quite clearly that people certainly do expect more from the health service (Department of Health 1997). Six key principles are identified in this document, including the need to get the NHS to work in partnerships and that by breaking down organizational barriers and forging stronger links with local health authorities the needs of the patient will be put at the centre of the care process. In the wake of *The New NHS: Modern, Dependable* people can expect easier and faster access to advice and information at home so that they may become better able to care for themselves and their families. The 24-hour advice line is one example of an attempt to provide people with a better information service to help them meet their health-care needs.

It has been recognized that people expect more from their health service and provision of information has been one response to that expectation. It has also been recognized that there is value in placing the patient firmly in the centre of the process of health-care provision. Recognizing the value of patients' involvement in their care empowers them and tends to encourage more active partnership in health-care provision.

Methods of enhancing partnerships

The consultation

The skills required to promote the active involvement of patients in their health care will be employed by nurse practitioners during the consultation process with their patients. Balint (1957) stated that by far the most frequently used drug in general practice was the doctor himself (or herself) which, by analogy, clearly emphasizes the importance of the nurse–patient relationship during the consultation process. Balint also stated that 'no guidance whatever is contained in any textbook as to the dosage in which the doctor should prescribe himself, in what form, how frequently, what his curative and maintenance doses should be and so on'. Livesey (1986) points out that for many doctors the outcomes of their consultations are regularly examined during medical school but the consultation process itself is rarely questioned. Nurse practitioners, however, are being examined on their history-taking process and their communication style during their courses. Patient participation can assist you in diagnostic reasoning and in making decisions relating to interventions. Tudor Hart (1988 p. 183) quotes Jean-Martin Charcot from the 19th century, who said: 'Listen to the patient, he is telling you the diagnosis'. Allowing patients the time and space to tell their story respects their autonomy and actively engages them in their health care.

Livesey (1986) suggests that we should consider the following points in consultations with patients:

- Expectations
- Welcome
- Patient's story
- Partners in care
- Physical examination
- Examination of the emotions
- Personalities and problems
- Simple explanations
- The farewell

The patient in Livesey's consultation process is clearly an active participant in the problem-solving process. Livesey points out that the patient's problem can be dealt with more effectively if the clinician has built up a clear idea of the patient's expectations and thoughts about the matter. If a thorough understanding of the patient's perspective has not been gathered during the consultation advice, medications and resources can all be misdirected. This failure, according to Livesey, is most commonly due to a communication breakdown between the patient and the clinician.

Anthony Clare (1991) provided a guide to help develop communication and interviewing skills for the consultation process. Clare suggests that clinicians should have a rough plan of the interview before meeting with the patient; persuade the patient to talk; control and guide him or her with encouragement and appropriate questioning; record salient features of the interview; arrive at a diagnosis and summarize and make decisions on treatment. Throughout the process the clinician should be aiming to elicit the patient's feelings and should be aware of the social, cultural and linguistic barriers to communication. Communication and interviewing skills can be developed with practice. A further discussion of communication and the therapeutic relationship can be found in Chapter 18.

A framework for practice

Much of the research relating to the consultation process has been carried out with doctors in the role of health-care professional. Nurse practitioners are now consulting with patients in a similar way and many of the lessons from medicine can be applied to our own practice. As with all nurse practitioner practice, it is essential that nurses do not lose sight of the benefits to the patient in delivering their care within a nursing framework. There are several nurse theorists who have considered the value of partnerships in care. Depending upon your area of practice and your own nursing philosophy you may find that a nursing model can provide a framework for your work.

One such nursing model is Dorothea Orem's self-care model for nursing (Orem 1985). The most fundamental belief, which underpins Orem's model, is that a need for self-care exists in each individual (Pearson and Vaughan 1986). Self-care is the personal care that human beings require each day and that may be modified by ill health, environmental conditions, the effects of medical care and other factors (Orem 1985). Ideally the person has the ability to meet this self-care need but sometimes the demand for self-care is greater than the individual's ability to meet it and this results in a self-care deficit. The inability to maintain a therapeutic level of self-care is the condition that validates the existence of nursing and this is how nursing relates to individuals. The goals of nursing are:

- to reduce the self-care demand
- to increase the self-care ability
- to enable relatives to give dependent care when self-care is impossible
- when none of these can be achieved, the nurse may meet the self-care needs.

The focus of the model is to help individuals view themselves as self-care agents. As individuals come to understand themselves in this way a process of personalization occurs (Orem 1985). Personalization is the potential fulfilment of wholeness, the health of body and mind and the experience of well-being. Nurse practitioners could utilize Orem's model of nursing to structure the assessment process and to focus interventions towards enhancing self-care activities and in this way a partnership in care can be developed. For a more detailed explanation of the assessment process and self-care requisites see Dorothea Orem's text *Nursing: Concepts of Practice* (1985).

Other nurse theorists who respect and encourage the active involvement of patients in their care include Sister Callista Roy, who made the client visible in the health-care process (Roy 1980; Meleis 1985), Imogene King, who identified a role of nursing as setting mutual goals with clients (King 1981) and Henderson, who identified the nursing role as complementary to and supplementing the patient's own knowledge (Henderson 1978). There are many more; frameworks such as the health belief model can also be utilized to involve the patient as a partner in health care (see p. 222). The value in turning to nurse theorists and health promotion models to underpin the work of the nurse practitioner is that it can guard against the dominance of the medical model. The medical model aims for biological homeostasis in patients and this can be achieved by diagnosing the cause of the disturbance and treating it. The individual patient plays a limited and mostly passive role within this framework; nurse practitioners who adopt this approach will be merely replicating the work of our doctor colleagues. It would therefore be difficult to suggest that nurse practitioners would be offering anything more than a substitute service when the whole purpose of implementing the role of the nurse practitioner should be to enhance the service we are currently offering our clients.

Quality assurance and service planning

If nurse practitioners are to suggest that offering patients health-care services within a nursing framework will promote partnerships in care and will enhance the quality of care we provide, how do we prove that these claims can be made and how do we ensure that the patient's voice is heard in the process? Many authors have pointed out the importance of actively involving patients in quality improvement programmes (National Association of Health Authorities and Trusts 1995) and identifying patients as major stakeholders in the provision of health-care services (Ham and Shapiro 1996). Toop (1998) states that there is not yet any solid evidence to prove that patient-centred care improves health outcomes. As patient participation is central to the current changes in delivery of health-care services in the UK, this is an area of practice that should be firmly on the research agenda.

Nurse practitioners can choose to research or audit their work in a variety of ways. The Dynamic Standard Setting System (DySSSy) is one method of setting standards of care and monitoring those standards (Royal College of Nursing 1990). This system is not only a method of evaluating the results of your work in practice but it also recognizes the value of engaging the patient in the standard-setting process. The DySSSy system is based on six key principles which were originally developed by a group of nurses in Oxford (Kitson 1989):

- Ownership: the standards are written by the practitioners delivering the care
- Participation: the practitioners must be involved with the process
- Patient-focused: the patient should be at the heart of the initiative
- Situation-based: it must be clear who the standards are for
- Setting achievable standards: the standards must be practical and realistic
- Multidisciplinary standard: the standards must transfer across disciplines

The patient is placed firmly in the centre of this process and the aim is always to improve quality from the patient's point of view (Poulton 1994). This requires active involvement from patients and willingness on the part of health-care professionals to work with patients to achieve quality. The DySSSy system is presented in three phases – defining, auditing and monitoring and taking action. Patients have an active role to play in defining the standards and it is in this phase that patients' views should be sought. There is evidence to suggest that the participative approach to improving quality which is exemplified by the DySSSy system improves patient outcomes and changes nursing practice (National Institute for Nursing 1994).

In practice, the DySSSy system can provide nurse practitioners with a framework to measure the quality of health care delivered to patients. Involving patients in the standard-setting process is a method of representing the patient's voice. This process ensures that the patient is not only a partner during individual consultations at the bedside or in the consulting room but also a partner in the planning and delivery of health-care services to the local population.

Conclusion

If you consider the concept of patient participation in your work as a nurse practitioner, you will broaden your perspective of the patient. You may find that some patients do not wish to be actively involved in the decision-making process or the management of their condition and you will need to be flexible to adopt the appropriate approach in each situation. It is without question, however, that your nurse practitioner role will always be an active one. Your energies will be directed towards assessing the patient's expectations and responding to them in a manner which respects the individuality of each human being in every consultation with your clients.

References

Association for Community Health Councils in England and Wales (1986) *Patient's Charter – Guidelines for Good Practice*, London, ACHCEW.

Balint M. (1957) *The Doctor, his Patient and the Illness*, London, Pitman.

Brearley S. (1990) *Patient Participation: The Literature*, London, Scutari Press.

Brownlea A. (1987) Participation: myths, realities and prognosis, *Social Science and Medicine*, **25**(6), pp. 605–614.

Burns R.B. (1980) *Essential Psychology*, London, MT Press.

Childress J.F. (1979) Paternalism and health care. In: Robinson W.L., Pritchard M.S. (eds.) *Medical Responsibility*. Clifton, New Jersey, Human Press. Cited in: Brearley S. (1990) *Patient Participation: The Literature*, London, Scutari Press.

Clare A. (1991) Developing communication and interviewing skills chapter 3. In: Corney R. (ed.) (1991) *Developing Communication and Counselling Skills in Medicine*, London, Routledge.

Department of Health (1989) *Working for Patients: The Health Service Caring for the 1990s*, London, HMSO.

Department of Health (1991) *The Patient's Charter*, London, HMSO.

Department of Health (1997) *The New NHS: Modern, Dependable*, London, Stationery Office.

Donaldson M., Yordv K., Vanselow N. (eds.) for the Institute of Medicine (1994) *Defining Primary Care: An Interim Report*, Washington, DC, National Academy Press. Cited in: Toop L. (1998) Primary care: core values. Patient centred primary care. *British Medical Journal*, **316**, pp. 1882–1883.

Downie R.S., Tannahill C., Tannahill A. (1997) *Health Promotion Models and Values*, 2nd edn., Oxford, Oxford Medical Publications.

Ham C.J., Shapiro J. (1996) Learning Curve, *Health Service Journal*, 18 January, pp. 24–25.

Henderson V. (1978) The concept of nursing, *Journal of Advanced Nursing*, **5**, pp. 245–260.

King I. (1981) *A Theory for Nursing: Systems, Concepts and Process*, New York, John Wiley.

Kitson A. (1989) *Framework for Quality*, London, Royal College of Nursing.

Kobasa S.C., Maddi S.R., Courington S. (1981) Personality and constitution as mediators in the stress-illness relationship, *Journal of Health and Social Behaviour*, **22**, pp. 368–378. Cited in: Lee H.J. (1983) Analysis of a concept: hardiness, *Oncology Nursing Forum*, **10**(4), pp. 32–35.

Lee H.J. (1983) Analysis of a concept: hardiness, *Oncology Nursing Forum*, **10**(4), pp. 32–35.

Leopold N., Cooper J., Clancy C. (1996) Sustained partnership in primary care, *Journal of Family Practice*, **42**, pp. 129–137. Cited in: Toop L. (1998) Primary care: core values. Patient centred primary care, *British Medical Journal*, **316**, pp. 1882–1883.

Livesey P.G. (1986) *Partners in Care: The Consultation in General Practice*, London, Heinemann.

Meleis A. (1985) *Theoretical Nursing: Development and Progress*, Philadelphia, JB Lippincott.

Millar B. (1991) 'I have in my hand a piece of paper', *Health Service Journal*, **101**(5277), pp. 12.

National Association of Health Authorities and Trusts (1995)

Improving Quality in Health Care – Partnership Agenda, National Association of Health Authorities and Trusts, Association for Quality in Healthcare and British Medical Association.

Naidoo J., Wills J. (1994) *Health Promotion. Foundations for Practice,* London, Baillière Tindall.

National Consumer Council (NCC) (1983) *Patient's Rights A Guide for NHS Patients and Doctors,* London, HMSO.

National Consumer Council (NCC) (1993) *Consumer Concerns 1993,* London, NCC. Cited in: Tschudin V. (1995) *Ethics: The Patient's Charter,* London, Scutari Press.

National Institute for Nursing (1994) *The Impact of the Dynamic Standard Setting System (DySSSy) on Nursing Practice and Patient Outcomes (the ODySSSy Project),* Oxford, National Institute for Nursing.

Orem D.E. (1985) *Nursing: Concepts of Practice,* 3rd edn., New York, McGraw-Hill.

Parsons T. (1951) *The Social System,* London, Routledge and Kegan Paul.

Payne S., Walker J. (1996) *Psychology for Nurses and the Caring Professions,* Buckingham, Philadelphia, Open University Press.

Pearson A., Vaughan B. (1986) *Nursing Models for Practice,* Oxford, Heinemann Nursing.

Poulton B. (1994) Setting standards of care, *Nursing Standard,* **8,** pp. 51 RCN Nursing Update 3–8.

Pritchard P., Pritchard J. (1994) *Teamwork for Primary and Shared Care: A Practical Workbook,* 2nd edn., Oxford, Oxford Medical Publications.

Roy C. (1980) The Roy adaptation model. In: Riehl J.P., Roy C. (eds.) *Conceptual Models for Nursing Practice,* 2nd edn., New York, Appleton Century Crofts.

Royal College of Nursing (1990) *Quality Patient Care: The Dynamic Standard Setting System,* London, RCN.

Seligman M.F.P. (1975) *Helplessness: On Development, Depression and Death,* New York, Freeman. Cited in: Payne S., Walker J. (1996) *Psychology for Nurses and the Caring Professions,* Buckingham, Philadelphia, Open University Press.

Stocking B. (1991) Patient's charter, *British Medical Journal,* **303**(6811), pp. 1148–1149.

Strong P.M. (1979) *The Ceremonial Order of the Clinic.* London, Routledge & Kegan Paul.

Strickland B.R. (1978) Internal–external expectancies and health related behaviours, *Journal of Consulting and Clinical Psychology,* **46**(6), pp. 1192–1211. Cited in: Brearley S. (1990) *Patient Participation: The Literature,* London, Scutari Press.

Szasz T.S., Hollender M.H. (1976) The basic models of the doctor–patient relationship, *Arch. Intern. Med.,* **97,** pp. 585–589. Cited in: Toop L. (1998) Primary care: core valves. Patient centred primary care, *British Medical Journal,* **316,** pp 1882–1883.

Thomasma D.C. (1983) Beyond medical paternalism and patient autonomy: a model of physician conscience for the physician–patient relationship, *Annals of Internal Medicine,* **98,** pp. 243–248. Cited in: Brearley S. (1990) *Patient Participation: The Literature,* London, Scutari Press.

Toop L. (1998) Primary care: core values. Patient centred primary care *British Medical Journal,* **316,** pp. 1882–1883.

Tschudin V. (1995) *Ethics: The Patient's Charter,* London, Scutari Press.

Tudor Hart J. (1988) *A New Kind of Doctor: The General Practitioner's Part in the Health of the Community,* London, Merlin Press.

Waterworth S., Luker K.A. (1990) Reluctant collaborators: do patients want to be involved in decisions concerning care? *Journal of Advanced Nursing,* **15,** pp. 971–976.

CHAPTER 18

Therapeutic communication and the nurse practitioner

Joy Duxbury

Introduction

The emotionally disturbed patient can present to the nurse practitioner in a host of ways, some of which are less obvious than others. Patients may be recently bereaved, the victim of domestic violence, under great stress as a result of social circumstances such as debt and unemployment, or have a range of personality problems. S/he may simply be angry and frustrated at what is perceived to be inadequate treatment or feel desperately insecure and become very demanding as a result. Every patient has the potential to experience emotional difficulties such as these, which makes the health-care environment a potential minefield of uncertainty, psychological disruption and personal vulnerability. The crucial skills of therapeutic communication are therefore as essential as a stethoscope for the nurse practitioner.

Therapeutic communication is the essence of nursing and involves a meeting of two people, the nurse and the patient. The priority of this meeting must be the individuals involved and not their roles or stereotypes. It has been described as an inter-subjective meeting in which the caring person (nurse practitioner) helps the cared-for person (patient) to 'be' and 'stay as' a person despite the challenges to personhood presented by disease and treatment. It keeps alive our humanity, and prevents the patient being reduced to an object. Therapeutic communication is a true and meaningful meeting between two people and therefore involves dialogue. This dialogue leads to open interpersonal communication between individuals, not objects, and as such has a measure of unpredictability built into it. Therepeutic communication therefore takes place with all patients and is particularly important in helping those who are emotionally distressed or disturbed.

As a nurse practitioner the development of basic communication skills that can take the heat out of potentially confrontational situations are vital. In addition, it is important to know when simple counselling interventions can help patients tell you their story and take responsibility for making decisions about their care. This can reduce problems of non-compliance. You also need to know when to refer patients for specialist counselling help over what may be a lengthy period. This chapter seeks to help you in these important aspects of your work and draws heavily upon the works of both Gerard Egan (1986) and John Heron (1990), together with the author's own personal experience.

Communication allows the nurse practitioner to get to grips with patient problems such as aggression, non-compliance, pain, fear, anxiety and reluctant collaboration (Luker and Waterworth 1990). It offers a way round the problem of stereotyping patients with labels (which tend to stick), such as manipula-tive, attention-seeking, uncommunicative, unco-operative, hysterical and other categories related to the patient's ethnic group, religion or sexuality. These were all factors that contributed to the concept of the unpopular patient, described by Stockwell (1984). Most nurses have encountered a difficult patient and sighed with relief when the individual has gone home or been referred on elsewhere to become somebody else's problem.

Emotionally disturbed patients present behaviour that creates a barrier to effective nursing. If behaviour is the presenting problem, nurses have the potential to be more effective by both understanding that behaviour and promoting more effective communi-cation. This chapter is aimed at finding communi-cation strategies that may assist the nurse practitioner in his or her therapeutic response, laying the foundation for the development of a therapeutic relationship. Although we can suggest principles, it is what you do with these principles that determines the success of the intervention. Feedback and ongoing evaluation of personal performance in our nurse–patient relationships is crucial to following these guidelines and selecting the right tools for the right situation. If one response does not work then there may be others.

Emotionally disturbed and 'difficult' patients

Patients with deep emotional needs undoubtedly make us feel uncomfortable and at times ineffective as nurses. Feeling uncomfortable may be the result of disliking an individual, feeling frustrated at the patient's progress or unsure of the behaviour we may encounter and the impact it may have. All of these things, in turn, may make us feel ineffective as nurses and unhappy with ourselves. Nurses like to be liked and to feel useful, and being effective as carers is part of the job satisfaction we see as inherent in our role (Rodwell 1996). To face patients on a regular basis who challenge our professional value, can wear down the most motivated of health-care workers.

Emotionally disturbed patients may be labelled as 'difficult' and hence become unpopular patients. Stockwell (1984) initially focused on the care given to hospital patients classified as 'difficult' by the nursing staff but her findings are equally applicable in primary health care. Personality and communication factors rated high when identifying patients who were deemed to be popular or unpopular. Nurses indicated that they least enjoyed looking after two main groups of patients: the first group included those who indicated that they were not happy to be on the ward or with what was being done to or for them. These were patients who grumbled, complained or demanded attention. The second group involved those whom the nursing staff felt did not need to be in hospital or who belonged elsewhere. Unpopular patients also had communication problems, such as individuals with a history of mental illness or violence or those who came from ethnic minorities (Stockwell 1984). Previous studies have produced similar findings (Ritvo 1963).

Peterson (1967) argued that a difficult patient is seen as demanding, unco-operative, unresponsive to treatment or unappreciative. In truth this patient is not having his or her needs met, be they emotional or physical. The patient's expressed needs, which s/he claims are not being met, may not be the real needs, which remain hidden. For example, a patient attending the surgery every week with a string of minor aches and pains which never seem to improve may actually be an isolated, depressed individual who needs human contact and support, rather than medication, Tubigrip and a course of physiotherapy.

Looking at the problem from a different angle may be necessary, Miller (1990) stresses that there are four ways in which a person can portray a degree of neediness which may, in turn, be perceived as being difficult. These may be summarized as withdrawal, passivity, manipulation, aggression and violence.

The act of withdrawal

This involves refusing to interact and may take the form of non-co-operation through disinterest, denial, fear, protest or refusal on moral grounds. Withdrawal must be recognized and worked through if a thorough history is to be obtained or if the nurse practitioner is going to be able to work with a patient who has a chronic disease requiring self-care such as diabetes. Withdrawal may not be a conscious decision and can result from a range of problems, including pain, anxiety, fear, lack of sleep and disorientation. It may be a reaction to a lack of knowledge, consistency in treatment or support. It could be that the patient is trying to come to terms with bad news and is engaging in denial as a coping mechanism. Withdrawal may be partial and/or intermittent and may be influenced by a variety of factors within the health-care setting.

Assumptions are commonly made on initial contact about an individual's ability to take in, comprehend and retain new information. This is particularly important in dealing with chronic disease management such as asthma and diabetes. Assumptions generally seem to be the most common culprit in precipitating problematic behaviour. They are often incorrect, overgeneralized, misconceived, non-person-centred and based on insufficient knowledge and understanding of the individual. They involve seeing the patient as a stereotype and hence there is a lack of therapeutic communication.

Passivity and the unco-operative patient

This, argues Miller (1990), is failure to take action and is different from withdrawal in that a passive person is often willing to allow interactions to take place and relies upon others to remain in a passive state. Passive patients, although seen today as problematic, are historically a product of the institution and were once valued as ideal patients. The patient may agree with everything you say in a consultation but then fail to put into practice any of the interventions discussed because s/he does not wish to take responsibility for his or her own condition or progress. Avoiding self-responsibility may also lead to obstructive behaviour such as active non-compliance or non-conformity.

The medical model has commonly perpetuated passivity in patients. Abdication of responsibility in such individuals is as problematic for the nurse as the patient who will not comply with treatment or who prolongs the need for health care by not being prepared to help him or herself sufficiently. Such patients may be perceived as demanding, as delaying the return to well-being means more care is required.

Passivity leads to others making decisions and taking action for the passive person. For years, the nurse–patient and doctor–patient relationship has been based upon such passivity. It is therefore the responsibility of the nurse practitioner to ensure that the patient's own active responsibility for his or her well-being is defined at the beginning of a therapeutic relationship. This sets the scene for negotiation and participation, as opposed to passivity and control. The nurse practitioner also needs to recognize the importance of culture and religion, as what may appear to western eyes as passivity may to those of other religions be an expression of faith in God's will.

Manipulation

This is the practice of using devious means to achieve an anticipated outcome. Some individuals resort to emotional blackmail and threats, such as: 'Unless you do this, I will do that...' sometimes culminating in an overdose or other act of self-harm. Manipulation also includes demanding or attention-seeking behaviour. Demanding patients may be perceived as noisy, complaining, 'clingy', overly emotional or dissatisfied. Staff may decide they are feigning illness or discomfort in order to prolong treatment. Attention-seeking behaviour may also include making unsubstantiated complaints, playing one member of staff against another and seeking constant attention that does not reflect the level of need. We should ask why the patient needs constant attention rather than why s/he is never satisfied with what we do for him or her.

Emotionally demanding individuals tend to make us feel uncomfortable. This is because we feel they are encroaching upon our time or we do not have the time needed. We feel uncomfortable because they appear intrusive and may overstep the boundaries we clearly lay for the nurse–patient relationship or we do not like the way such patients make us feel about ourselves and our ability to work effectively.

The main problem with manipulative behaviour is that it is stressful and can distract the nurse's attention away from the patient's real problem (Miller 1990). Nurses commonly avoid patients who make excessive demands, fearful that when they encounter the patient again a new or additional demand will be made. If not actually avoiding patients, there is an increased display of detachment or gradual withdrawal (Smith and Hart 1994). This in turn may make the patient more needy and a vicious circle emerges, with both nurse and patient the losers.

Effective communication is all about honesty, and it is therefore dishonest to fail to address a client problem in order to avoid discomfort for ourselves. Most patients welcome the opportunity to talk and be listened to, as they have a story to tell. The process of making patients feel worthwhile and valued begins and ends with giving a little time and listening carefully to what is being said and, in many instances, what is not (Egan 1986). In the health-care setting, manipulation is not a useful term for patients, nor is it one that inspires closer and more fruitful nurse–patient relationships. Some individuals need more support and reassurance than others and it is possibly when such basic needs are not being met that emotional disturbance presents. Often sharing, explaining and negotiating mutual expectations can be the crucial ground work to avoid escalation of demanding and later attention-seeking behaviour which may then progress to maladaptive forms of communication in a patient, such as feigning illness, refusing to co-operate, extreme displays of emotion, including anger and aggression, or making demands that may appear unreasonable and obstructive. The emphasis must be upon recognizing the patient's needs.

Aggression and violence

Aggression and violence are forms of confrontation and are more directly threatening than passivity, withdrawal or manipulation (Miller 1990). As such, they are the most feared form of behaviour experienced by nurses in all specialities. Although it appears true that some areas such as A&E departments and mental health settings have a more widely reported incidence of violence (HSAC 1987), all nurses are at risk and report episodes of expresssed patient anger that may escalate into something more violent (Duxbury 1999). Irrespective of place of work, nurses are increasingly likely to face confrontation from patients and their kin. Confrontation is usually caused by a combination of factors such as unrealistic expectations, stretched resources and increased waiting times, the effects of stress and lowered morale on staff, impaired communication, alcohol and other drugs.

Any person-centred activity can be a minefield of anxieties, complaints, fears and frustrations which can result in confrontation if not recognized and addresssed. When dealing with confrontation, communication is largely both the problem and the solution. Questions regarding prognosis, waiting times, information about treatment and even questions which relate to the nurse's knowledge, skill and ability can appear challenging and confrontational. The need to communicate effectively and understand the difficulties of being a patient are essential steps in reducing the incidence of aggression and confrontation.

The confrontational patient poses a range of real and potential problems for the nurse practitioner, the biggest of which is the degree of threat that confrontation involves. Aggression is mostly the expression of anger with an implication of violence. Violence is the actual physical act against another, self or property which is intended to cause damage. Often it is simply not enough to feel an emotion, there is also the urge to express it in some form which is unknown until it happens. Past experience will influence our concern about an aggressive encounter with a patient while our responses will play a crucial part in determining the course of an aggressive outburst. The following key points will help reduce the risk of an aggressive person becoming violent (Walsh 1996):

- Do not raise your voice in response to shouting or give any other non-verbal cues to the individual which might provoke further confrontation (e.g. facial expressions, body posture)
- Avoid direct eye contact: this can be threatening and challenging in these circumstances
- Stand slightly more than arm's length away from the individual. This avoids crowding his/her personal space and also reduces the risk of you being grabbed or punched suddenly
- The ideal posture is slightly oblique to the individual (square-on is confrontational) with your weight on your dominant leg, which should be slightly behind you and your arms by your side. This is least threatening but gives you the best chance of taking defensive action in the event of a sudden attack
- Try and find out what is causing the aggression and try to make the person understand that you want to help
- If the person is with others, try and talk to him or her alone. Removing the group usually reduces the risk of violence, although if one individual is having a calming effect on the patient, try and retain that person's involvement
- It is easier to repair damaged property than damaged staff, therefore if the person starts breaking things, do not physically intervene

In many cases, speaking in an even tone, establishing what the problem is and that you are there to help will calm things down and allow for a successful outcome. If the situation does escalate out of control the police should be called and as a matter of policy assaults upon staff should result in prosecution.

Although the confrontational patient is feared for his or her potential to become aggressive, other forms of confrontational behaviour are possible. This may include:

- The lodging of a formal written complaint
- A disagreement over care which may lead to non-compliance. Such confrontations are particularly common in mental health or in patients with chronic problems who may see no need for therapeutic interventions which have no immediate effect
- Patients who refuse to co-operate when their values do not conform to those of the health professionals. This may range from the strong beliefs held by certain religious groups regarding various medical interventions to unhealthy or high-risk lifestyle choices. Patients may also not wish to follow traditional medical care but opt instead to follow a course of alternative therapy of no empirically demonstrated benefit
- Assertive patients who make reasonable demands upon our service by requesting information may still be perceived as a threat to our authority
- Patients who display emotive behaviours such as fear, sadness, anxiety and neediness. Many nurses find it difficult to cope with displays of emotion, be it their own or that of the patients they care for (Burnard and Morrison 1991)
- Patients who overstep the nurse–patient relationship boundaries. This may include patients who are sexually intrusive

All these individuals may be viewed as emotionally disturbed clients. No one set of behaviours is more problematic or distressing for the nurse than another. Each will be rated and perceived by different nurses in different ways depending upon experience, personality, knowledge and confidence. What may be perceived as a threat one day may appear less troublesome in the light of a new day. Personal variables and situational context are important in our experience of emotional patients, whether withdrawn, passive, demanding, confrontational or generally unco-operative.

Emotionally disturbed patients will also experience a level of threat; therefore there must be joint exploration, discussion and negotiation about the way forward. In order to be most effective, the degree of non co-operation, the reasons behind it and the behaviour it leads to must be determined. It may be a deliberate act to block progress, a personal attack against an individual practitioner, a protective defence mechanism or a genuine lack of knowledge and awareness. Only when these issues are explored and determined can an effective therapeutic programme be initiated.

The most beneficial approach to ensuring that the needs of the emotionally disturbed patient are met is to focus on the positive challenge facing the nurse and the ultimate difference s/he can make.

To view such patients in a solely negative light can only do harm and perpetuate the need. Nurses must try to put subjectivity to one side and objectively seek to intervene, on the understanding that here you have an individual in distress. Recognize the distress and the underlying thinking and feelings of the individual and a therapeutic connection may be possible.

The basics of effective therapeutic communication

Therapeutic communication should be goal-directed, involving focused dialogue between nurse and client, and be tailored to the needs of the client (Severtson 1990). This process involves the exchange of ideas, feelings and attitudes related to desired health-care outcomes. As such it is a two-way process in which both parties must be actively engaged (Arnold and Boggs 1995). When this engagement fails and is not pursued by either patient or nurse then communication problems can result, which in turn will damage the therapeutic relationship.

Egan's model of helping

Egan's model offers a framework for working with the patient to achieve exploration, understanding and action on his or her problems. Originally geared towards the world of counselling, Egan (1986) argues that his model is applicable to any context in which people need help and as such can easily be translated to the health-care setting (Duxbury and Brown 1997). The approach is essentially a general framework for helping people to help themselves (Davis and Fallowfield 1994) and is suitable for nurse practitioners helping patients with complex personal problems over a period of time. It consists of three stages: problem clarification, setting goals and facilitating action.

Stage 1: problem clarification

In order to address problems effectively it is necessary to have a full picture of the individual's experience and needs. This requires exploration of how you as a nurse perceive the situation and also full exploration of the presenting problem from the client's viewpoint. Egan commonly refers to this as encouraging the person to 'tell their story' and the nurse practitioner will be familiar with the importance of this in history-taking. Allowing the individual to outline these feelings takes time and an ability on the part of the helper to establish a trusting and supportive atmosphere (Davis and Fallowfield 1994). This stage also involves the early initial phases of bonding.

How the practitioner manages this early stage will lay the foundations for future progress. In order to establish a fruitful therapeutic relationship, Egan (1986) suggests certain fundamental qualities. These include active listening skills, the use of reflection in portraying empathy, probing to explore certain areas more fully and the ability to respond appropriately ensuring consistency in both your verbal and non-verbal communications. Above all it is crucial that the individual feels valued by the helper, which requires a style that gives messages of respect, genuineness and trust. The ability to show your patients that you are interested in them, accepting of their needs and willing to help requires an effective combination of verbal and non-verbal communication skills. These qualities will be invaluable even if your consultation is with a straightforward patient who has a problem which is mainly physical (e.g. asthma). If your patient has multiple social and emotional difficulties then the model suggested by Egan is even more beneficial. Your assessment and problem clarification work lead logically to the second and third stages, described below.

Stage 2: setting goals

We do not always recognize our own problems or the part we can play in solving them. Sometimes our view of what has happened is distorted, therefore the helper can enable clients to develop a more realistic understanding of their situation (Davis and Fallowfield 1994). This can be achieved because, as practitioners, we are able to stand outside a situation which may for the client be loaded with pain, anxiety or disappointment. We can also identify potential weaknesses and untapped resources, giving a much fuller picture of the individual's situation beyond his or her own subjective view.

Once a better understanding has been gained we can help the person decide what s/he would like to achieve by way of managing the problems identified. This in turn may involve setting a single goal or a series of subgoals, leading to a final desired outcome for more complex problems. Goals must be clear, specific, measurable, realistic, achievable and owned by the individuals themselves (Egan 1986; Davis and Fallowfield 1994). If goals are not set in this way then often the patient will have difficulty moving on to the third stage of Egan's model.

Stage 3: facilitating action

The aim of this final stage is to put into operation ways of achieving goals set in stage 2. This is a crucial stage and requires the nurse practitioner to be a catalyst rather than a doer. This is where nurses historically have tended to fall into difficulties as they have traditionally done things for patients. By doing everything for our patients there is little need to give information, explain, promote health or educate and as a result patients struggle once discharged from hospital. Today we are more aware of the need to promote self-caring philosophies and behaviours, yet facilitation skills are still under-developed and underused. This was highlighted by Burnard and Morrison (1991), who consider that most nurses relied heavily on prescriptive and informative skills, although more facilitative support skills were also present. Evaluation of client progress is essential as it leads to the beginning of a new cycle of therapeutic intervention.

Example

Mrs X weighed 100 kg but claimed that, despite following a 1000 cal/day diet rigorously and taking exercise, she could not lose any weight. The nurse practitioner realized that conventional patient teaching and information-giving techniques were not working and so began to explore the situation with Mrs X using Egan's framework. The first stage of exploration was used to analyse the patient's situation. With gentle probing she revealed that she did take a mug of Horlicks and a ginger biscuit before going to bed as this helped her sleep. Having shared this with the nurse practitioner, Mrs X immediately said, 'I suppose I could cut out the Horlicks and biscuits'. Attending and listening skills had helped the patient to start to solve her own problem. It transpired that since the death of her husband a year previously she had found sleeping difficult. This knowledge allowed the nurse practitioner and Mrs X to explore other strategies to help her sleep. Subsequent sessions revealed other digressions from the 1000-calorie diet that she had not mentioned at the first meeting and on each occasion it was Mrs X who came up with a solution which allowed her to adhere to the correct diet more consistently. The exploration, understanding and action stages of Egan's model were all in evidence in helping Mrs X.

Therapeutic communication skills

In order to use Egan's model, or simply to get the patient to tell you the full story during a history-taking session, there are certain skills which are invaluable. The most fundamental communication skill involves the ability to attend to patients fully and to listen actively. Patients rate the need to be listened to highly and these skills involve both verbal and non-verbal behaviour.

Attending skills

Attending skills involve being receptive to another person both verbally and non-verbally. This includes displaying non-verbal signals that show constant attention and being able to communicate the same to another by means of eye contact, head nods, facial expression and appropriate verbal encouraging clues.

Active listening

Active listening includes the process of attending but takes the concept of hearing and showing you are hearing to a much deeper level. Arnold and Boggs (1995) argue it is an interpersonal skill essential to therapeutic communication. It is a dynamic process whereby one person hears a message, decides upon its meaning and conveys an understanding about the meaning to the sender. It involves a supportive response and is sometimes referred to as listening with the third ear (Stewart 1993). It includes the integration of factors such as non-verbal cues, tone of voice, intuition and previous conversations. Above all, in listening to a person, you must be sure that you really hear that person's voice rather than respond to a stereotype which may be quite discriminatory (Thompson 1996).

Passive listening requires far less time and energy and largely involves lying back and letting something happen (Dainow and Bailey 1992). It is highlighted by non-attending and is often without response or with an inaccurate response. Dainow and Bailey (1992) argue that active listening is disciplined listening and that listening and speaking should be on a ratio of 2:1.

Egan (1986) advocates the use of the SOLER framework for guiding active listening skills. Although a basic recipe, it incorporates the crucial elements of attending effectively:

S: *sit* squarely to your patient
O: Adopt an *open* posture
L: *lean* slightly forward
E: Maintain good *eye* contact
R: Endeavour to portray a *relaxed* approach

The key is to show concern and interest in an accepting and relaxed atmosphere. It is not about putting yourself into positions that feel unreal and unnatural to you, but about recognizing the importance of what you say and do in establishing a trusting relationship. SOLER largely emphasizes the non-verbal elements of actively listening, yet when you are listening, the intermittent verbal messages you give back to the patient must also be recognized and valued for their importance. Verbal skills will assist the active listening process and prompt patients to open up more, allowing you to listen more effectively. Nelson-Jones (1994) suggests the following combination of skills: openers, small rewards and open-ended questions. Each requires the use of only a few words as well as good and accurate voice and body messages.

Openers

Openers indicate 'I'm interested and prepared to listen' and an example would be 'You seem a bit down today, is there something on your mind?' Your tone of voice and body message must be congruent with your verbal messages in order to be effective. Some clients may find it difficult to talk straightaway, therefore an encouraging comment such as 'Take your time' might be useful. Setting the scene in any relationship is all-important and first impressions really do count. Persuading a patient to open up on that initial meeting, even though feeling vulnerable, is a crucial step forward.

Small rewards

These are brief verbal expressions of interest designed to encourage the speaker to continue once started. Examples are 'Go on' or 'And...'. Another form of small reward is to repeat the last word or last few words back to someone in the form of a question. So, for instance, if a patient said to you 'I feel so angry with him for what he did', you might want to turn this into a question 'What he did?' This shows you are both listening attentively and interested and encourages the individual to expand upon something that is obviously painful.

Open-ended questions

These encourage individuals to elaborate their internal viewpoints or get them to expand into an area you feel is important. They cannot be answered by yes, no or a one-word response and usually begin with ' In what way ... ?' or 'Can you tell me ... ?' They are the how and why questions.

Empathy

Empathy in its most fundamental sense involves understanding the experience, behaviours and feelings of others as they experience them. The concept was developed by Rogers (1957) who defined empathy as the ability 'to sense the client's private world as if it were your own without ever losing the "as if" quality'. Empathy should not be confused with sympathy, which involves *sharing* the same feelings as another person as opposed to *recognizing* these feelings (Thompson 1996).

Price and Archbold (1997) consider empathy to be a natural gift which develops as we mature but which can be enhanced by learning a range of communication skills (such as those mentioned in this chapter) and appreciating how they can be used in the helping process. Empathy therefore consists of natural basic empathy and trained empathy which we can learn to use therapeutically (White 1997). A crucial point made by Baillie (1997) is that empathy is useless unless the nurse communicates back to the patient that s/he is empathizing with them – there has to be an external expression of empathy. This should not be a glib remark such as 'I know how you feel', when clearly a young female nurse practitioner aged 30 cannot know how a 70-year-old widower, who has just been discharged after major surgery for rectal cancer, really feels.

Entering into the other person's world is a difficult and challenging task, requiring skills that have to be learnt, but it can be rewarding therapeutically. For instance, a client talks about his anger at his wife, but as he talks, the helper hears not just anger but also hurt. It may be that someone can talk with relative ease about anger but not about feelings of hurt. Empathetic listeners ask themselves questions such as 'What is this person only half saying?'

A key skill involved in the process of empathy is reflection, which involves rewording the client's statements, reflecting feelings and the reasons that might lie behind them. Skilled helpers are very sharp at picking up clients' feelings. Reflecting feelings is built upon the ability to reword. Both reflecting feelings and rewording involve taking what the patient has said to you and rephrasing the gist of the meaning in your own words. It is not about parroting or just repeating.

Rewording alone has distinct limitations. The nurse practitioner must look beyond superficial words to find feelings and reasons. The client may say 'I'm OK' yet be speaking with tearful eyes. A good reflection of feelings picks up these messages and reflects them back to the client.

A simple example of rewording might be:

Mother: I told my kids to go to hell.
Nurse practitioner: You were really angry with them.

A good rewording of verbal content can provide mirror reflections that are clearer than the original statements. Clients may show appreciation and feel that you are in tune with them and say something like, 'That's right'. A simple tip for rewording is to start your responses with 'You ...'.

Rewording is a basic technique used mainly to reflect verbal content. However, the language of feelings is not just words. Reflecting feelings is seeing a client's flow of emotions and being able to communicate this back to him or her. Inadequately distinguishing between thoughts and feelings can be a problem for both clients and helpers. The distinction is important both in reflecting feelings and also when helping clients to influence how they feel by altering how they think. Constant reflective responding focusing on feelings runs the risk of encouraging clients to wallow in feelings rather than to move on to how best to deal with them (Nelson-Jones 1993).

A useful formula is: 'I think I hear what you're saying. It sounds like you ... Am I right?' Further clarification might still be needed, such as: 'I'm not altogether clear what you're saying to me.' This is the core skill of clarification and is an ongoing and integral part of reflection. When reflecting feelings there are two key stages:

1   Decode the overall message accurately using any of the above techniques

2   Formulate an emotionally expressive reflective response that communicates back the crux of the client's feelings

A useful variation on reflective responding is to reflect both feelings and the reasons for them. This does not mean that you make your own interpretation or offer an explanation from your external viewpoint but instead use the client's reasons for a feeling.

Here the helper's 'You feel ... because' response shows greater understanding. This helps clients tell their stories and reveals how the client's thinking contributes to unwanted feelings.

Egan (1986) suggests the following tips for improving the quality of empathy:

• Give yourself time to think – don't jump in!
• Use short responses – it is the client you want to engage in dialogue
• Gear your responses to the individual client – share emotional tone

Advanced empathy is a term highlighted by Egan (1986) and involves giving expression to that which the client only implies. This is particularly in relation to finding feelings and meanings that are buried or beyond the immediate reach of the client. It is an ongoing process that involves piecing together relevant information and experience from the helping relationship. The nurse practitioner has to beware of putting words in the client's mouth, however. Advanced empathy can be communicated in a number of different ways:

• Expressing what is only implied once rapport has been established
• Identifying themes – patterns of behaviour and/or emotion, e.g. poor self-image, helplessness
• Connecting islands – building bridges and helping clients to make connections or fill the gaps between emotions and behaviours. It may be that you notice they become angry or upset at certain times or when discussing certain people or situations
• From the less to the more – unclear issues are clarified and built upon. Greater understanding may be achieved as you explore issues with them and ask for clarification or check out uncertainties. Don't be afraid to get the clearest possible picture you can. If you don't understand, say so. This also means that you role-model good foundations, whereby the client will feel more able to ask questions when unsure

Sundeen *et al.* (1984) outline a model for the application of the process of empathizing in the nurse – patient relationship. They describe four steps in the process: identification, incorporation, reverberation and detachment. The process is often spontaneous and rapid with a great deal of overlap between stages. The following example illustrates the point:

Example
On New Years Eve, a local publican presented at the health centre with a history of chest pain. Examination and an ECG were carried out leading to a provisional diagnosis of a myocardial infarction. Arrangements were made for admission to hospital. At this point the man became very distressed and asked if the admission could be delayed until after New Year. The nurse practitioner was aware that this was the busiest time of the year for a publican and checked her understanding of this fact with the patient by stating 'It seems you are feeling really worried about how your pub will cope without you over New Year'. The subsequent dialogue involved the patient expressing his disbelief that this was happening to him as well as his fears of what would happen to the business at this crucial time of the year in his absence. A critical component of actively empathizing with the patient is detachment and the nurse practitioner was careful to retain her own identity during the dialogue, which concluded with the patient agreeing to admission. Without this therapeutic communication, involving the nurse practitioner empathizing with the patient, it is possible he may have refused admission, with tragic consequences.

Empathy can be inhibited by prejudice or by identifying too closely with the patient (Jones 1990). In counselling a patient with AIDS, for example, Jones points out the danger of unconsciously thinking 'I am unlike this person and therefore will never get AIDS' as a self-defence mechanism. Conversely, the nurse practitioner working with a young woman who has breast cancer might think: 'I am the same age as this woman, this could be me'. Such close identification with the patient can distort judgement and the empathic process. We must lay our own feelings aside in order to achieve full empathic understanding.

Heron's six-category intervention analysis (SCIA) framework

Heron provides the practitioner with an array of valuable tools to choose from and utilize throughout each stage of Egan's model. He established this framework for counselling interventions in the mid 1970s. He revised and enlarged the model to incorporate a range of intervention approaches and tools that apply to a range of occupational groups (Heron 1990). The framework can be used by any practitioner offering a professional service to a client. Between practitioner and client there is a mutually agreed voluntary contract implicit in the relationship. The nurse–patient relationship is a good example of this.

Heron's model comprises six categories, each with suggested interventions. The six categories fall naturally within two much broader headings – authoritative and facilitative. The first three are termed authoritative interventions because the nurse largely takes a lead role in the care. They are:

- Prescriptive, offering advice and making recommendations
- Informative, health education and teaching
- Confronting, challenging and raising awareness

They require the nurse practitioner to take the initiative and responsibility when patients are not able to do so for themselves, due to lack of knowledge, ability or motivation. Authoritative interventions may be more commonly used in the early stages of the nurse practitioner–patient relationship depending on the level of need or disability, moving to more facilitative approaches later on.

Facilitative interventions seek to enable clients to become more autonomous and take greater responsibility for themselves. This may involve giving them the knowledge, information and skills to do this, by affirming their worth and value as human beings or by releasing the emotional pain that appears to be blocking their personal power (Heron 1990). They are classed as:

- Cathartic, helping the client to release pent-up emotions and feelings
- Catalytic, helping self-discovery and self-directed living in the client, leading to the person taking more responsibility for their life
- Supportive, encouraging and affirming the worth of the client

As an example of these six categories in action, consider a patient with diabetes. The nurse practitioner will initially recommend adherence to a medication regime (prescriptive) and give information about diet, medication and the long-term complications of the disorder (informative). Several months later the nurse practitioner may find blood glucose levels are too high and that the patient is gaining too much weight. This now requires the nurse practitioner to explore the situation with the patient and discuss his or her cooperation, presenting him or her with the clinical data regarding blood glucose levels and weight gain (confrontation). Subsequently the patient may express fear and anger at the diagnosis, in which case the nurse practitioner can facilitate expression of these anxieties (catharsis). By moving the patient on to discuss the future the nurse practitioner is using a catalytic intervention. If there is then progress towards better co-operation with treatment then the nurse practitioner should encourage the continuation of such behaviour (supportive).

The nurse practitioner who wishes to work with emotionally troubled clients is recommended to undertake a counselling course to learn and develop the skills required. To help you gain insight, cathartic strategies are briefly outlined below as they can be helpful in getting the client to deal with painful and repressed emotions which can in turn lead to guilt, displays of 'difficult' or unco-operative behaviour and a range of health-related problems. As healthcare professionals, we are often afraid to allow others to unleash their emotions for fear that the patients will then become out of control. It may be that we are in turn afraid of our own emotions. If the consultation is well-managed it is uncommon for the client to escalate out of control.

Suggested cathartic interventions for emotionally troubled patients

Create a warm and accepting atmosphere conducive to trust, whereby exploration of distress can be facilitated. This will be achieved through the skills of active listening and empathy addressed earlier but also with the timely use of silence. Some diversional tactics may be useful in the initial stages of trying to create a bond with a distressed patient. Patients are often withdrawn because they are afraid of what they think or feel or what is happening to them. You will know from your relationships generally that we tend to disclose details to others when we are ready and when we feel it is safe to do so. As nurses, we often make the mistake of assuming that the nurse–patient relationship is somehow different and that we have a right to certain information. This is not the case. Most people will eventually respond to warmth, time and an approachable nurse.

Patience is a crucial key. Several short meetings with the patient may be necessary in order to build up a level of rapport. The skills outlined in SOLER should be used. Additionally, touch is a useful approach if appropriate. This may involve reaching out to touch an arm lightly in a supportive way or possibly embracing the client if s/he begins to express emotion. Such are the complex cultural meanings attached to touch that it should only be used with great care and only when you are sure it is appropriate. Advanced empathy gives some indication as to when it is OK to invade your patient's personal space.

Having gained the confidence of a patient, catharsis can be encouraged by working with the content of the person's problems. This involves getting the person to describe the problems in his or her own words and staying with the client's version, using narrative and bringing the person's account into the present tense to give it a sense of here and now. Slips of the tongue can be useful clues as to how a patient is feeling and may warrant attention in encouraging greater expression, e.g. 'I noticed you just said … can you tell me more?'

The person's silence or reluctance to express him or herself may be an indication that s/he feels it is not good to open up. The person needs to feel valued and that s/he has permission to open up and express emotion. This is an extremely important general point, outside the context of any counselling work, because nurses often appear to be very busy. We should try and allow time for patients to talk and express emotions, but we must be prepared to be supportive and available for a while once the patient has released pent-up fears and emotions.

For the more experienced practitioner, the advanced cathartic skills of repetition with amplification, lyrical release, psychodrama and monodrama are further possible options, but not to be undertaken lightly and without appropriate training. There is no real need to be afraid of emotion as it is largely self-limiting.

Summary and guidelines for practice

Counselling and therapeutic communication skills can be of immense value to the nurse practitioner, whether to enhance history-taking, achieve more effective patient teaching, defuse confrontational situations or to assist in working with clients who have multiple complex psychosocial problems. The common theme that emerges from such skills is that the nurse practitioner comes to see the patient as a person and therefore avoids the pitfalls of labelling, especially if that person is experiencing social and emotional difficulties which translate into behavioural problems. In this way a therapeutic relationship may be established which benefits both patient and the nurse practitioner. The nurse practitioner is not a counsellor and should know when to refer on to another professional such as a community psychiatric nurse or counsellor. However, the use of counselling skills can greatly enhance nursing practice in general, and the work of the nurse practitioner in particular.

The following guidelines for practice summarize many of the points made in this chapter:

- Be approachable and warm but stand back and let patients come to you. Allow patients to open up to you and facilitate the discussion of their concerns by being approachable and accessible
- Patients require advice, guidance, assistance and support at different times depending upon need. They may not always ask for help, therefore you must be sensitive to their needs
- Patients value honesty, genuineness and people taking time to listen to them (Hargie et al. 1994; Sundeen et al. 1994)
- To nurse effectively we do not have to remain detached, uninvolved and distant from our patients. As nurses we are humane carers and must be allowed to connect
- As nurses we work in an environment that is familiar to us. However, many patients know little of health care and may find hospitals and other health care settings places filled with alien sights and sounds which generate feelings of fear and insecurity. Therefore as carers it is our duty always to be welcoming, to explain what is happening to the patient and to assume nothing
- The patient's perception is different to yours, therefore you must try and see things from his or her point of view and negotiate common ground. Empathy is understanding someone in such a way that you feel able to put yourself into his or her shoes
- Only make promises you know you can keep. If subsequently you are unable to keep a promise, explain why you did not meet your original commitment
- Patients are often unsure of what to expect and what will be expected of them. It is our role to ease patients into their new roles and guide them along the way, explaining and negotiating as we go
- There are many situations when an apology coupled with an adequate explanation could mend bridges and avoid the escalation of patient anxiety and dissatisfaction into emotional outbursts and anger
- Know yourself. Reflect and recognize your good and bad points
- No matter how hard we try, there will be times when things do not work out. If this happens, don't be disillusioned and don't give up. Reflect on the situation and learn for next time

References

Arnold E., Boggs K. (1995) *Interpersonal Relationships*, London, W.B. Saunders Company.

Baillie L. (1997) A phenomenological study of empathy, *Journal of Advanced Nursing*, **24**, pp. 1300–1308.

Burnard P., Morrison P. (1991) *Caring and Communicating*, London, Macmillan.

Dainow S., Bailey C. (1992) *Developing Skills with People*, Chichester, John Wiley.

Davis H., Fellowfield L. (1994) *Counselling and Communication in Health Care*, Chichester, John Wiley.

Duxbury J., Brown A. (1997) Day surgery – communicating and interviewing skills, *British Journal of Theatre Nursing*, **7**(4), pp. 10–15.

Duxbury J. (1999) An Exploratory Account of Registered Nurses' Experience of Patient Aggression in Both Mental Health and General Nursing Settings, *Journal of Psychiatric and Mental Health Nursing*, **6** (2), pp. 107–14.

Egan G. (1986) *The Skilled Helper*, California, Brooks/Cole Publishing.

Hargie O., Saunders C., Dickson D. (1994) *Social Skills in Interpersonal Communication*, London, Routledge.

Health Service Advisory Committee (1987) *Violence to Staff in the Health Care Service*, London, HSAC.

Heron J. (1990) *Helping the Client*, London, Sage Publications.

Jones A. (1990) Empathy in the counselling process, *Nursing Standard*, **4**(44), pp. 53–55.

Luker K.A., Waterworth S. (1990) Reluctant Collaborators: Do patients want to be involved in decisions concerning care?, *Journal of Advanced Nursing*, **15**(8), pp. 971–976.

Miller R. (1990) Managing Difficult Patients, London, Faber and Faber.

Nelson-Jones R. (1993) *You can Help*, London, Cassell.

Nelson-Jones R. (1994) *Practical Counselling and Helping Skills*, London, Cassell.

Peterson D.I. (1967) Developing the Difficult Patients. *American Journal of Nursing*, p. 522. Cited in Stockwell F. (1984) *The Unpopular Patient*, London, Croom-Helm.

Price V., Archbold J. (1997) What's it all about, empathy?, *Nurse Education Today*, **17**, pp. 106–110.

Ritvo M. (1963) Who are the Good and Bad Patients?, *Modern Hospital*, **100**(6), pp. 79.

Rodwell C.M. (1996) An analysis of the concept of enpowerment, *Journal of Advanced Nursing*, **23**(2), pp. 305–313.

Rogers C. (1957) The necessary and sufficient conditions of therapeutic personality change, *Journal of Consulting Psychology*, **21**, pp. 95–103.

Severtsen B.M. (1990) Therapeutic communication demystified, *Journal of Nursing Education*, **29**(1), pp. 190–192.

Smith M.E. and Hart G. (1994) Nurses' Responses to Patient Anger. From disconnecting to connecting, *Journal of Advanced Nursing*, **20**, pp. 643–651.

Stewart W. (1993) *An A-Z of Counselling Theory and Practice*, London, Chapman and Hall.

Stockwell F. (1984) *The Unpopular Patient*, London, Croom-Helm.

Sundeen J.J., Stuart G.W., Rankin E.A.D., Cohen S.A. (1994) *Nurse Client Interaction*, London, Mosby.

Thompson N. (1996) *People Skills*, London, Macmillan.

Walsh M. (1996) *A & E Nursing: A New Approach*, Oxford, Butterworth-Heinemann.

White S. (1997) A literature and concept analysis, *Journal of Clinical Nursing*, **6**, pp. 253–257.

Part two

PROFESSIONAL AND LEGAL ISSUES

CHAPTER 19

Development of the nurse practitioner role

Shirley Reveley

The title nurse practitioner was first used in the USA in the 1960s to describe a level of advanced nursing practice in the area of paediatrics in primary health care. The role was supported by a programme of education at the University of Colorado, pioneered by Loretta Ford, a nurse, and Henry Silver, a doctor. Since 1965 the title has been used extensively in the USA to describe an advanced nursing role in both primary care and hospital settings. The nurse practitioner movement became prominent in the USA during the 1960s and 1970s and in the UK during the 1980s and 1990s when nurse practitioner development was pioneered by Barbara Stilwell (Stilwell 1982) working in two general practices in Birmingham in the early 1980s, and Barbara Burke-Masters (1986) working with homeless people in London. Fawcett-Henesy (1991) states that the nurse practitioner role developed from inadequacies in providing medical care. She cites the USA, Scandinavia and some developing countries in support of her contention, and suggests that in the UK the development of the role has occurred for the following reasons:

- Lack of appropriately qualified and experienced medical practitioners, for example in A&E departments
- Patients' dissatisfaction with the quality of care, including consultation time and choice of available treatments, as in primary health care
- Difficulties in access to primary health care

Alongside the changes in established community nursing organization and shifting role boundaries in the UK, the nurse practitioner movement has developed, attracting attention nationally and locally. It is a role that impacts significantly on the work of both nurses and doctors, and has developed in a range of health-care settings such as mental health care, learning disabilities, hospitals (both inpatient and outpatient), alternative community settings and general practice (Watson *et al.* 1994). That the nurse practitioner role should become a feature of primary health care was highlighted in the *Report of the Community Nursing Review Team (Cumberlege Report)* which stated:

> We believe that community nurses who have, or acquire, the necessary skills in health promotion and the diagnosis and treatment of disease among people of all ages should have the opportunity to practise those skills in the setting of a clinic or neighbourhood (Department of Health and Social Security 1986).

The review team's vision was that the nurse practitioner would be managed by the neighbourhood nursing manager and assigned to a general practice where s/he would be accountable to the GP for carrying out agreed medical protocols. The Tomlinson Report (1992) and the NHS Executive Committee (1993) also supported the concept of the nurse practitioner in primary health care. Key government proposals for the future of care in the community from 1987 onwards led to a political climate in which nurses are seen as a resource which should be used effectively and factors within nursing such as the *Scope of Professional Practice* (United Kingdom Central Council 1992, Department of Health 1992) have enabled the development of new nursing roles.

It was the government's white paper *Promoting Better Health* (Department of Health and Social Security 1987) that set the agenda for primary health care in the 1990s. This document places general practice firmly at the centre of health-care delivery outside hospital. A major factor resulting from the GP contract (Department of Health and the Welsh Office 1989) is the enormous rise in the number of practice nurses in general practice. Many nurse practitioners in primary care come from the ranks of practice nurses, whilst in hospital the role has developed from areas of specialist practice and changes to the conditions of work of junior doctors.

It has been argued that, as doctors are an expensive

labour resource, skill mix reviews must also include doctors and not be confined to nurses (Adams and Bond 1997). Tudor Hart, for example, says that doctors must rethink their role; the ideology of medicine has perpetuated the image of the doctor as 'responding to the complaints of individual patients suffering from disease or the fear of disease' (Tudor Hart 1984). There are some doctors, of course, who are involved in the health of populations, but according to Tudor Hart the group general practice could take responsibility for both the health of a local neighbourhood as well as personal care of patients. The expanded primary care team would be involved in searching out health needs, screening for preventable disease, planning chronic disease management, and collecting morbidity and mortality statistics for the local population to use. This would also mean that patients/clients would be involved in decision-making and professionals would be more accountable to them. The nurse practitioner role would expand, with some nurse practitioners combining health-visiting and district nursing roles, and a nurse practitioner would undertake community development such as setting up local health forums, providing health promotion and education in schools and involving the local community in decisions as to the provision of health care. Such changes would utilize the skills of all team members and entail an active role for GPs instead of the passive 'shop-keeping inheritance' wherein they meet the public only in times of health breakdown (Tudor Hart 1984).

These developments have important implications for the ethos of the primary health care team. Much has been written about the roles and functions of the primary health care team and leadership within it; for example the *Cumberlege Report*. (Department of Health and Social Security 1986.)

There has been a philosophical shift (if not an actual shift) from seeing the GP as the natural team leader to a vision whereby the leader becomes the individual whose knowledge and expertise are required in a particular situation. Locating primary health care – and money – around a practice population may mean that the GP once again assumes the leadership mantle and has control over other team members. This is especially true of the core team working closely with the GP in terms of the GP employing them, as is the case with practice nurses and nurse practitioners, where the role is seen to align closely with the medical model of care.

There have been many opportunities afforded by the NHS reforms and changing health care needs for nurses, both in hospital and primary care settings, to develop new roles and advance the standing of the profession. However, the progression of the nurse practitioner movement has not been straightforward. As Butterworth (1991) points out, the British government has been giving mixed messages about the role of nurses. Some government reports have supported the development of nurse practitioners' potential, but others have undermined or ignored it. Butterworth concludes that nurse practitioners appear to confuse government, worry our medical colleagues and heighten expectations in some parts of the nursing profession (p. 55). Much of the confusion surrounds the level at which nurse practitioners practise and whether they practise autonomously.

Advanced nursing practice

The concept of advanced nursing practice is highly contentious and this has direct implications for the role and education of nurses. Although the literature on nurse practitioners sees the role as being an advanced nursing role, other nursing roles are also described as advanced.

Sparacino and Durand (1986) state the following attributes are needed for an advanced practitioner. The advanced practitioner must:

- Portray sophisticated use of clinical knowledge
- Demonstrate high levels of accountability
- Carry out systematic assessment and intervention
- Demonstrate independent clinical decision-making
- Participate in risk-taking
- Portray autonomy and independence
- Expand the boundaries of nursing practice

Mitchinson (1996) defines advanced practice as:

Professional practice which is defined, negotiated and developed by individual practitioners who are solely responsible and accountable to the patient and their professional body for their actions and omissions (p. 34).

She draws a distinction between advanced practice and independent practice by stating:

Independent practice can be defined as practice which is assigned to and developed by individual practitioners who are then responsible and accountable for their actions which are undertaken without direct supervision or monitoring from any other practitioner or manager (p. 34).

The United Kingdom Central Council's (UKCC's) report *Standards for Education and Practice Following Registration* (1994) state that those practitioners with a first degree in their area of practice are specialist practitioners, and that there is another level of nursing practice that constitutes advanced practice:

Advanced nursing practice is concerned with adjusting the boundaries for the development of future practice, pioneering and developing new roles responsive to changing needs and, with advancing clinical practice, research and education to enrich professional practice as a whole (United Kingdom Central Council 1994).

However, there was no statement about how nurses may become registered as advanced practitioners, and standards for education and practice for advanced practitioners were not elucidated in this document. Rather, there was an intimation that advanced practice would be at masters level, and the profession itself would decide how advanced practice was to be defined. These views have now been superseded by a discussion document entitled *A Higher Level of Practice* (United Kingdom Central Council 1998), published in the summer of 1998, which outlined plans for a number of nurses to practise at a higher level. These nurses would have to meet certain criteria, such as being educated to first degree level, and be assessed. Successful individuals would have the suffix H added to their name on the professional register. The word advanced is deliberately omitted from the document and the terms nurse practitioner and clinical nurse specialist are not protected. Nor did the UKCC specify training programmes or define standards for these roles. It remains to be seen what the profession will decide regarding the higher-level practice, but it leaves nurse practitioners in the same position they were before, that is, with no prescribed training programme and no protected title. To add to the confusion, in September 1998, the Prime Minister announced that some nurses (unspecified) would bear the title 'consultant'. Advanced practice and the position of nurse practitioners was again passed over without discussion.

Castledine (1991) states that many of the skills of the advanced practitioner appear similar to those used in the practice of medicine. He suggests that:

> The advanced practitioner will be able to explore the differences and significance of nursing as opposed to medical techniques. Not only will physical assessment be used, but psychosocial assessment and advanced counselling skills will also be crucial (p. 34).

Castledine (1991) argues that the question is not which jobs should be created for advanced practitioners, but which existing jobs fulfil the criteria for advanced practice.

The nurse practitioner movement and the UKCC

Under the Nurses, Midwives and Health Visitor's Act 1979, the UKCC for Nursing, Midwifery and Health Visiting was created as the statutory body for governing standards of education and practice in nursing. Four National Boards were created: one each for Northern Ireland, Scotland, Wales and England. Subordinate legislation set out in the Statutory Instrument 1983 No. 873 embodies the statements on the competence required of first- and second-level registered nurses. In addition, the Council has a code of professional conduct which is 'both a statement of the values of the profession and an explicit expression of the primacy of patients and clients' (Ralph 1991, p. 122).

The UKCC has been slow to give official recognition to nurse practitioners, preferring to await the outcome of research into the effectiveness of the role and to enter into consultation with the profession as a whole through a series of meetings held in various parts of the country during 1996. Frustration among the ranks of nurse practitioners and the Royal College of Nursing continues as, despite the demonstrable success of nurse practitioners in a range of settings (Stilwell *et al.* 1987; Salisbury and Tettersell 1988; Chambers 1994; Read and Graves 1994; Touche Ross 1994; Marsh and Dawes 1995; Coopers and Lybrand 1996), the UKCC is reluctant to affirm the nurse practitioner role as a legitimate role within nursing.

The reasons for this, it can be argued, are several. First, the nurse practitioner role now covers such a wide range of practice in both hospital and community settings that it is difficult to decide which of these roles fits the criteria for a nurse practitioner. Second, much confusion abounds as to the difference between a nurse practitioner and other nursing roles such as that of the clinical nurse specialist. This debate has been raging for several years, both in the UK and in the USA. Third, there is a wide range of educational provision for nurse practitioners from in-service training programmes to first degree and masters level and it is debatable which of these should be officially recognized.

Colin Ralph, UKCC registrar until 1995, appears to be concerned about the boundaries of nursing practice. Nursing legislation establishes boundaries of practice and denotes spheres of activity and responsibility to practitioners. Therefore, Ralph (1991) argues:

> The impact of extending the boundaries of nursing practice will often influence the boundaries of medicine or other practice. Similarly, expansions in medical practice, or the negotiated delegation of some medical activities to nurses by doctors will have an impact on the boundary of nursing practice (p. 122).

Ralph (1991) suggests that another impediment to progress is semantics. He illustrates the confusion that can arise by citing the titles practising nurse (a nurse whose name appears on the professional register held by the UKCC), practice nurse (a nurse employed by a GP of a medical practice) and nurse practitioner (used to denote a level of clinical activity and responsibility that goes beyond the conventional role of nursing practitioners (p. 121). Ralph is here talking about nurse practitioners and a *level* of clinical activity. He goes on to say that the discussion is moving away from semantics to a more fundamental one of professional practice and the scope and boundaries between professions.

Castledine (1993) agrees with the UKCC view that the title nurse practitioner is ambiguous and misleading. He is opposed to the term, stating it is ambiguous because all nurses practise and this term can be restrictive when used to describe one discrete area of practice by an individual. However, he contributes to the ambiguity by talking about 'the advanced nurse practitioner' (1991; p. 35). If nurse practitioners are exemplars of advanced nursing, then prefixing the title nurse practitioner with the descriptor advanced is unnecessary.

The UKCC, along with the Royal College of Nursing, has been involved in a project to professionalize nursing since the early 1980s with the introduction of the nursing process which was to provide a scientific basis for nursing practice and promote the autonomous practitioner role (Keyzer 1985). The emphasis on holistic – rather than task-centred – care is also seen as an ideology on which a claim for professional status can be based, as can the introduction of specialist nurses and the extended nursing role (MacKay 1993). Another move towards professionalization was the restructuring of pre-registration education (United Kingdom Central Council 1986), which placed nurse education in the higher education sector (Walby and Greenwell 1994). Post-registration education and practice also came in for reform, placing responsibility on nurses to keep up-to-date by introducing mandatory updating, and introduced the concept of the live register (United Kingdom Central Council 1994).

It has been argued that the drive for professionalization comes mainly from education (Melia 1987; MacKay 1993) and that the professionalizing group wish to maintain stronger links with medicine by losing the 'dirty work' (MacKay 1993, p. 243). But for some, dirty work is seen as an essential part of nursing and passing this on to others creates a distance between patient and nurse (Johnson 1978, p. 112). There is a danger of two tiers of nursing developing from the professionalization project, and some argue there should not be a distance between qualified and unqualified colleagues (Salvage 1985; MacKay 1993). MacKay argues that:

> Within nursing there is less than wholehearted support for the pursuit of professionalization which senior nurses are pursuing which may arguably reduce the force of claims for professional status, because for many nurses, it is not professional status but respect and appreciation of their skills that is sought (p. 221).

There are many nurse specialisms in both hospital and community settings, but the UKCC has yet to specify outcomes for those clinical nurse specialists working in hospital settings. Eight areas of specialist practice have been identified for community nursing: public health nursing (health visiting), community nursing in the home (district nursing), community children's nursing, school nursing, community mental health nursing, general practice nursing, occupational health nursing and learning disabilities nursing.

It is of interest that the outcomes for general practice nursing set out by the UKCC in the 1994 document parallel closely those outcomes set out in the Royal College of Nursing Institute nurse practitioner diploma in 1989. The community specialist roles outlined above share a core of competencies which may comprise up to two-thirds of the whole programme and indeed, on examination, the competencies set out for all the specialist routes within the community nursing programme are extremely similar, which begs the question as to why the UKCC did not take the opportunity when overhauling educational preparation for community nurses to introduce the generic community nurse practitioner as recommended by the National Health Service Management Executive (1993) in its booklet *Nursing in Primary Health Care: New World, New Opportunities*. We may speculate that it had something to do with keeping intact traditional roles and role boundaries in order to satisfy the interests of the various groups within nursing.

Nurse practitioners and clinical nurse specialists

There is currently much confusion about nurse practitioner and clinical nurse specialist titles and the level at which each works. Read and Graves (1994) state that over the past 20 years new nursing roles in the UK have developed into two streams – the nurse practitioner stream and the clinical nurse specialist stream. They argue that 'both streams may rightly be called advanced nursing practice' (p. 9) If, as Read and Graves (1994) state, the *level* of practice for both streams is advanced, then the specialist component of the clinical nurse specialist title must come from a specialist *area* of practice which derives from the clinical specialities of medicine, for example diabetes nurse specialists, rheumatology nurse specialists and many more.

The nursing profession seems to be overly concerned with establishing and maintaining discrete areas of nursing which have their own specialist title. Ascribing a title to a discrete area of nursing practice assumes that each of these specialisms has its own body of knowledge and skills for which some kind of expertise and/or specialist education is required. The problem is that there is such a plethora of nursing specialisms and titles that the profession itself is confused, let alone commissioners of health care and patients. Stilwell, in recent (unpublished) work done in a south of England hospital, noted over 50 specialist nurse titles (International Nurse Practitioner Conference Heriot-Watt University, Edinburgh, August 1996), and Walsh (1996) reports over 40 nurse specialist titles in one regional health authority (Nurse Practitioner Study Day, Lancaster, September 1996).

Some clinical nurse specialists work in a particular clinical sphere; others are specialists at specific techniques rather than specialities. Occupational health nurses, for example, are described as community specialist nurses (United Kingdom Central Council 1994), yet many work autonomously and independently from doctors, offering a full range of health care and able to prescribe some medicines. On the other hand, some nurse practitioner's work is difficult to distinguish from the nurse specialist (Watson *et al.* 1994, p. 46). In the *Future of Professional Practice* report (United Kingdom Central Council 1994), recommendation 7 points out that there is a fundamental difference between being engaged in advanced practice and simply working in a speciality. Only those nurses who have advanced their knowledge and skills through education and experience can exercise increasing clinical discretion and accept greater responsibility through advanced practice.

Sutton and Smith (1995) argue that a rethink of specialist practice is needed. They state that advanced nursing practice differs from expert and specialist nursing practice which is 'evident in the different ways in which advanced nurse practitioners think, see and experience nursing practice' (p. 1040). Advanced nurse practitioners, they argue, focus their efforts on the patient and situations which enhance positive outcomes for the patient (client). Thus the practitioner's actions are 'purposeful, directed towards excellence (in client terms) and pragmatic'. The advanced practitioner is reflective and recognizes that the contribution s/he makes to client care makes a difference. Nurse practitioners also, importantly, 'give of themselves' and are willing to bend the rules. They locate themselves in the immediacy of client situations and are consistently stretching the boundaries of nursing practice. Specialist nursing practice, suggest Sutton and Smith, developed from a different set of premises and focuses on different elements associated with experience. As nursing grew alongside medical specialities and 'nurses worked for longer periods of time with specific client groups they developed additional specialised knowledge and skills grounded in the scientific knowledge of medicine … this resulted in nurses coming together within their speciality field' (p. 1039).

These authors are discussing advanced nursing practice in Australia, but in the USA there is also a problem of distinguishing between clinical nurse specialists and nurse practitioners and it is suggested that the two roles are blurring (Kitzman 1989). Indeed, several courses of preparation in the USA for clinical nurse specialists and nurse practitioners are blending. Page and Arena (1994) say that in the USA the clinical nurse specialist and nurse practitioner roles were created with different goals in mind. The clinical nurse specialist role was meant to improve quality of nursing care delivered to patients and to keep the expert, specialized nurse at the bedside. The clinical nurse specialist's client, they argue, is the nurse and his/her focus is on nursing staff, education, systems analysis, and providing direct and indirect nursing care. On the other hand, the nurse practitioner's client is the patient and the focus of the nurse practitioner is providing direct patient care. In the USA, nurse practitioners have the greatest effect on the quality of care by delivering direct patient care and increasing access for clients to primary care providers. The clinical nurse specialist role uses consultation to address patient care and systems; much of his or her time is spent consulting with and educating others who provide direct care to patients. Clinical nurse specialists influence health care quality by their interactions with health-care providers, improving quality by providing direct care or through work with nurses at the bedside.

Advantages in combining the two roles include increased political power, public acceptance of the advanced practitioner role and the independence of the advanced practice nurse (Page and Arena 1994, p. 316). The authors point out that there has been less discussion on the possible disadvantages but a single title is not viewed favourably by nurse practitioners. Driving the merger of the two roles, according to Page and Arena, is academia, mainly because of the difficulty and cost of maintaining two separate routes of education and at the same time maintaining quality (p. 317). They go on to say that nursing has created confusion by not making clear what entitles an advanced practice nurse to be called a nurse practitioner or a clinical nurse specialist and if the profession itself does not reach a consensus on titles, education and functions then decisions may be purely financial.

This lack of clarity over roles makes it difficult for policy makers to state what nursing is, let alone what distinguishes nurses from others. The *Report of the Work of the Expert Committee on Nursing Practice* (1995 cited in Stilwell 1996) for example, states:

> The ad hoc development of nursing practice … has meant that it has become more difficult for policy makers and planners to describe the nature and scope of nursing practice, and at times to differentiate it from the practice of other health workers (Stilwell 1996, personal communication).

The Royal College of Nursing

The nursing profession in Britain has a strong voice in the Royal College of Nursing, and this body has made its position on nurse practitioners plain, both in official documents (*Boundaries of Nursing* (1988a), *Specialties in Nursing* (1988b)), and in the development of the first formal course for nurse practitioners in the UK. The Royal College of Nursing also endorses its support of nurse practitioners by providing cover against legal liability after accepting that the scope of practice is a legitimate extension of the nursing role.

The formal course of preparation for nurse practitioners began as a diploma course run at the RCN Institute in 1990 (Simon 1992). Within 2 years, it was realized that the level of practice for nurse practitioners was more than diploma level and the course was developed into an honours degree programme. The Royal College of Nursing course has received much support throughout the country, and there are now seven institutes of higher education nationwide that franchise the programme from the Institute. Those institutions operating the Royal College of Nursing nurse practitioner programme have formed a national forum for promoting the education of nurse practitioners which links with an American National Organization of Nurse Practitioner Faculties (NONPF).

One way of giving official recognition to the nurse practitioner role would be to outline minimum standards for nurse practitioner practice, whether at specialist or advanced level. However, the debate surrounding nurse practitioners is also concerned with whether they really are advanced practitioners or doctor substitutes.

Nurse practitioners: advanced-level nurses or substitute doctors?

Nurse practitioners create a problem for the UKCC: a decision needs to be made as to whether there is a role for nurse practitioners which can be separated from other nursing roles and how the role relates to the role of doctors. Is it merely an extended nursing role, in which nurses learn to take on delegated medical tasks, thereby rendering them assistant doctors? Or is it a new role that will become the norm of tomorrow (MacGuire 1980)?

In August 1996 the UKCC reported in a discussion paper that the consultation exercise it had undertaken with members of the nursing profession had recommended that nurse practitioners who practise the role like doctor substitutes should not be defined as advanced practitioners. The UKCC's comments provoked a storm of protest when the paper was leaked at the International Nurse Practitioner Conference held in Edinburgh in August 1996. A letter of complaint was sent to the UKCC Registrar setting out the Royal College of Nursing's dismay at an apparent lack of understanding and support for the nurse practitioner role. The letter was signed by senior nursing representatives from several countries, including the USA and Australia. It is clear that nurse practitioner role as doctor substitution creates concern, and there appears to be a division between those commentators who see the role of the nurse practitioner as no more than substitute doctors and those who see it as an advanced nursing role. MacGuire (1980) in her work on extended and expanded nursing roles has described two models which underlie the literature and these may help to illuminate the debate:

Model A

Nursing and medicine are two distinct disciplines; commentators are concerned about the possibility of nursing functions being lost from the new role in favour of the assumption of medical tasks.

Model B

There are many tasks to be carried out to maintain the health of communities and to care for patients. Who does what is immaterial provided they are trained for the task, competent, acceptable to patients and achieve the same standards.

Thus there are those advocates of the nurse practitioner role who stress the nursing element and deny any accusations of acting as doctor substitutes (Robinson 1993, Cable 1994); on the other hand are advocates of the role who emphasize the extended aspects of the role and see nothing wrong in being doctor substitutes. Indeed, Burke-Masters (1986), and early pioneer in the UK, regards herself as a nurse with an extended role into medicine. She states she is not about 'constructing models of nursing … but … in meeting health needs'. She realized that a nursing role without diagnostic skills or autonomy would not meet the health needs of her patients.

The issue of doctor substitution was brought to the fore in a debate that took place in London in December 1995 organized by Professional Nurse and the Queen's Nursing Institute entitled *Are nurse practitioners merely substitute doctors?* Pearson proposed the motion: 'This house believes that current nurse practitioners are no more than substitute doctors'. Pearson (1996) argues that nurse practitioners seem to be 'flavour of the month' and there is money available for nurses to expand their roles. She states that 'ultimately there is a constantly shifting balance between the extension of a nurse's role and the adoption of a medical role. We must judge whether that balance falls on the side of nursing or medicine' (p. 325). She goes on to argue that in North America nurse practitioners filled a clear gap, as there is very little specialist community nursing provision in the USA and that in the UK the nurse practitioner role may be about developing a clear structure for nurses to remain in clinical practice. However, Pearson fails to expand on what criteria we can use to make the judgement where the balance between nursing and medicine falls. Nor does she offer an explanation as to why the nurse practitioner role should be the way nurses remain in clinical practice when there is currently a proliferation of clinical nurse specialist roles and eight community nursing specialisms.

The motion was opposed by a nurse practitioner, who argued that:

> Nurse practitioners see themselves as a complementary service, which increases patient choice, adds diversity to patient care, enhances collaboration with the medical profession and enhances the scope of the skill mix across the primary health-care team (Emmerson 1996, p. 326).

The motion was overwhelmingly defeated but the debate highlights the dichotomy that exists between protagonists and antagonists of the nurse practitioner role. An issue that has added fuel to the fire of doctor substitution is the reduction in junior doctors' hours (Loveland 1992). 'Making better use of ... support staff and mechanisms' and 'Making the best use of the skills of nurses and midwives' were included in the new deal (Read and Graves 1994). The new deal can be seen as exploiting nurses by delegating tasks to them that were previously undertaken by junior doctors in order to fulfil the recommendations that junior doctors' hours be reduced. Thus, what is essentially a problem for doctors became a problem for nurses (Keyzer 1996). Others, such as Pickersgill (1993), see the new deal as a tremendous opportunity for nurses, and other commentators hold the view that if nurses don't fill the gap left by the reduction in junior doctors' hours, then someone else will; thus, rather than an imposition on nursing, the new deal for junior doctors should be seen as an enabling development to enhance nursing roles (International Nurse Practitioner Conference, 1996).

Watson *et al.* (1994) argue that a new ecological niche is appearing in the division of health labour that is located between doctors' and nurses' traditional work. This new role requires a level of education and skills that not all nurses will wish to obtain. They say that: 'whatever this called, some nurses in some areas will be recruited to it. If they do not colonise it for whatever reason, some other group will' (p. 63).

Morley (1992) saw night duty as being an appropriate area where night nurse practitioners could relieve junior doctors of many of their tasks, whilst McKee and Black (1992) looked at how midwives might be used to reduce the night-time work of junior doctors in obstetrics. The Greenhalgh report (1994) suggested that some areas of junior doctors' work could be taken on by nurses and the following activities could be shared by both during the day, and particularly at night; taking a patient history; venous blood sampling; inserting peripheral intravenous infusions; referring a patient for investigations; writing discharge letters; administration of drugs.

Richardson and Maynard (1995) in an influential discussion paper talk of 'doctor–nurse substitution'. They undertook a review of the literature and tell us that in a variety of settings (mostly primary care) some tasks may be performed by nurses, or other health professionals, at a comparable level to that provided by the doctor or physician. They state that the results of studies suggest that between 30% and 70% of doctors' tasks could be carried out by nurses, though they warn us that the studies suffer from a lack of external validity. Despite this, the authors argue, substitution has occurred to a significant degree in the UK. The answer to the question: fewer doctors? more nurses? they say appears to be 'yes' in terms of practice in the USA. In the USA and the UK there are changes in the use of assistants, aides, counsellors and other types of skill. Richardson and Maynard (1995) say the evidence base to support fewer doctors and more nurses is poor and the changes cannot be justified from the literature. They argue that 'it is unfortunate that decision-making in this area of health policy, as in others, is not "confused" by the results of well-designed evaluative studies' (p. 18).

> The cost-effectiveness of substituting nurses for doctors cannot be demonstrated without the measurement of the quality of the services provided... To estimate the level at which doctors can be substituted with nurses in the UK would require a randomized control trial with careful measurement of costs and patients' outcomes and an adequate follow-up period... the costs of a properly controlled trial may be small when compared to the potential savings available by substituting nurses for doctors and the potential costs (including damage to patients) of changing skill mix 'on the hoof' and in the absence of a sufficient knowledge base. It is inefficient, but usual, for the NHS and other health care systems to alter skill mix and pay little regard to the evaluation of such policies (p. 16).

Discussion papers such as this can only serve to confuse policy makers like the UKCC, which is perhaps what Richardson and Maynard would wish. However, their paper continually talks about tasks and doctor substitution rather than holistic care and doctor–nurse collaboration. Moreover, the studies reviewed may be small-scale, single-site and evaluating short-term outcomes, but their cumulative effects – especially added to which are the Touche Ross (1994) and Coopers and Lybrand (1996) studies published after Richardson and Maynard's paper – are impressive in their support of the effectiveness of the nurse practitioner role, especially in general practice settings. Richardson and Maynard's stance on nurse practitioners may be seen as taking too narrow a view of the role. Nurse practitioners certainly take on some tasks previously located within the domain of medical practice, but studies (for example, Stilwell 1988) demonstrate that nurse practitioners bring something extra to the consultation, and that something extra, it is argued, is a nursing focus.

Furthermore, the doctor is used as the gold standard for professional health-care delivery and it is taken for granted that 'damage to patients' will only happen with doctor substitution. McKee and Black (1992) also suggested that, rather than achieving improvements in patient care, detriments will occur if tasks are delegated. This is of course an important consideration, especially if skill mix and delegation from doctors to nurses occur in an *ad hoc* fashion. Statutory regulation of nurse practitioners and standardization of competence through a formal education programme will help to ensure safe practice and minimize the risk to patients.

Read and Graves (1994), in their study of the nursing contribution to the reduction of junior doctors' hours in the Trent region, state after a review of the literature that the nursing profession's response to performing some tasks currently undertaken by junior doctors is mixed. There are fears that nurses will become 'pseudo medical assistants' or 'super trained technicians'. However, they argue that 'NHS workforce planning must not be undertaken in the watertight compartments of medicine and nursing but that decisions as to who does what in patient care should be considered within a multidisciplinary and multiprofessional forum with carefully planned research testing different ways of doing things' (p. 5). Watson *et al.* (1994) state that in an effort to emphasize the nursing rather than the medical aspects of the nurse practitioner role, writers assume current nursing orthodoxies. They cite the following example from the literature:

> To write of the nurse practitioner is to write of the nurse – for every nurse who practices his or her profession is a nurse practitioner (Robinson (1973) quoted in Studner and Hirsch 1986).

This chapter has examined the development of the nurse practitioner role in the changing political and professional context of health care in the UK. It is clear from scrutiny of relevant literature and commentaries that the role of the nurse practitioner is quickly becoming a key feature of health-care delivery in both acute and primary care settings. The role is, however, a contentious one in that debates at several levels are ongoing. Until nursing's statutory body, the UKCC, clarifies its position on standards for nurse practitioner education and practice, uncertainty will reign. Clarification of the role is far from straightforward, as the foregoing discussion has pointed out. Questions are still to be answered as to whether the role comprises a *level* of practice, be it specialist or advanced, or a discrete set of characteristics and tasks that only nurse practitioners undertake.

There is also the issue of extended and expanded roles; if nurse practitioners extend their role into the medical domain, is this because the interests of patients will be better served? because it will facilitate the professionalization of nursing? or because it will help answer a crisis in medicine brought about by the new deal for junior doctors and recruitment problems of general practice? Perhaps all of these factors interrelate and the proponents of the nurse practitioner role have seen the opportunities afforded by the NHS reforms to carve out a niche for themselves.

That the role (or title) is becoming increasingly popular is clear, and the nursing profession must ask why this is occurring and why existing roles such as the clinical nurse specialist role and the community specialist nursing roles are not answering the needs of nurses. It may be that courses of preparation for such nursing roles do not adequately prepare nurses to meet the health-care needs of patients as well as they might. For example, professional rhetoric espouses holistic care, yet the fact that nurses cannot prescribe medication, perform a physical assessment, take a complete history and manage straightforward illness flies in the face of holism. Moreover, as nurses become more involved in nurse-led interventions such as assessment clinics and chronic disease management, it is uneconomic and inefficient to refer to medical colleagues those aspects of clinical care that can be managed well by appropriately educated nurses.

The issue of power and vested interests is of course central to the debate on nurse practitioners. Territorialism within nursing is rife and the boundaries between medicine and nursing, though blurring, are fraught with medicolegal pitfalls that need to be urgently addressed. Government white papers and reports urge interprofessional collaboration and interdisciplinary team-working, yet until nurses have a strong voice and the knowledge and political awareness to be advocates for themselves as well as patients, the profession's subservience to medicine will continue. Nurse practitioners undergoing a formal course of education are encouraged to be politically and professionally aware, to be clinically competent, to develop their interpersonal skills and to be confident to express their views and needs. All this, together with the additional skills of assessment and diagnosis, makes nurse practitioners eminently marketable as members of the health-care team – though not as a cheap alternative to doctors.

It is clear that full acceptance of the nurse practitioner role in the UK will not be possible without the support of key stakeholders in both the nursing and medical professions, government and patients. Acceptance by the medical profession is paramount and it has been demonstrated (Hupcey 1993) that the main barrier to nurse practitioner practice was resistance from physicians and other health-care workers, particularly staff nurses. Prevailing ideologies of medicine and nursing within the organization of health care may prove to be a barrier to the further development of the nurse practitioner role, and the role must be negotiated within this context. It therefore seems pertinent to draw on the body of work on the theory of negotiation in social interactions to help illuminate the process of integrating a new role into the already established social order of the group general practice. Chapter 22 in this volume utilizes the theoretical framework of the negotiated order perspective developed by Strauss and his colleagues (1963) to explain how the new role of the nurse practitioner is becoming part of the social organization of health care in the UK.

References

Abbott. A. (1988) *The System of Professions: An Essay on the Division of Expert Labour*, Chicago, University of Chicago Press.

Adams, A., Bond, S. (1997) The human factor, *Health Service Journal*, **6**, pp. 30–1.

Burke-Masters, B. (1986) The autonomous nurse practitioner: an answer to a chronic problem of primary care, *Lancet*, **1**(8492), pp. 1266.

Butterworth, C.A. (1991) Getting our professional house in order In: Salvage J. (ed.) *Nurse Practitioners, Working for Change in Primary Health Care Nursing*, London, King's Fund Centre.

Cable, S. (1994) What is a nurse practitioner? *Primary Health Care*, **4**(5), pp. 12–14.

Castledine, G. (1991) The advanced nurse practitioner (part two), *Nursing Standard*, **5**(44), pp. 33–36.

Castledine, G. (1993) Nurse practitioner title: ambiguous and misleading, *British Journal of Nursing*, **2**(14), pp. 734–735.

Chambers N. (1994) *The Derbyshire Nurse Practitioner Project*, Derby, Derbyshire Family Health Services Authority.

Coopers and Lybrand (1996) *Nurse Practitioner Evaluation Project Final Report*, London, NHS Executive.

Department of Health (1992) *The Extended Role of the Nurse/ Scope of Professional Practice (EL/CNO(92)4)*, London, Department of Health.

Department of Health and Social Security (1986) *Neighbourhood Nursing – A Focus for Care: Report of the Community Nursing Review Team (Cumberlege Report)*, London, HMSO.

Department of Health and the Welsh Office (1989) *General Practice in the National Health Service: A New Contract*, London, HMSO.

Department of Health and Social Security (1987) *Promoting Better Health: The Government's Programme for Improving Primary Health Care*, London, HMSO.

Emmerson P. (1996) Are nurse practitioners merely substitute doctors?, *Professional Nurse*, **11**(5), February.

Fawcett-Henesy A. (1991) The British scene. In: Salvage J. (ed.) *Nurse Practitioners: Working for Change in Primary Health Care Nursing*, London, King's Fund Centre.

Greehhalgh and Company Limited (1994) *The Interface between Junior Doctors and Nurses: A Research Study for the Department of Health*, Macclesfield, Greenhalgh and Company.

Hupcey J.E. (1993) Factors and work settings that may influence nurse practitioner practice, *Nursing Outlook*, **41**, pp. 181–185.

International Nurse Practitioner Conference, Heriot-Watt University, Edinburgh, August, 1996.

Johnson M.L. (1978) Big fleas have little fleas – nurse professionalization and nursing auxilliaries In: Hardie M., Hockey L. (eds.) *Nursing Auxilliary in Health Care*, London, Croom Helm.

Kitzman H.J. (1989) The CNS and the nurse practitioner. In: Hanric A.B., Spross A., Spross J. (eds) *The Clinical Nurse Specialist in Theory and Practice*, New York, Grune and Stratton.

Keyzer D.M. (1985) *Learning Contracts, the Trained Nurse and the Implementation of the Nursing Process: Comparative Case Studies in the Management of Knowledge and Change in Nursing Practice*. Unpublished PhD thesis, London University, Institute of Education.

Keyzer D. (1996) Keynote speech. *Making a World of Difference: Nurse Practitioners: A Global Perspective*, 4th International Conference and Exhibition on Nurse Practitioner Practice, Edinburgh, Heriot Watt University, August 22–24. Unpublished.

Loveland P. (1992) The new deal: an account of progress in reducing junior hospital doctor's hours in England, *Health Trends*, **24**(1): pp. 3–4.

MacGuire J. (1980) *The Extended Role of the Nurse*, Project Paper RC3 London, King's Fund Centre.

MacKay L. (1993) *Conflicts in Care: Medicine and Nursing*, London, Chapman & Hall.

Marsh G.N., Dawes M.L. (1995) Establishing a minor illness nurse in a busy general practice, *British Medical Journal*, **310**, pp. 778–780.

McKee M., Black N. (1992) Does the current use of junior doctors in the United Kingdom affect the quality of medical care?, *Social Science and Medicine*, **34**, pp. 549–558.

Melia K. (1987) *Learning and Working: The Occupational Socialization of Nurses*, London, Tavistock.

Mitchinson S. (1996) Are nurses independent and autonomous practitioners?, *Nursing Standard*, **10**(34), pp. 34–38.

Morley B. (1992) The role of the night nurse practitioner, *British Journal of Nursing*, **1**: pp. 719–721.

National Health Service Management Executive (1993), *Nursing in Primary Health Care: New World, New Opportunities*, London, HMSO.

Page N.E. Arena D.M. (1994) Rethinking the merger of the clinical nurse specialist and the nurse practitioner roles, *Image Journal of Nursing Scholarship*, **26**, pp. 315–318.

Pearson, P. (1996) Are nurse practitioners merely substitute doctors?, *Professional Nurse*, February, **11**(5), p. 325.

Pickersgill F. (1993) A new deal for nurses too?, *Nursing Standard*, **7**(35), pp. 21–22.

Ralph, C. (1991) The role of the regulatory body. In: Salvage J. (ed.) *Nurse Practitioners: Working for Change in Primary Health Care Nursing*, London, King's Fund Centre.

Read S., Graves K. (1994) *Reduction of Junior Doctors' Hours in Trent Region: The Nursing Contribution*, NHS Executive, Leeds, Trent Regional Health Authority.

Richardson G., Maynard A. (1995) *Fewer Doctors? More Nurses? A Review of the Knowledge Base of Doctor-Nurse Substitution* Discussion paper 135, York, York Centre for Health Economics, York Health Economics Consortium, NHS Centre for Reviews and Dissemination.

Robinson D. (1973) *Patients, Practitioners and Medical Care*, London, Heinemann.

Robinson D. (1993) Nurse Practitioner or Mini Doctor?, *Accident and Emergency Nursing*, **1**, pp. 53–55.

Royal College of Nursing of the United Kingdom (1988a) *Boundaries of Nursing: A Policy Statement*, London, Royal College of Nursing.

Royal College of Nursing of the United Kingdom (1988b) *Specialties in Nursing: A report of the working party investigating the development of specialties within the nursing profession*, London, Royal College of Nursing.

Salisbury C.J., Tettersell M. (1988) Comparison of the work of a nurse practitioner with that of a general practitioner, *Journal of the Royal College of General Practitioners*, **38**, pp. 314–316.

Salvage J. (1985) *The Politics of Nursing*, London, Heinemann.

Simon P. (1992) Pioneer spirit, *Nursing Times*, **88** (30), pp. 16–17.

Sparacino P., Durand, B. (1986) Editorial on specialisation in advanced nursing practice, *Momentum*, **4** (2), pp. 2–3.

Stilwell, B. (1982) The nurse practitioner at work, *Nursing Times*, **78**(43), pp 1799–1803.

Stilwell B. (1988) Patient attitudes to a highly developed role – the nurse practitioner, *Recent Advances in Nursing*, **12**, pp. 82–100.

Stilwell B., Greenfield S., Drury V.W.M., Hull F.M. (1987) A nurse practitioner in general practice: working style and pattern of consultations, *Journal of the Royal College of General Practitioners*, **37**, pp. 154–157.

Strauss A., Schatzman, L., Ehrlich D., Bucher R., Sabshin M. (1963) The hospital and its negotiated order. In: Freidson E. (ed.) *The Hospital in Modern Society*, New York, Free Press.

Studner J., Hirsch H. (1986) Nurse practitioners: functions, legal status and legislative control, *Medicine and Law*, **5**, pp. 61–75.

Sutton F., Smith C. (1995) Advanced nursing practice: new ideas and new perspectives, *Journal of Advanced Nursing*, **21**, pp. 1037–1043.

Tomlinson B. (1992) *Report of the Enquiry into London's Health Service, Medical Education and Research*, London, HMSO.

Touche Ross (1994) *Evaluation of Nurse Practitioner Projects*, London, Touche Ross Management Consultants.

Tudor Hart J. (1984) A new kind of doctor. In: Black J. (ed.) *Health and Disease: A Reader*, Buckinghamshire, Open University Press.

United Kingdom Central Council (1986) *Missing Title*, London, United Kingdom Central Office.

United Kingdom Central Council (1992) *The Scope of Professional Practice*, London, United Kingdom Central Council.

United Kingdom Central Council (1994) *The Future of Professional Practice: The Council's Standards for Education and Practice Following Registration*, London, United Kingdom Central Council.

United Kingdom Central Council (1998) *A Higher Level of Practice: Consultation Document*, London, United Kingdom Central Council.

Walby S., Greenwell J. (eds.) (1994) *Medicine and Nursing: Professions in a Changing Health Service*, London, Sage Publications.

Walsh M. (1996) *Nurse Practitioner: To Be or Not To Be*, Paper presented at a nurse practitioner study day, Lancaster, University College of St Martin. Unpublished.

Watson, P., Hendey N., Dingwall R. (1994) *Role Extension/Expansion with Particular Reference to the Nurse Practitioner*, Nottingham, School of Social Studies, University of Nottingham.

CHAPTER 20

The professional and legal framework for the nurse practitioner

Shirley Reveley

Introduction

The nurse practitioner movement in the UK has developed in the midst of political, professional and legislative changes. Nurse practitioners and their employers are concerned with the issues of accountability for practice and legal issues relating to this expanded nursing role. Nurse practitioners are pushing forward the boundaries of nursing practice and are in the front line of innovation, therefore they sometimes feel vulnerable and question their legal position. It is vital that nurse practitioners feel they have a secure base from which to practise, and this requires a strong foundation of knowledge derived from education and experience, together with a contract of employment and a good grasp of the professional/legal framework within which to function. This chapter is concerned with that legal and professional framework and, although these issues will be discussed under separate headings, of course the two are inextricably linked.

Accountability

The UK Central Council (UKCC) rightly insists on personal and professional accountability for nurses in the interests of public safety and professional development (UKCC 1992a, 1992b, 1996). In 1990 the Welsh National Board issued a discussion paper on the topic of professional responsibility and extended roles which added fuel to the debate about extended nursing roles and the need for certificates of competence. In 1992 the Chief Nurses of the UK Health Departments withdrew previous guidance on the extended role, requesting instead that all nurses and managers act in accordance with the *Code of Professional Conduct* (UKCC 1992a) and the

Scope of Professional Practice (UKCC 1992b). According to the UKCC, accountability means answering for one's actions and the opening statement in the booklet *Guidelines for Professional Practice* (1996) is as follows:

> As a registered practitioner, you hold a position of responsibility and people rely on you. You are professionally accountable to the UKCC, as well as having a contractual responsibility to your employer and accountability to the law for your actions (p. 8).

The UKCC (1992a) document *The Code of Professional Conduct* underlines each nurse's professional accountability:

> As a registered nurse, midwife or health visitor you shall act, at all times, in such a manner as to: safeguard and promote the interests of society; justify public trust and confidence and uphold and enhance the good standing and reputation of the professions.

Accountability means obligations and liabilities that arise from several areas of regulation:

- Regulations of the UKCC for Nursing, Midwifery and Health Visiting
- The law on civil wrongs to patients (a civil wrong is known as a tort)
- Employment law which covers the relationship between employer and employee

Figure 20.1 illustrates how these different lines of accountability affect the nurse. Sometimes they can be pulling in different directions and set up real conflicts, especially between accountability to your employer and the UKCC.

Accountability involves giving an account of your actions with rationales and explanations for why you did what you did. You have to be prepared as a nurse or nurse practitioner to justify your actions at all times if necessary.

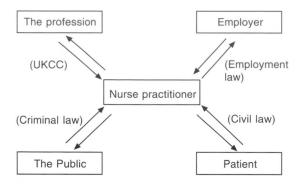

Figure 20.1 Patterns of accountability. The arrows show the two way nature of accountability. The possible involvement of the law is shown in brackets. Nurse practitioners are also accountable through the process of critical reflection on practice and ultimately their own conscience

Accountability may be:

- Personal: the individual is accountable
- Goal-related and therefore measurable: a person cannot be held accountable unless there are written goals to be achieved (standards of care, critical pathways, for example). Clinical audit therefore has a key role in accountability
- About a two-way contract: the employer must make resources available and agree goals before holding the employee accountable
- Motivational for staff: success brings rewards but underperformance brings sanctions

To be accountable the nurse practitioner needs to be in possession of all the facts and information (education and communication), and have the power (authority) to act as s/he sees fit with proper mechanisms for measuring outcomes in place (audit). Having the power to act is the link between accountability and autonomy. Freedom to act (autonomy) always means freedom to act within the boundaries of competence as well as other external constraints. Autonomy is therefore a relative concept, as nobody has complete autonomy. Even the most powerful medical consultant is constrained by factors such as the General Medical Council, NHS trust management (e.g. expenditure limits) or limitations on drugs that can be prescribed on the NHS.

Responsibility is a word which is often and mistakenly used interchangeably with accountability. Responsibility means that a person is responsible for following orders, doing what s/he is told and acknowledging when s/he is out of his or her depth. A health-care assistant or pre-registration student is responsible in law and to his or her employer for the care given, but it is the registered nurse who is ultimately accountable. The nurse practitioner should therefore think carefully before delegating tasks to staff who do not hold a nursing registration as the NP will be held professionally accountable for the care received by that patient even though s/he did not carry it out.

Extended and expanded roles

The publication of the *Scope of Professional Practice* document made clear an important difference between extended and expanded roles. Extension is acceptance of new tasks which are usually delegated by others, whilst expansion refers to the practitioner's decision as to which new roles or tasks to take on. Extension therefore implies dependence and expansion implies independence. This led Vaughan (1989) to make an important distinction between the two terms: 'If expansion does not ocur, the unique function of nursing will be lost' (p. 54).

However, there are certain considerations involved in expanding nursing roles. For example, Colin Ralph (1991), until fairly recently Registrar of the UKCC, accepted that informal adjustments to role boundaries change in response to patient need. He also agreed that working arrangements between nurses and doctors leading to improvements in treatment and practice were required. However, he warned of the consequences: 'when a nurse strays into territory formerly bounded by medical practice' (p. 123). Ralph suggested that there were several consequences. For example, will the primary caring role of nursing be compromised if a new element of the nursing role is accepted and is this a logical extension of the caring role? The personal liability of the practitioner accepting the new element of practice, and the liability of the practitioner who may have authorized the assumption of new responsibilities must be considered, as must the interests of the patient or client.

Another consequence identified by Ralph is that there is always an unavoidable delay between the occurrence of developments and their formalization because developments in clinical practice and care usually happen in the clinical setting before policies and the curriculum can be revised. This supports the point made by Abbott: 'By the time a profession has won its legal position, it has usually won its public position long before" (Abbott 1988, p. 64). Ralph argued that this phase–the 'pioneering' phase – is when patient, client and practitioner are most vulnerable. He stressed the need to focus on making clear those elements of the nurse practitioner role that are different from those of existing nursing roles before the new role became a blueprint.

The Scope of Professional Practice (UKCC 1992b) is an important document in helping doctors and nurses decide which activities are appropriate to share, and under what circumstances. It moved nursing on from tasks delegated by doctors for which an endless series of certificates of competence had to be obtained. However the political circumstances of the time cannot be ignored. As West (1995) points out:

> Whilst the literature is suggesting that there are opportunities for nurses to extend their scope of professional practice at night (and at other times) in order to facilitate the reduction in junior doctors' hours, it is necessary to consider the results of these studies in order that nursing does not automatically take for itself the previous practice of the medical profession but rather learns from these and develops the scope of professional practice within clear parameters which provide the optimum support mechanisms, appropriate educational opportunities and adequate manpower resources (p. 7).

In summary, *The Scope of Professional Practice*:

- Makes nurses arbiters of their own competence to expand their role
- Emphasizes accountability
- Negates the need for certification for new roles and tasks
- Requires nurses to delegate appropriately
- Insists that expansion must not compromise existing practice
- Offers the potential for expansion of practice in a professional way

However, there are certain problems with this approach that the nurse practitioner must recognize, starting with the awkward question: how can nurses assess their own competence? The suspicion remains that it was merely a means of resolving medical staffing shortages which might have the paradoxical effect of stimulating conflicts with other professions such as radiography, let alone medicine. The key question of whether nurses can be held truly accountable when they have so little power and therefore autonomy remains. Nurse practitioners are caught up in all these issues and need to be thinking through strategies with colleagues and employers to work around these problems.

Autonomous nursing practice

Most commentators who try to describe the nurse practitioner role refer to the concepts of autonomous practice and accountability without defining what is meant by these terms. Kendrick (1995) argues that the use of such terminology is useless in the face of medical dominance. He argues that:

> to use terms such as 'autonomous', 'responsible' and 'accountable' in relation to nursing practice seems facile when the medical model holds such influence over the approach used for the delivery of care. Nurses must accept a degree of culpability for the level of inertia

which has allowed this position to continue and prosper (p. 242).

Doctors, unlike nurses, are trained to work on their own and to rely on their own independent judgement. 'The need for autonomy in their clinical decision-making is fundamental to the dominance of the medical profession' (Elston 1977, p. 27). Recent management changes and financial restraints imposed upon the NHS have limited the autonomy of doctors to prescribe treatment and medication. The medical profession does not enjoy the degree of autonomy it once used to. Autonomy is therefore a relative concept. Doctors and nurses have degrees of autonomy but nobody has absolute autonomy to do whatever they please as they are limited by their employers, health authorities and their professional bodies, not to mention the law of the land.

Nurse practitioners are aiming for higher degrees of autonomy than traditional nurses. It is clear that the more autonomy a nurse practitioner enjoys, the more authority she will have to determine practice and therefore the more accountable s/he may truly be said to be. The reverse is also true and this calls into question the concept of accountability for many nurses as they have little authority over practice.

How easy is it for the nurse practitioner to claim a high degree of autonomy? Data from the study by Reveley (1997) which was carried out to evaluate the nurse practitioner role may shed light on this area. The work was done in primary health care in a large group practice and involved interviews with patients, nurse and doctors on their perceptions of the nurse practitioner role. The question of autonomy was a key issue. The nurse practitioner working in the practice herself felt she had a lot of autonomy:

> it (nurse practitioner role) has evolved into me seeing all the acute GP patients who need to be seen and assessing them and diagnosing them and deciding on treatment and deciding on the prescription and again it's how far do you go? I have a lot of freedom; a lot of responsibility. I have a lot of support and I think I'm very careful about where I stand legally ... There's a lot of clinical issues that come up that I ask the doctors about and they haven't got the answer to and there aren't protocols for them either. And again it's just making a clinical decision based on what you know and what the patients tell you (CNP).

There are commentators who are concerned about nurse practitioners working autonomously in this way as they lack the ability to deal with the full range of symptoms that may present at the surgery. Kassirer (1994) feels that common sense alone argues that the shorter training of nurse practitioners will limit their capacity to deal with diagnostic uncertainty and complexity. As a result they will be unable to reason from first principles and handle probabilistic reasoning. The limited exposure of nurses to these concepts is likely to find them unprepared for certain diagnostic and therapeutic tasks. As a result, Kassirer feels that nurse practitioners may not always appreciate the seriousness of a clinical problem. The GPs in the case study practice were well aware of this issue; one agreed with Kassirer's statement (1994) in so far as this GP believed that:

> the beauty of a good GP is that he has all the skills and is doing it all the time so he can ... go from very simple concepts to very complex concepts; a GP can combine them all, a nurse practitioner by definition can't. If she is going to do that then she's a doctor so the weakness of the role is that you can't combine all the skills necessary for holistic care (GP).

Kassirer does concede that nurse practitioners can play a major role in primary care, particularly in collaborative work with GPs, and much recent research has demonstrated that nurse practitioners can provide high-quality care within this setting (Ashburner *et al.* 1997).

GPs in the study practice were well aware of the medicolegal implications of the ambiguous nature of the nurse practitioner role. One GP talked about the buck stopping with the GPs, and doctors having to live with uncertainty. Nurses, GPs and some patients concurred that the lack of direction from the centre (Department of Health, statutory bodies) as to what a nurse practitioner actually was constituted a major problem. As one GP said:

> We have a problem because there's no such definition of what a nurse practitioner is, is there? Anyone can say they're a nurse practitioner ... but there's nothing to recognise them is there? On balance I think we can accept that she does a lot of work, takes a lot of our work, but there are a few issues that need ironing out aren't there? More at a structural level than a clinical level really. Because on the clinical confidence side of her, you know, she's fine, there's not a problem at all. (GP in Case Study Practice).

The future role of the nurse practitioner within the case-study practice was couched in terms of her being the first point of contact for patients and referring to the GP as a second service for patients who needed purely medical skills. This triage role differs from some areas where the nurse practitioner takes on more chronic disease management. One GP in the research described a vision of the nurse practitioner in these terms:

> 'The first point of contact for patients would be the nurse practitioner and they would become the primary health care physician, the GP dealing more with follow-ups and complicated problems; things that again might generally be followed up traditionally in outpatient departments in hospital. In other words they [GPs] would take on things they have already done like diabetics with help from the nurse practitioner which is already well established, but there's cardiology, complicated patients in so many ways – the first point of contact for the nurse practitioner would be the GP who would have more of a specialist interest in particular fields (GP).

This statement implies a great deal of autonomy for nurse practitioners in primary health care. However, there is a major limitation to this autonomy and that is the prescribing of medication. It is difficult to imagine how any group of nurses can be autonomous when they do not have the power to prescribe medicines but have to rely on another professional to sanction their treatment decisions. The Community Nursing Review recommended that the Department of Health and Social Security should agree a limited list of items and simple agents which may be prescribed by nurses as part of a nursing care programme, and issue guidelines to enable nurses to control drug dosage in well-defined circumstances. (Department of Health and Social Security 1986.)

Nurse prescribing has finally been made legal (the Medicinal Products: Prescription by Nurses etc. Act 1992). However, though the eight pilot sites in GP fundholding practices throughout the country reported favourable outcomes, there was a further delay in extending nurse prescribing powers to all community nurses when another pilot was ordered. The town of Bolton was designated a further test site for a period of one year from April 1996. Furthermore, nurse prescribing was originally only permitted to those nurses holding a recognized community nursing qualification, thus a nurse not holding such a qualification (including many practice nurses and nurse practitioners) were effectively barred from this professional activity. Commentators also write of the severe limitations of the formulary which contains little more than dressings and minor drugs. Many would wish the formulary to be extended and some would like to see nurses having prescribing rights which extend to the full *British National Formulary* (Jones and Gough 1997). In these circumstances, the principles laid down in the *Scope of Professional Practice* document (UKCC 1992b) would regulate safe practice.

There is some scope for an extension to prescribing rights for nurses, as was announced in a government white paper, *Primary Care: Delivering the Future* (Department of Health 1996) that existing nurse prescribing pilots will be extended to another 500 general practices and 1500 nurses from April 1997. A professional working party will meet over a year to develop consistent practices for the administration and supply of medicines by professionals other than doctors. The implications for legislation and professional training will also be considered. At the Royal College of Nursing Congress in May 1998, Frank Dobson announced a rolling out of the nurse prescribing project.

It can be seen that the question of the nurse practitioner's autonomy is a difficult one. With regard to seeing patients with undifferentiated conditions and making management decisions from a range of options, the nurse practitioner can be said to be working autonomously. As a qualified nurse she is also accountable for those decisions. Yet that autonomy is limited by the absence of prescribing rights and also by the fact that others exert a large degree of control over the content of her work.

Furthermore, a question hangs over the relationship between autonomy for nurses and their role as patients' advocate. Porter (1991) contends that the justification for nurses being a patient's advocate is that doctor–patient relationships are biaised in favour of doctors so that nurses need to speak up for patients. This is based on the idea that the nurse does for the patient what s/he would do for him/herself if s/he were well enough. As the nurse practitioner takes on a more active and autonomous role in managing a patient's health problems and the doctor slips into the background, might not the patient need an advocate to intervene between nurse and patient? Clearly the nurse practitioner cannot advocate against him/herself on behalf of the patient. In mental health, lay practitioners have evolved to take on the advocacy role and nurse practitioners may well find the same problem in their evolving practice.

Professional discourse emphasizes the power of practitioners expressed through notions of autonomy, accountability, responsibility and decision-making (Pashley and Henry 1990; Porter 1991). But there exists a tension between nurses being partners in care with patients, acting as their advocate on the one hand, whilst being autonomous decision-makers on the other (Witz 1994). Also, in their relationship with doctors and managers nurse practitioners cannot be truly autonomous any more than autonomous practitioners can work successfully as part of a multidisciplinary team. How far can any health professional claim to be truly autonomous in the light of government policies on teamwork and interagency collaboration? The best that can be said is that autonomy for nurse practitioners, as for everyone else, is relative.

Legal issues surrounding the nurse practitioner role

Within the legal system there are two main aspects – criminal and civil law. Criminal law refers to that system wherein offences are punished by the state and the action is brought by the Crown against a defendant. A case of criminal law is referred to as *Regina* versus (the defendant), usually written as R v. (the defendant's name) e.g. R v. *Brown*.

This section is largely concerned with civil law as legal issues surrounding nursing are usually related to civil rather than criminal law. The possible consequences of accountable expanded practice involving greater degrees of autonomy mean that in order to practise safely, the nurse practitioner must understand some of the basic principles which govern civil law. In civil law an action is brought by a person (the plaintiff in England; the pursuer in Scotland) against another person or organization (the defendant). An action is usually brought because a person has suffered some harm or loss and is seeking compensation. The type of civil law action nurses are most likely to be involved in are claims for damages as a result of the tort of negligence (McHale *et al.* 1998). A tort is a civil wrong and can refer to negligence or a battery.

As well as being accountable to patients via the UKCC *Code of Professional Conduct* (UKCC 1992a), nurses are also accountable in law, as are all other professionals. A nurse has a legal duty to act carefully towards patients and malpractice could lead to a civil action or, in extreme cases, criminal prosecution. A nurse who fails to act with sufficient care towards a patient and thus causes harm may be held accountable in the tort of negligence. The standard legal definition of negligence dates from the 19th century and it is:

> The omission to do something which a reasonable man, guided upon these considerations which ordinarily relate the conduct of human affairs would do – or to do something which a prudent and reasonable man would not do (*Blyth* v. *Birmingham Water Works* 1891, cited in McHale *et al.* 1998).

Put simply, therefore, negligence involves not doing something that you should have done, doing the right thing wrongly or doing completely the wrong thing. The tort of negligence has five elements:

1   There must be a duty of care owed to the person
2   The standard of care appropriate to that duty must be broken
3   That breach must cause the loss complained about
4   That loss must be of a kind that the courts can recognize and compensate
5   That loss must have been reasonably foreseeable

Only if all five elements are present will there be liability for negligence – the absence of any one element will prevent it (*Donaghue* v. *Stevenson* 1932). The plaintiff normally has to prove his or her case on the basis of probabilities. A nurse practitioner who is alleged to be in breach of a duty of care would have his or her conduct viewed from the perspective of what is known as the Bolam test (see below) which can be summarized as what the 'ordinary skilled nurse in her speciality would have done in the circumstances of the case'. In addition, the nurse would have been expected only to take precautions against reasonably known risks.

Dimond (1994) tells us that currently the law does not prescribe who is to perform certain health tasks but leaves it to the statutory bodies to determine their own rules. Further, she tells us that in determining competence the primary focus of the courts is not whether a task is carried out by a nurse or a doctor unless there is a statutory requirement to that effect. Rather, the courts will want to determine from experts in the field what standards of care the patient should expect to receive and whether there are any acceptable reasons why they were not present.

Thus lawyers would take advice from nurses in the same speciality as the defendant and if the case went to trial, the judge would draw conclusions from expert evidence as to the standard of professional practice. The legal principles have their basis in the case of *Bolam* v. *Friern Hospital Management Committee* (1957 - 1WLR 582), cited in McHale *et al.* (1998, p. 19), and this has become known as the Bolam test.

> The test is the standard of the ordinary skilled man exercising and professing to have that special skill. A man need not possess the highest expert skill; it is well established in law that it is sufficient if he exercises the ordinary skill of an ordinary competent man exercising that particular art.

The term nurse practitioner can be substituted for man in the above definition. The recent growth of the evidence-based practice movement has not gone unnoticed by the legal profession and sheds new light on how the traditional Bolam test might be interpreted. The nurse practitioner will be on safer ground in justifying practice upon the basis of evidence which demonstrates clinical effectiveness rather than opinion as to what constitutes 'the ordinary skill'.

But what of nurses expanding their roles? Does the nurse practitioner taking on tasks that traditionally belong in the medical domain have to work to the same standard as the ordinary doctor? In *Wilsher* v. *Essex* (1986), it was determined that 'the inexperienced doctor needs to realise his own incompetence and seek supervision'. In the case of *Nettleship* v. *Weston* (1971), Lord Denning said that:

> The learner's incompetent best is not good enough. A junior doctor should have a minimum of competence necessary for the safety and proper treatment of the patient, regardless of his actual level of competence and experience.

Nurse practitioners taking on doctors' tasks need to remember that if doctors are used as the 'gold standard' by which to measure competence, the medical standard of care is the standard of a reasonably skilled and experienced doctor (Bolam test). This begs the question – reasonable by whose standards?

> In my view the law requires the trainee or learner to be judged by the same standard as his more experienced colleagues. If it did not, inexperience would frequently be urged as a defence to an action for professional negligence (Glidewell in the Court of Appeal Judgement, *Wilsher* v. *Essex AHA* 1986).

In other words, a nurse is likely to be judged by the professional standard of the post s/he is performing at that time, 'regardless of the innovative nature of the post', rather than by his or her own standards as a nurse (Dowling *et al.* 1996, p. 1212). This leads logically to the view that:

> If a nurse undertakes a task for which s/he knows s/he has insufficient training, this in itself may constitute negligence, even if she is acting on the orders of a doctor … if a nurse takes on the doctor's role s/he will be judged by the standards of the reasonable doctor (Kloss 1988, pp. 41–47).

To paraphrase Glidewell, the nurse practitioner, if called upon to perform a specialist skill, should as part of that skill seek the advice and help of someone more experienced. Glidewell was referring to junior doctors and said: 'If he does seek such help, he will often have satisfied that test, even though he may himself have made a mistake' (Kloss 1988, p. 43). Kloss adds that 'a nurse who accepts instruction from the doctor is not negligent unless the instructions are patently wrong, because it is usually reasonable to rely on someone more expert than oneself' (p. 43). However, the liability of a doctor does not necessarily exclude the liability of the nurse.

This complex issue may be summarized as follows:

- The best legal advice to nurse practitioners is that whenever you are practising in an expanded role which was once medical territory, you have to be as competent as a reasonable doctor
- All nurses are aware that it is no excuse to say: 'I only did what the doctor told me' when such instructions were obviously wrong, such as in a drug error. That principle also applies to nurse practitioners – such is the nature of accountable practice

Vicarious liability

Earlier in this section we saw that the person responsible for the commission of a tort is the person held to be liable. It is possible, however, that another person who has not personally committed the tort may be held to be liable in addition to the person who did commit it. This is referred to as the doctrine of vicarious liability. In such a situation there has to be a clearly recognized relationship between these two individuals such that in law it can be accepted that one person has responsibility for the other person who committed the tort in question. Relationships of relevance in vicarious liability are:

- Master and servant relationship
- Principal and independent contractor relationship
- Principal and agent relationship
- Parent and child relationship

A contract of service usually involves a close relationship between the parties whereby one can hire or fire the other and where he or she has greater control over the actions of the other person – is the master and servant relationship. In more modern language this translates as employer (e.g. NHS trust or GP) and employee (nurse practitioner). The master and servant relationship is is the one that most vicarious liability actions tend to involve. A legal maxim: *qui facit per alium facit per se* is applied; this translates into: 'he who does a thing through another does it himself'. The relationship that exists between master and servant is defined in the following rather arcane legal language:

- The master controls his servant
- The master chooses his servant
- The master and servant are a group
- The master profits from the servant's work for him

Translating these terms into a modern health-care setting shows that the employer fulfils the criteria for vicarious liability for the nurse practitioner. There is a let-out for the employer, however; he is not liable if the nurse practitioner was working for his or her own personal gain when the incident occurred. As long as the nurse practitioner was working for the employer and not for personal gain, the employer remains liable, however inappropriate the employee's actions may have been. Situations where the employer may be liable include:

- The employer authorizes the act
- The employer is negligent him/herself
- The work involves certain serious risks of damage
- The employer is under a statutory or strict liability

In summary, the employer is liable for the civil wrongs of the employee during the course of employment, providing those acts are not for personal gain. The UKCC *Code of Professional Conduct* (1992a) para 4 states that: 'In taking on new work registered nurses must acknowledge any limits in their competence and decline duties unless able to perform them in a safe and skilled manner'. In order to fulfil their accountability to the patient and to the UKCC, nurses must ensure they are really competent before expanding their roles. They have to be equally sure of their ground in declining new roles on the grounds of limitations in competence (Lunn 1994).

In certain circumstances, Kloss (1988, p. 43) points out that 'in fact it may constitute gross misconduct justifying dismissal for a nurse to refuse to obey a doctor's instructions'. Obvious examples include a patient resuscitation attempt or refusal to help a patient as a result of some personal view held by the nurse. No nurse can pick and choose which patients s/he will or will not care for. The principle of professional accountability means each nurse is personally accountable; nobody else will take the blame. All vicarious liability means is that lawyers for the plaintiff will always sue the employer as the employer can be held liable for the tort of negligence and higher damages can be recovered from the employer rather than an individual. Vicarious liability does not mean that doctors can cover nurses, although this notion is still evident, as in the following fairly typical quote from a practice nurse interviewed in a recent research study undertaken by the author (Reveley 1997).

> Well, you're always going to have the GP to back you, aren't you? You're never going to make a decision on your own. Someone's always going to have to check at some point, I always feel reassured when there's someone to back you and I guess it's the same for the nurse practitioner.

The problem is that it is not the same for the nurse practitioner. If you are practising in a true role with a high degree of autonomy, you cannot ask the GP to check every decision. The need expressed in this quote to have all decisions verified by another profession really calls into question in a fundamental way nurses' aspirations to full professional status.

Trespass

Trespass is a civil law concept and can apply to land, property or to the person. Trespass to the person has several aspects: assault is an attempt at, or threat of, unlawful force being applied to the person. Battery is the actual application of force to that person where physical contact occurs (Young 1994). Touching a patient without consent is battery and, unlike negligence, harm does not have to ensue for damages to be awarded. There is no trespass to the person however if there is no intention. Accidental contact is not battery (although it may be negligence!).

The major legal defence against the civil torts of assault and battery is consent (Young 1994), therefore the nurse practitioner must be careful to gain consent to care whenever possible. Consent can be obtained in different ways. The Medical Defence Union (1986) holds that for most physical contact between doctor and patient consent is implied by the voluntary actions of the patient and legally the nurse's position is similar (Young 1994). Consent can be oral or written; the oral method is used most by nurses. Where investigations or treatments carry a special risk, written consent should be obtained and this is the responsibility of the doctor. However, nowadays nurses are becoming involved in gaining written consent from patients and these special circumstances are beyond the scope of this chapter. The nurse practitioner involved in gaining written consent from patients should act in accordance with local policy and at all times be aware of the limits to his or her competence.

A person can give a legally valid consent if s/he has the capacity to understand and come to a decision on what is involved and to communicate that decision (Skegg 1984). Informed consent is: 'The process whereby explicit communication of information is provided and included. In this are not only details of the treatment to be carried out but also of the risks involved' (Young 1994, p. 13). A difficult area concerns how much information constitutes sufficient for consent to be informed. The view in the UK is that the doctor decides how much is sufficient, which means that the doctor is not obliged to discuss every possible complication, however remote the possibility. Not all patients wish for detailed information and the nurse practitioner must respect this, but it must be remembered that legal action may follow if the patient feels s/he was given incomplete information and harm ensued as a result. This is where a note communicating what the patient was informed of should be put on the patient's records as this will be crucial in any subsequent legal action.

Consent to touching by one person or profession does not act as consent to touching by any other person or profession (Dowling et al. 1996). Without explaining to the patient that she is a nurse, the nurse practitioner may invalidate the patient's consent if the patient assumes by the nature of the task and the way the nurse practitioner 'held herself out' that she is a doctor.

In determining standard of care, the court will take account of a range of things, including the task and the way in which the nurse 'holds herself out'– her dress, language, name badge, and so on. According to Dowling et al. (1996, p. 1212), if a task is usually performed by a doctor and the patient expects it to be performed by a doctor, the nurse practitioner must explain her status to the patient. In these circumstances, it is possible that the patient may not consent to the task being performed by a nurse. In her early pioneering days Stilwell approached the Medical Defence Union for insurance cover and, after much negotiation, a 10-point agreement was reached to safeguard patients. One of the points stated that: 'it is essential, both ethically and for the credibility of the project, that the patients realise that they are consulting a nurse, not a doctor, and

there will be considerable emphasis on conveying this information' (Stilwell 1988, p. 86).

If the patient gives consent to a procedure and the nurse practitioner's title and role are carefully explained, there is no civil case to answer for assault, battery or trespass upon the person.

Criminal proceedings would only be likely in extreme cases, for example, where a patient died as a result of gross negligence, when a charge of manslaughter might be brought. For a criminal charge of assault leading to actual or grievous bodily harm, the prosecution has to prove intent to inflict harm on the part of the assailant. This explains why doctors or nurses are rarely prosecuted under this section of the criminal law as, however incompetent they may have been, to prove that harm was intentional is extremely unlikely. One final point about the criminal law is that if the victim consents to having violence inflicted upon him or her, this does not constitute a defence for the accused.

Record-keeping

The UKCC document *Standards for Records and Record Keeping* (1998) states that record-keeping is an integral and essential part of care and not a distraction from its provision. The Patient's Charter (Department of Health 1991) allows for the right of patients and relatives to have their complaints investigated promptly. The first line of complaint is to the health-provider organization; then the ombudsman (Health Service Commissioner) becomes responsible for investigating patient complaints that have not been satisfied by the appropriate health authority. There are approximately 1000 such cases each year, of which 70% are related to problems of communication; often this is an omission in the records (NHS Training Directorate 1996). Poor record-keeping featured prominently in the ombudsman's annual report for 1996–97 (Stokes 1997). Legal action can be taken up to 3 years after an alleged incident, which means that unless the nurse practitioner has kept good records, s/he is unlikely to have any recollection of a patient subsequently bringing a complaint.

Good record-keeping promotes good-quality patient care, safeguards the nurse in case of legal or disciplinary action and empowers nurses to practise to the highest standard of care. In the event of a patient complaint about the care given by a nurse practitioner, the complaint could be heard in a number of places: a local disciplinary hearing, a UKCC hearing, a Health Service Commissioner's enquiry or a court of law (NHS Training Directorate 1996). The nurse practitioner should ask him- or herself whether his or her records would stand up in a court of law or disciplinary hearing, and whether another health professional could use the notes to provide continuity of care.

One of the most common cases that coroners oversee is the person who dies in the A&E department or soon after leaving it. In such an instance an important part of the inquest is the nurse's initial observation record and triage decisions (NHS Training Directorate 1996). It is clear from this that accurate documentation is vital. Records should be written legibly and should include the date and time and a full signature (not initials). Abbreviations should not be used unless they are approved and unambiguous. An entry, once made, should not be altered, nor should an addition be disguised and clinical notes should be made at the time of treatment or as soon as possible afterwards (Norwell 1997). A good record should be understandable, accurate, confidential, legible, concise, objective, unambiguous, contemporaneous, consistent, complete and up-to-date (NHS Training Directorate 1996).

Confidentiality

Confidentiality is an important consideration in record-keeping, as in any other area of professional practice. The *Code of Professional Conduct* (UKCC 1992a) states that the nurse must:

> Protect all confidential information concerning patients and clients obtained in the course of professional practice and make disclosure only with consent, where required by the order of a court or where you can justify disclosure in the wider public interest.

In Scotland, a breach of confidence comes under the law of torts; therefore a person who breaches a confidential relationship can be sued if a breach of that confidence results in injury. However, in England, Wales and Northern Ireland the only route a patient can take is to sue for defamation (Young 1994, p. 114).

Oral and some written information remains fairly free of legal control but written records about patients or clients are subject to controls. The law provides some rights of access to information and also makes sure that only those people entitled to it have access to such information. Relevant statutes are the Access to Health Records Act 1990, the Access to Personal Files Act 1987 relating to Social Services files, and the Access to Medical Reports Act 1988.

The Data Protection Act 1984 covers automatically processed data. An employee is personally liable under the Act for damage caused by inadequate security of personal data (Young 1994, p. 115). A person whose records are held on computer can apply to see her or his records. If it is believed that the data is erroneous, the patient can ask for these to be amended and if the patient has suffered damage or distress from this erroneous data then s/he is entitled to compensation (McHale *et al.* 1998). If a patient is incapable due to mental disorder or incapacity, a request can be made on his or her behalf. Children can request to see their records if they are deemed to be mature enough to do so but parents do not have a right to see their child's records.

Schedule One of the Data Protection Act requires personal data to be:

- Obtained fairly and lawfully
- Held only for one or more lawful purposes specified in the data user's registry entry (a requirement of the Act is registration by applying to an independent Data Protection Registrar)
- Used or disclosed only in accordance with the data user's register entry
- Adequate, relevant and not excessive for these purposes
- Accurate and where necessary up-to-date
- Not kept longer than is necessary for the specified purpose
- Made available to data subjects on request
- Properly protected against loss or disclosure

The doctor may refuse to divulge any or all personal health data if requested by a patient on the grounds that it may be possibly harmful to the patient's physical or mental health (McHale *et al.* 1998). Under the Access to Health Records Act 1990, similar restrictions apply to written records. Another limitation on access to records is that there is a fee payable.

Keeping up-to-date

The law expects that professionals keep up-to-date with current practice. This does not mean that if a nurse practitioner fails to read one article or use equipment that is newly invented and not widely available s/he will be held to be negligent. But it does mean that where new information is widely available the nurse practitioner should read it and act on it. Department of Health and health authority circulars are examples of this (Young 1994), together with evidence-based practice publications such as *Effective Health Care Bulletins*. There is a responsibility by employers with regard to this also, particularly in relation to health and safety, such as moving and handling techniques. The nurse practitioner therefore has a legal and professional duty to update his or her knowledge: ignorance is no defence in law. A lack of knowledge or experience is not an excuse for incompetent care (Tingle 1988).

Delegating to others

A more senior nurse or manager can be negligent in delegation. This leaves him or her liable in any law suit and also accountable to the UKCC (if a nurse) for malpractice. Before delegating any tasks, a nurse practitioner therefore should satisfy him- or herself on the following:

- The extent of the nurse's knowledge
- How skilful the nurse is at the delegated task – a verbal check may be sufficient
- Supervision of the nurse while s/he carries out the delegated function. This should take place over time and follow teaching of knowledge and skill as appropriate to compensate for any deficiencies. This is important in the case of an unregistered nurse – supervision should be on-going (Young 1994, p. 58).

In nursing there is a hierarchy of authority which may be reinforced in job descriptions and grading criteria. Thus, a postholder may be expected to supervise junior staff and teach qualified or un-qualified staff, a Project 2000 student is responsible for giving good-quality care, but it is the registered nurse who is accountable to the UKCC (Young 1994).

The General Medical Council's guidance *Good Medical Practice* (1995) permits the delegation of medical care to nurses if they are certain the nurse is competent to undertake the work. However, the doctor remains responsible for managing the patient's care. When accepting a task the nurse must be sure s/he is competent to perform it. Negligent delegation and negligent acceptance of a task are both liable for any resultant harm to the patient (Kloss 1988).

Summary

This chapter has outlined the legal and professional position of the emerging nurse practitioner role. As a result of the newness of the role, we have had to extrapolate from existing principles to offer a discussion of the likely situation. It is in the nature of the civil law that precedents have to be set before principles become firmly laid down in law, therefore important changes to the guidance offered in this chapter may occur in the future. The fundamentals for safe practice remain those of personal account-ability, the basic tests surrounding the tort of negligence, and the advice that if you cannot do something as well as a reasonable doctor, you should not be doing it at all. Above all, keep the patient informed of who you are and what you are about to do. Good communication will eliminate many potential problems.

References

Abbott A. (1988) *The System of Professions: An Essay on the Division of Expert Labour,* Chicago, University of Chicago Press.

Ashburner L., Birch K., Latimer J., Scrivens E. (1997) *Nurse Practitioners in Primary Care: The Extent of Practice and Research,* Keele University, Centre for Health Planning and Management.

Department of Health (1991) *The Patient's Charter,* London, Stationery Office.

Department of Health (1996) *Primary Care: Delivering the Future,* London, Stationery Office.

Department of Health and Social Security (1986) *Neighbour-hood Nursing – A Focus for Care: Report of the Community Nursing Review* (Cumberlege Report), London, HMSO.

Dimond B. (1994) *Legal Aspects of Nursing,* London, Prentice Hall.

Donaghue v. *Stevenson* (1932) AC562. Cited in: Dimond B. (1990) Legal Aspects of Nursing, Hemel Hempstead, Prentice-Hall.

Dowling S., Martin R., Skidmore P., Doyal L., Cameron A., Lloyd S. (1996) Nurses taking on junior doctors' work: a confusion of accountability, *British Medical Journal,* **312**, pp. 1211–1214.

Elston, M. (1977) Medical autonomy: challenge and response. In: Barnard K., Lee, K. (eds.) *Conflicts in the NHS,* London, Croom Helm, p. 27.

General Medical Council (1995) *Good Medical Practice,* London, GMC. Cited in: Kloss D. (1988) Demarcation in medical practice: the extended role of the nurse, *Professional Negligence,* March/April.

Jones M., Gough P. (1997) Nurse prescribing – why has it taken so long? *Nursing Standard,* **11**(20), pp. 39–42.

Kassirer J.P. (1994) What role for nurse practitioners in primary care?, *New England Journal of Medicine,* **330**.

Kendrick K. (1995) Codes of professional conduct and the dilemmas of professional practice. In: Soothill K. Mackay L., Webb C. (eds.) *Interprofessional Relations in Health Care,* London, Edward Arnold.

Lunn J. (1994) The scope of professional practice from a legal perspective, *British Journal of Nursing,* **3**(15), pp. 770–772.

McHale J., Tingle J., Peysner J. (1988) *Law and Nursing,* Oxford, Butterworth-Heinemann.

Medical Defence Union (1986) *Consent to Treatment,* London, Medical Defence Union.

National Health Service Training Directorate (1996) *Keeping the Record Straight: A Guide to Record Keeping for Nurses, Midwives and Health Visitors.*

Nettleship v. *Weston* (1971) 2QB 691. Cited in: Dawling S., Martin R., Skidmore P., Doyal L., Cameron A., Lloyd S. (1996) Nurses taking on junior doctors' work: a confusion of accountability, *British Medical Journal,* May, pp. 1211–1214.

Norwell N. (1997) The ten commandments of record keeping *Journal of the Medical Defence Union,* **13**(1), pp. 8–9.

Pashley G., Henry C. (1990) Carving out the nursing nineties. *Nursing Times,* **86**, pp. 45–46.

Porter S. (1991) The poverty of professionalisation: a critical analysis of strategies for the occupational advancement of nursing, *Journal of Advanced Nursing,* **17**, pp. 720–726.

Ralph C. (1991) The Role of the Regulatory Body. In: Savage J. (ed.) *Nurse Practitioners: Working for Change in Primary Health Care Nursing,* London, King's Fund Centre.

Reveley S. (1997) *Introducing a Nurse Practitioner into General Medical Practice; The Maryport Experience.* A Report for North Cumbria Health Authority in association with Celeste College, Carlisle, St Martin's College.

Skegg P.D.G. (1984) *Law, Ethics and Medicine*, Oxford, Clarendon Press.

Stilwell B. (1988) Patient attitudes to a highly developed role – the nurse practitioner, *Recent Advances in Nursing*, **12**, pp. 82–100.

Stokes B. (1997) Setting the record straight, *Nursing Standard*, **11**, pp. 14.

Tingle J.H. (1988) Negligence and Wilsher, *Solicitor's Journal*, **132**(25), pp. 910–911. Cited in: Young A.P. (1994) *Law and Professional Conduct in Nursing*, London, Scutari Press.

United Kingdom Central Council (1992a) *The Code of Professional Conduct for Nurses, Midwives and Health Visitors*, London, United Kingdom Central Council for Nurses, Midwives and Health Visitors.

United Kingdom Central Council (1992b) *The Scope of Professional Practice*, London, United Kingdom Central Council for Nurses, Midwives and Health Visitors.

United Kingdom Central Council (1996) *Guidelines for Professional Practice*, London, United Kingdom Central Council.

United Kingdom Central Council (1993) *Standards for Records and Record Keeping*, London, United Kingdom Central Council for Nurses, Midwives and Health Visitors.

Vaughan B. (1989) Autonomy and accountability, *Nursing Times*, **85**(3), pp. 54–55.

Welsh National Board for Nursing, Midwifery and Health Visiting (1990) The Extended Role of the Nurse, Cardiff, WNB.

West B.J.M. (1995) *Health Service Developments and the Scope of Professional Nursing Practice: A Review of the Pertinent Literature*, Edinburgh, National Nursing Midwifery and Health Visiting Advisory Committee.

Wilsher v. *Essex Health Authority* (1986) 3AII ER 80. Cited in: Dimond B (1990) *et seq.*

Witz A., (1994) The challenge of nursing. In: Gabe J. Kelleher, D. Williams G. (eds.) *Challenging Medicine*, London, Routledge.

Young, A.P. (1994) *Law and Professional Conduct in Nursing*, London, Scutari Press.

CHAPTER 21

Working with others: the nurse practitioner and role boundaries in primary health care

Shirley Reveley

Although this chapter is about research in primary health care, the lessons are equally applicable to a hospital environment. Introducing a nurse practitioner into a general practice or hospital department alters the pattern of consultations; it adds another element that otherwise would not be there. The usual pattern of doctor–patient and doctor–nurse interaction is disturbed as power relations and role boundaries shift. Discussions about role boundaries are a consistent feature in the debates about nurse practitioners who are rapidly being introduced into a variety of health-care teams with seemingly little research being undertaken into the effects on established role boundaries within teams. Kaufman (1996) and Stilwell (1989) reported team disruption as a factor in their own experiences of working as nurse practitioners in primary care. It is therefore important to discover the impact on other staff members of introducing the nurse practitioner. This issue will be discussed in the context of research investigating the introduction of a nurse practitioner with a predominantly triage function in one group general practice. Particular attention will be paid to the perceptions of doctors, nurses and patients concerning the work of the nurse practitioner in relation to the work of other staff. Data collected over a period of $2^{1}/_{2}$ years forms the basis of the chapter and the lessons learnt should be considered when introducing a new nurse practitioner role in either a primary health or hospital setting.

Background to the research

In November 1993 a health authority in the north of England funded a 2-year pilot project for a nurse practitioner post within a group general practice. The practice was looking at new ways to deliver health care, and it was expected that the nurse practitioner would carry out a triage role which involved seeing patients with undifferentiated diagnoses and making decisions about their management and treatment. She would work within protocols for acute presentations and also manage the care of a range of patients with chronic illness. It was suggested that the introduction of a nurse practitioner would mark a significant shift from the current conventional GP-run service, and would improve waiting times and access, as well as releasing GP time to treat those attenders in need of pure medical expertise.

The practice is the only one in a small town which, with surrounding villages, has a total population of 15 000. The nearest general hospital with a 24-hour A&E service is 18 miles away, requiring two bus journeys for those without a car. The local population is declining in numbers and suffers from severe deprivation linked to geographical isolation and a high unemployment rate which is several times the national average. Demands on the practice are increasing and there is a high consultation rate which is linked to the high incidence of disease, socio-economic factors and an associated dependency culture. Analysis of practice activity between 1987 and 1992 revealed that in addition to those patients with appointments, an average of 35 extra patients are seen daily. In the winter months this figure can rise to 50. There are eight doctors in the practice, three practice nurses, 15 clerical/reception staff, five attached district nurses, two attached health visitors and two midwives serving a practice population of 14 376 patients.

Research questions to be answered

The introduction of yet another role within the practice, that of the nurse practitioner, brings another set of skills which must be integrated into the practice team. But how could this be done? How would existing staff react to another nurse trained to practise at a new and advanced level? How would patients view this new role? In order to answer these questions an evaluative study was designed with the following aims:

- To evaluate the effectiveness of the nurse practitioner triage role in this general practice
- To explore the perceptions of staff in the primary health care team and patients concerning the role of the nurse practitioner
- To investigate the extent to which the introduction of the nurse practitioner role affects traditional role boundaries
- To identify the professional activities undertaken by the nurse practitioner

Data were collected at several stages, beginning with semistructured interviews with doctors, practice nurses and attached community nurses, midwives and health visitors (22 respondents). These interviews were undertaken during the first 6 months of the pilot project to elicit, among other things, how respondents perceived the nurse practitioner role would be viewed by patients, and how their own particular role might be affected. During the first year of the study perceptions of patients (or their carers) about the effectiveness of the nurse practitioner were also sought, using a semistructured questionnaire which yielded both quantitative and qualitative data. This was followed by unstructured interviews with a volunteer sample of patients from those who completed the questionnnaire.

In the second year a comparison of the work of the nurse practitioner with that of GPs in the practice was undertaken over a 5-day period. Twenty surgeries were studied, 10 held by the nurse practitioner and 10 by the GPs. A range of activity data was collected using a proforma sheet designed for the purpose. During the 5-day period a sample of 60 patients was interviewed immediately following their consultation; 30 were consulting the nurse practitioner and 30 the GPs. The interviews utilized a semistructured interview schedule designed to elicit their perceptions of the consultation. The schedule included questions on what the patients perceived the role of the nurse practitioner to be.

The perceptions of doctors and nurses concerning changes in service provision, effects on roles and working practices resulting from the introduction of the nurse practitioner role were elicited in the second year of the project by use of unstructured interviews. In all, 189 patient questionnaires, 90 patient interviews and 42 interviews with doctors and nurses were undertaken.

Results of the study

Role boundaries and the perceptions of nurses

At the beginning of the study the nurses perceived little impact on their role. However, they were largely of the opinion that it was too early to predict how their roles might be affected as the nurse practitioner had been in post for less than 6 months when most of the interviews took place. The practice nurses were the group of nurses whose role would be most likely to be affected. However, they did not seem to think there was much overlap, mainly because these nurses felt there was a well-defined division of labour operating among the practice nurse team which at this early stage had not been destabilized by the introduction of the nurse practitioner.

The three practice nurses each had their own separate sphere of activity but helped each other out during busy times and holiday periods; one nurse dealt mostly with treatment room work; one, who had a district nursing qualification, undertook screening of the elderly population as well as running certain clinics for chronic disease management; and a third was mainly employed to undertake health promotion work. The nurse practitioner was perceived to be a triage nurse, and this was viewed as yet another sphere of activity which was more aligned to the work of the GPs, and more to do with acute or urgent work rather than overlapping with the practice nurses' area of work. The organization of nursing work within the practice was explained by a practice nurse:

> There is no effect on the practice nurses' role because clinics are well-used and well-established. These clinics are practice nurse-led with a GP in attendance. Practice nurses in this practice are using different skills, e.g. health promotion, elderly screening. Nurses have individual skills between them; they ask each other.

The GPs were also of the opinion that the nurse practitioner's role did not impinge on the work of the practice nurses; moreover, they didn't seem to think it should. For example:

> It's more what the partners do rather than the practice nurse's role. Practice nurses have a traditional role; they work to protocols in specific roles to do with chronic disease management so they are extending their role. They don't extend beyond limited things whereas the

nurse practitioner is examining hearts and chests which practice nurses don't (GP).

This statement echoes that of the practice nurses and highlights a division of labour arising from areas of competence, which can be said to erect demarcation boundaries for the various activities of doctors and nurses. However, the role of the practice nurse has changed a great deal over recent years and will continue to do so. The outline of the general practice nurse's role set out in the UK Central Council's (UKCC) *Standards for Post Registration Education and Practice (PREP)* document (1994) includes being able to:

> Assess, diagnose, and treat specific diseases in accordance with agreed medical/nursing protocols: provide direct access to specialist nursing care for undifferentiated patients within the practice population and to undertake diagnostic health screening, health surveillance and therapeutic techniques applied to individuals and groups within the practice population.

It can be seen that this role specification corresponds closely to that described by the Department of Health and Social Security (1986) and Pearson *et al.* (1995) maintain that: 'many of these aspects of practice fit within current ideas about the role of nurse practitioners' (p. 157).

In these first interviews health visitors and midwives were inclined to see the effect on their roles in terms of referrals they may get from the nurse practitioner, or the other way round, as referrals from themselves to the nurse practitioner. Not much of this activity was in evidence, however, which was thought to be due to the newness of the nurse practitioner role. Health visitors were happy to accept that the nurse practitioner would be able to diagnose and treat minor ailments like rashes and respiratory infections in children but they would prefer her to refer to them those problems of childhood that health visitors traditionally regard as their 'turf' such as feeding problems, sleep problems and potty training. Midwives were of the opinion that, as the nurse practitioner was not a midwife, all pregnant women consulting the nurse practitioner should be referred to the midwifery service.

When first interviewed the district nurses were also waiting to see what would develop, and there were few referrals in either direction at these first interviews. One district nurse thought that home visits by the nurse practitioner might be a possibility, and didn't see this as a problem as there was overlap between team members anyway:

> There's no effect on my role at the moment. She might refer someone to us – say a leg ulcer. She might do home visits to check drugs if we're not going in. I think there's overlap between primary health care team members.

The topic of home visits was also raised by a GP at the first interview in the context of clinical freedom of the nurse practitioner:

> There's no reason why she shouldn't do home visits – most home visits are a waste of time.

All the community nurses, midwives and health visitors had met the nurse practitioner and talked briefly to her about her role during her period of orientation to the community and practice. Relations had been helped by the fact that she was 'such a nice person'.

At the end of the study there had been little or no change concerning perceptions of role boundaries. The nurse practitioner and practice nurse roles rarely overlapped and there was no discernible impact on the practice nurses' workload as a result of having the nurse practitioner running surgeries. There was an impact however on the perceptions some of the GPs had of other nursing roles. At the second interviews one practice nurse explained that her role had changed to take on some triage work. However, this practice nurse was undertaking the BSc (Hons) Nurse Practitioner course incorporating the Royal College of Nursing Nurse Practitioner Diploma. The other practice nurses believed that they would also be expected to undertake some triage work:

> The doctors are wanting all the nurses to take on a triage role. We are asking, is it a nursing role or a practitioner role? One doctor is very keen on the nurses taking on a triage role but wants to do it on a simpler basis – taking blood pressures rather than diagnosis. There's no way practice nurses could listen to chests. We have no training. Practice nurses would take the pulse, take the history, take the temperature and the peak flow then refer them on to the doctor. There are different levels of triage, the nurse practitioner examines patients and makes a diagnosis (practice nurse).

Two years on, and with two new health visitors in post, there was no noticeable role overlap and extremely few referrals from health visitor to nurse practitioner and vice versa. However, there was change in the increased involvement of health visitors at the practice. At the doctors' request, the health visitors were operating an open-access clinic for families for 1 hour each afternoon Monday to Friday. This clinic, which deals mainly with common complaints in the under 5s, receives patients with undiagnosed undifferentiated conditions and the health visitors assess and manage them themselves, or refer them to the doctor on duty. The conditions most commonly dealt with are chest infections, otitis media, nappy rash, gastroenteritis, feeding problems and other minor ailments. Thus the health visitors are undertaking a triage role similar to that of the nurse practitioner. The two health visitors felt they needed extra training for this role as basic clinical examinations and diagnostic skills were not covered in their training. GPs also felt the health visitors needed extra training such as in the area of ear, nose and throat conditions. A GP is available during these clinics but the health visitors felt that the nurse practitioner would be an equally appropriate person to refer on to for some of the more straightforward ailments children present with. This seems to accord with the perceptions of the practice nurse who said there are 'different levels of triage'.

In the second round of interviews with district nurses, they reported that the doctors had suggested that district nurses could do home visits to assess patients and see if there was a need for the doctor to go. One doctor had started to refer patients for the district nurse to see:

> like hypertensions and also to check on patients after a hospital admission. The doctors tend to be using all the nurses in this respect whereas I thought it would be more of the nurse practitioner's role (district nurse).

Other district nurses stated

> I think the doctors would like all the district nurses and all the nurses to be nurse practitioners. What she is doing in the surgery the GPs would like doing in the community as well. I think if we'd gone on the course that would be fine. I don't think we're trained sufficiently to do what nurse practitioners do.

and:

> The GPs are quite keen about her role and what she's able to do. I think they'd actually like to see more nurses doing more.

One of the GPs explained this encouragement of nurses to expand their roles in this way:

> I don't know how much of it is a reflection of what's going on in the outside world as what's happening internally. It [the NP role] has certainly shown the partners that nurses can take on an increased role in assessment of patients, and the practice is now moving forward in getting the other nurses to triage patients potentially at particular times (GP).

All the district nurses agreed that their own role had not been affected by referrals form the nurse practitioner and there was no duplication or overlap of work. However, there was a feeling that the nurse practitioner was moving nursing forward:

> I think it's the way that nursing is going. There's a lot of nurse practitioner jobs advertised. I think we're very capable to work as junior doctors; I think it's your nursing background that gives you such a good background to do that job (district nurse).

The survey of nurse practitioner pilot projects undertaken by Touche Ross (1994) demonstrated that one of the key factors influencing effective and early implementation of the nurse practitioner role included a clearly defined scope of operation. From the interviews it seems that, in this case study practice, the role of the nurse practitioner is clearly defined in its scope of operation. Moreover it does not appear to increase the work of other nurses to any noticeable extent; the only work that had passed to other members of the nursing team from the nurse practitioner were a few patients to the practice nurses, two to the health visitors and two to the midwives. The reason why there were so few referrals at the outset of the pilot study was possibly because the role was so new and all staff were feeling their way slowly, the nurse practitioner may not have felt able to refer to her nursing colleagues until they had accepted her into the practice. However, the situation had not changed by the end of the pilot study and well into the first year of the nurse practitioners' post as a qualified professional. The reason is likely to be that the nurse practitioner is seeing many patients with minor self-limiting conditions that do not require follow-up. Those patients who require further investigation, treatment or follow-up are transferred to the GPs, and therefore referrals for district nursing services are more likely to come from the doctors.

There was slightly more feeling that the nurse practitioner may relieve the work of other nurses rather than increasing it, and this was more evident in the surgery staff than the community staff. As one practice nurse explained:

> Practice nurses are not seeing as many patients in a day since the nurse practitioner came. I think in some respects it will cut down on the practice nurse's work because, whereas when doctors see patients they automatically send them to the practice nurse but the nurse practitioner might deal with them herself.

This was echoed by a GP:

> In some ways it may relieve them [practice nurses] somewhat in that the nurse practitioner is having more time with patients and is able to carry out some nursing functions doctors would push the practice nurse's way.'

These predictions turned out to be correct. The nurse practitioner does undertake her own clinical procedures, with the exception of administering injections. The traditional nursing skills of the nurse practitioner are being used as well as the newly acquired skills of physical assessment and diagnosis. Where she is losing skills, however, is in the area of chronic disease management which is no longer a part of her particular role, though of course many nurse practitioners undertake chronic disease management.

The Touche Ross study (1994) and several others (see, for example, Bowling and Stilwell 1988) demonstrated that patients valued the styles of nurse practitioners, in particular the more wide-ranging focus on well-being as well as illness. But what about the effects of the nurse practitioner role on that of

GPs? It is to this question that the discussion now turns.

Role boundaries and the perceptions of GPs

In the early days of the pilot study, the GPs' workload was not affected and in fact may even have increased with the need to supervise the nurse practitioner's work. This was remarked upon by several people:

> It's not reduced the GPs' workload because the nurse practitioner has to keep disturbing the GPs, so their lists are cut to accommodate that. The doctor is seeing less patients but the others have to see more. I think that is temporary; when she finds her feet and doesn't have to consult as regularly (practice nurse).

Interestingly, the GPs who were most closely involved in supervising the nurse practitioner acknowledged the extra pressure on them but didn't seem to mind this too much. For example, one GP stated:

> It's a bit of a hassle sometimes, supervising, but I think it's far outweighed by the interest of teaching and the help. There are occasions when you don't want to be bothered, but it's the same in any job.

There was the perception that there was a blurring of roles between doctor and nurse, which was well expressed by a GP:

> There's a blurring of roles of doctors and nurses as specialist skills increase. Properly so. There are no major disadvantages but we all have to be certain that the nurse practitioner does acquire skills that a GP has. There are no more objections from patients seeing the nurse practitioner than we would get from a new partner; less actually, which is interesting. It's more what the partners do rather than the practice nurse's role (GP).

There are several issues implicit in this one statement: blurring of roles; increase in specialist skills; no disadvantages; nurses acquiring doctors' skills. During the interview this doctor appeared comfortable with his own role, and did not give any hint, either by demeanour or verbally, that nurses acquiring doctors' skills would prove a threat to medicine. On the contrary, this doctor seemed to favour it, providing the correct training was given. Again there was the notion that there was a clear distinction between the role of the nurse practitioner and the practice nurses.

This GP, it seems, was not at all threatened by the spectre of a nurse practitioner taking over the GP role, going on to say:

> I would be entirely happy that nurse practitioners come to have as much clinical freedom as a GP. It's true of all of us that that we've got to know our limitations and when to give up and seek advice, so I'm sure nurse

practitioners could take on the role of part of the work the GP does (GP).

The nurses interviewed were not as clear as the doctors about where the role of the nurse ended and that of the doctor began. Some saw it as a continuum: 'It's a sort of halfway point really; more than a nurse, but not a doctor; a specialist nurse' (midwife). A district nurse thought that: 'The nurse practitioner role is a bit of nursing and a bit of medical. More aligned to GPs; no hands-on nursing'.

The views of these doctors and nurses reflect several aspects of the nurse practitioner's role, such as the skills of diagnosing, clinical skills, examining, health promotion, extra knowledge, observation, referral, responsibility, accountability, identifying signs and symptoms, listening, counselling, competence. Whilst some respondents seemed to think that these skills could be achieved through education and training, others thought of them more in terms of the individual nurse practitioner's aptitude for the job, mental attitude and previous experience. Not surprisingly, there was much emphasis on those skills traditionally perceived as being in the medical domain, and how the acquisition of those skills marks the difference between nurse practitioners and other nurses. The following quotes illustrate the point:

> The nurse practitioner has extra training in diagnosis (practice nurse)

> Examination skills, referral skills, knowledge of how society can affect health. We just identify need, we can't diagnose (health visitor).

The following lengthy quote sums up the views of one of the GPs.

> There are certain areas where one has to recognise that a nurse practitioner is better qualified to make decisions than a doctor, such as family planning and cervical cytology. Ninety-eight per cent of interactions with a GP here are non-life-threatening so it doesn't really matter too much. I would certainly want to examine myself someone with chest pain or breathing difficulties, someone with pyrexia of unknown origin, or someone who looks very ill. The age of the patient is less important than the condition. Chronic attenders might be better seen by the nurse practitioner because of more time, more counselling, and altering their expectations. Family planning – but only if she's specially trained in that, or conditions where the patient does not expect a prescription but advice. The nurse practitioner is better equipped than the practice nurse because she sees a wider range of conditions (GP).

Several GPs saw no limit to the amount of clinical freedom the nurse practitioner should have, whilst others did restrict the role, pointing out that there had to be limits which would be negotiated as roles evolved. Trust between nurse and doctor was seen as an important aspect of such an evolutionary process, with the key question in the doctor's mind being whether the nurse can recognize those problems which she can manage and those which need referral to the GP.

Though all the doctors and nurses felt the nurse practitioner was practising a nursing role, there was a view that the role had developed from triage to something more:

> I think she's a different being, she really is. I mean, she may not like it but she is becoming very much more a medical role. That's because of her experience. She is probably taking on far more responsibility than other nurses opposite her – it's experience (GP).

There was also a raising of awareness among nurses in the practice that they could take on more in relation to patient care. The nurse practitioner was of the view that several nurses responded to her post by realizing that their role does not stop if they have decided a patient should be seen by the doctor. They can become involved in taking a history and carrying out an exam, leading to a possible conclusion concerning what is wrong with the patient and discussing this with the doctor as they present the patient. The nurses realized that their practice can move on from merely deciding that patient X needs to see the doctor, then 'switching off', before attending to patient Y.

A study of role boundaries in health-care teams would not be complete without eliciting the views of consumers of the service and, as stated in the introduction, this was undertaken by means of questionnaire and interviews. The data presented here are derived from interviews undertaken with a volunteer sample of 30 patients who had completed the questionnaire and agreed to be interviewed in their own homes about their experience of their consultation with the nurse practitioner. During the course of the interviews respondents were asked to explain how they saw the work of the nurse practitioner in relation to the work of other nurses and GPs.

Patients' comparisons of the role of the nurse practitioner with that of other nurses

Patients saw definite differences between the roles of nurse practitioners and practice nurses, and were more inclined to compare the nurse practitioner role to that of the GP. By and large, the GP was the yardstick by which the nurse practitioner was judged, not nurses. All respondents perceived practice nurses to be there for 'technical' procedures. They felt practice nurses had less time than nurse practitioners. 'You are in and out' was a frequent comment. This was seen to be the way things are and to be accepted. Respondents were asked whether they saw the nurse practitioner as having different skills to other nurses

and there was a clear perception of differences between the nurse practitioner and practice nurses. For example, one woman explained the difference as:

> You see the other nurses for stitches and things, whereas the nurse practitioner to me was just like a doctor you know, so that's the differences sort of thing.

Another woman agreed with this, saying:

> Practice nurses are there for routine tasks. Nurse practitioners are there for individual problems. I've been with the little one for his injections. That's their job, not to talk and find out. With the nurses you don't actually go with a problem, it's just sort of general health checks and blood test where the nurse practitioner's there for individual problems. If you want stitches out you'd go to the nurse where the nurse practitioner is there to give you medicine if you need it. Just double check what the doctor's to sign for.

Another woman thought the nurse practitioner practised a more specialized role:

> I was aware of the difference because she was more knowledgeable, she knew what she was doing. I thought it was something like that carrying on from where the general nurse leaves off.

There was a general feeling across these interviews that practice nurses were busy, had less time to spend with patients than the nurse practitioner and were task oriented. It was the practice nurse's job to take bloods, give injections, remove stitches and do general health checks. There was no perception of the roles of the nurse practitioner and the practice nurse overlapping, and, interestingly, other nurses were not mentioned except for the health visitor.

Patients' comparisons of the role of the nurse practitioner with that of the GP

Where patients saw considerable role overlap was with the GPs. Sometimes there was ambiguity about the nurse practitioner's role in relation to GPs and in general she was seen to be 'like a doctor but not a doctor'. A few people thought she was less well-qualified than a doctor, some thought she was a locum or a trainee, but after consulting her, most respondents realized she was a nurse. Most people were loyal to the GP they saw regularly but it was remarked upon that patients could see a different GP each time they went to the surgery. In general, the vast majority of respondents would consult the nurse practitioner with any illness/condition, though one woman said that she would not go with anything 'death-defying'. The following views are typical:

> There's no difference between the nurse practitioner and the doctor because the nurse practitioner done exactly the same as the GP when I visited previously with the same complaint.

No different than seeing a doctor. An extra person that's the same as a doctor. Like an apprentice, just the same as the others.

I thought she was sort of, you know, in between a nurse and a doctor which, you know, it probably is that sort of thing. She seems to know everything and the only difference is she got the prescription signed by the doctor. She's more a family person, more on a nursing level.

I thought it was someone who took over instead of a doctor. I knew she was a nurse with it being nurse practitioner, it was obvious it was a nurse. Signing the prescription is the only difference between the GP and the nurse practitioner. She's just like an extra doctor.

I just felt as if I'd been treated by a doctor. It didn't bother me that she wasn't a real doctor. She's more than a nurse I think, more like a doctor. She just filled forms out like a doctor and I don't think nurses can give treatment out like doctors do and she did. But it's just how it came across. Why should there be a nurse practitioner and not another doctor?

I'll be honest with you, I didn't think she was a nurse. I thought she was a doctor. She was very knowledgable for a nurse, but I don't see the nurses either so I don't know how much knowledge they have. But I felt at the time I was talking to a doctor. She definitely had plenty of knowledge of the ailment.

There are certain structures and processes operating that provide clues for patients but may also be confusing for them, in that the nurse practitioner role is a departure from the traditional image of a nurse. Such clues include a room of her own, which differentiates her from the practice nurse, a desk rather than a trolley or couch in the treatment room, and also the nature of consultation. For example, the way 'she asks questions' and 'she looks a bit like a doctor'. The manner in which other practice staff referred to or behaved towards the nurse practitioner was another factor. As one person explained:

Nobody made any difference between them. When you go in to her you treat her exactly like a doctor, so it was obvious she can do exactly what a doctor can do.

In the staff interviews several nurses had suggested that the patients would be confused by yet another nurse in the practice, and would think they were seeing a doctor. This was certainly borne out in the patient interviews. Several patients did not know the difference between a nurse practitioner and a doctor before the consultation, and there was some evidence that several still did not know the difference when they came out of the consulting room. This has implications for publicising the role more widely, and may have legal implications (Dowling *et al*. 1996).

That there is a qualitative difference between consultations with doctors and the nurse practitioner is apparent in many respondents' perceptions. The difference in consultations centred around time (not feeling rushed) and interpersonal skills such as listening, talking, giving full explanations and being easy to talk to. These were the factors most people mentioned, but clinical competence was also highly valued.

Several respondents felt that doctors would benefit from the nurse practitioner role as it would take the pressure off them. Two respondents questioned whether the introduction of the nurse practitioner role was a cost-cutting exercise. They seemed to be viewing cost-effectiveness in terms of the number of patients seen by the nurse practitioner, not the longer consultation or any qualitative differences between nurse practitioner and GP consultations. There was a recognition by several respondents that not all consultations need to be with a doctor; some things can be dealt with by the nurse practitioner, thereby freeing up the doctor's time for more serious things requiring special skills. It is difficult to ascertain exactly what the special skills are, but things requiring hospitalization, or 'death-defying things' and 'lumps' were mentioned.

Implications of the data

Until fairly recently it would not have been possible for nurses to take on the role of physical assessment of patients, making a medical diagnosis, instigating treatment or management regimes for episodes of illness. All of these were firmly located within the medical domain. Several interrelated factors have contributed to this shift in roles and responsibilities, such as:

- The increased knowledge base of nurses
- Demographic changes in society, leading to an increase in demand for health care from an ageing population
- Changes in the patterns of disease in our society that have led to an emphasis on management rather than cure
- The shortage of doctors in primary health care and moves to reduce the working hours of junior doctors in hospital
- The consumer movement
- *The Scope of Professional Practice* (United Kingdom Central Council 1992)
- The GP contract (Department of Health and the Welsh Office 1989)
- Research into the role of the nurse practitioner in the UK and USA
- The concern of many GPs about use and abuse of their services

Like many nurse practitioners in primary health care settings (Burke-Masters 1986; Poulton 1995; Kaufman 1996), the nurse practitioner in this study is seeing a large number of patients with a greater degree of autonomy than traditionally enjoyed by nurses. She makes diagnostic and treatment decisions and consults GP colleagues or refers to other health-care or social agencies as appropriate. This particular nurse practitioner utilizes a wide range of knowledge and skills in order to provide a holistic service to patients. Of course it could be argued that the nurse practitioner in this situation is practising in a way more akin to a doctor rather than a nurse. The nurse practitioner role as doctor substitution creates concern and there appears to be a division between those who see the role of the nurse practitioner as no more than a substitute doctor (Pearson 1996) and those who see it as an advanced nursing role (Department of Health and Social Security 1986; Cable 1994; Emmerson 1996). MacGuire (1980) in her work on extended and expanded nursing roles described two models which underlie the literature.

Model A

Model A sees nursing and medicine as two distinct disciplines. Commentators are concerned about the possibility of nursing functions being lost from the new role in favour of medical tasks.

Model B

Model B states that there are many tasks to be carried out to maintain the health of communities and to care for patients. Who does what is immaterial, provided they are trained for the task, competent, acceptable to patients and achieve the same standards.

The debate will no doubt rage for a while yet. However, as far as the case-study practice is concerned, the introduction of the nurse practitioner has been a success. Introducing the nurse practitioner into the health-care team must be done with care if existing role boundaries are not to be disrupted too much. The study has highlighted the fact that, with regard to role boundaries with other nurses, the nurses in the practice and those working in the community did not experience any infringement on their own roles and there was little overlap in nursing roles. Where referrals were made from nurse practitioner to other nurses these were thought to be appropriate.

There was seen to be considerable overlap with the work of the GPs with regard to consulting with 'urgent' patients, but the sphere of practice of the nurse practitioner had been clearly defined and few instances of conflict were reported. The nurse practitioner in this particular practice was an experienced practice nurse with a wide range of knowledge and skills which she brought to the nurse practitioner role. This, together with well-organized teaching and supervision in the practice setting and a structured programme of formal education, resulted in a highly effective practitioner.

Some of the GPs, however, felt that not all nurses are suitable to take on the role of nurse practitioner but some would have an aptitude for the job. All agreed that the nurse practitioner had made a difference to their workload, particularly in relation to the number of extras they were seeing at the end of surgeries. Several GPs remarked that patients were getting a better service because there was less pressure to stick to time in surgeries and there was more flexibility in the appointment system.

Patients did see a difference between nurse practitioners and doctors and this difference mainly relates to consultation style, accessibility and length of consultation. They also saw a difference between nurse practitioners and practice nurses; the practice nurses were perceived as being concerned with technical aspects of care, whilst the nurse practitioner was seen to have a wider remit, closer to that of the doctor. Patients value her availability, interpersonal skills, the time she has available, her educative function and her clinical competence. Almost all the patients would consult her again with minor ailments, women's problems and 'anything'. However, most patients did not wish to see the nurse practitioner replacing the doctor but rather acting in a complementary role. There was some confusion initially for some patients as to who they were consulting and this needs to be continually reinforced.

There is a good deal of consensus about the success of the nurse practitioner in this project. If there is a dearth of discussion about conflict it is because there is no evidence of this; all parties agreed that the nurse practitioner role had brought great benefits to both patients and GPs and, whilst there was no evidence of benefits to practice and community nurses, there were no diasadvantages either. Why is there then such broad agreement and very little tension and disruption? There are probably many reasons but one of the doctors felt it was because of the way the nurse practitioner post was set up in this particular practice; the role was clearly defined, with everyone knowing what it was about so that there was little blurring of boundaries between the nurse practitioner and other nurses. The role was also fit for purpose in that it met the needs of the patient population – high morbidity, much acute minor illness and high patient demand for same-day appointments.

The survey of nurse practitioner pilot projects undertaken by Touche Ross (1994) demonstrated that one of the key factors influencing effective and early implementation of the nurse practitioner role included a clearly defined scope of operation. Integrating the role of the nurse practitioner into this general practice seemed to involve the use of strategies of integration, such as:

- *Risk limitation* whereby GPs check patients after the nurse practitioner has seen them in order to confirm diagnosis and/or treatment. Signing prescriptions (a medicolegal requirement), checking diagnoses and management plans, authorizing referral letters to consultant and liaising over the ordering of clinical investigations are examples of risk limitation. These procedures were closely adhered to at first, but lessened in intensity as the nurse practitioner gained experience and confidence, and as trust developed between doctor and nurse practitioner. Now clinical supervision takes place on a daily basis and consists of a doctor randomly selecting a sample of patients' notes from the nurse practitioner's surgery and discussing them with her. These are documented and kept

- *Locating the nurse practitioner nearer to the GP end of the doctor–nurse continuum* seems to reduce the threat to existing nursing roles as the nurses do not see their established roles being eroded. However, aligning the nurse practitioner to the GP reinforces the medical rather than the nursing aspect of patient care, and because technical skills are emphasized may give rise to ambiguity as to the nature of the role, resulting in confusion in the minds of consumers of the service

- *Using the nurse practitioner as an access route to the GP* this sometimes involved nurses asking the nurse practitioner for a second opinion about a patient, or referring patients to her knowing they would be seen sooner than if an appointment with a GP was requested. In this way the nurse practitioner is seen as an asset rather than a threat

- *Emphasizing differences in skills amongst nursing specialties;* this allows nurses to maintain their specialist focus and thus their sense of professional identity. Providing the nurse practitioner doesn't cross the boundary line into health visiting, midwifery, district nursing or practice nursing, and providing she makes appropriate referals to these professionals, boundary lines and therefore role stability can be maintained

- *Using the nurse practitioner as a consultant in the nursing team* was initially slow, but as the nurse practitioner became established and trusted within the team, nurses began to ask her advice about patients' problems they were unsure about themselves, such as 'lumps and things', and areas of practice they felt were beyond their own sphere of competence and for which there were no practice protocols, such as emergency contraception

Summary

The nurse practitioner role was successfully introduced in this primary health care environment primarily because there was good interpersonal communication between all involved, absolute clarity of boundaries and role definitions from the outset and the nurse practitioner role was fit for purpose in that it matched the needs of the population served. This study suggests that in order to introduce a nurse practitioner service successfully elsewhere, whether in primary health care or a hospital environment, the following points are essential:

- There should be a close match between the job description (which should be agreed in advance of making an appointment) and the health need of the target group
- Ensure all staff clearly understand and agree where the boundaries of practice lie
- Good communication between team members is essential

References

Bowling A., Stilwell B. (eds.) (1988) *The Nurse in Family Practice: Practice Nurses and Nurse Practitioners in Primary Health Care,* London, Scutari Press.

Burke-Masters B. (1986) The autonomous nurse practitioner: an answer to a chronic problem of primary care, *Lancet,* **1**(8492), p. 1266.

Cable S. (1994) What is a nurse practitioner?, *Primary Health Care,* **4**(5), pp. 12–14.

Department of Health and Social Security (1986) *Neighbourhood Nursing – A Focus for Care: Report of the Community Nursing Review (Cumberlege Report),* London, HMSO.

Department of Health and the Welsh Office (1989) *General Practice in the National Health Service: A New Contract ,* London, HMSO.

Dowling S., Martin R., Skidmore P., Doyal L., Cameron A., Lloyd, S. (1996) Nurses taking on junior doctors' work: a confusion of acccountability, *British Medical Journal,* **312**, May, pp 1211–1214.

Emmerson P., (1996) Are nurse practitioners merely substitute doctors? *Professional Nurse,* **11** (5), p. 326.

Kaufman G. (1996) Nurse practitioners in general practice: an expanding role. *Nursing Standard,* **11**(8), pp. 44–47.

MacGuire J. (1980) *The Extended Role of the Nurse,* Project paper RC3, London, King's Fund Centre.

Pearson P. (1996) Are nurse practitioners merely substitute doctors?, *Professional Nurse,* **11**(5), p. 325.

Pearson P., Kelly A., Connolly M., Daly M.O., Gorman F. (1995) Nurse practitioners, *Health Visitor,* **68**(4), pp. 157–160.

Poulton B. (1995) *Keeping the Customer Satisfied, Primary Health,* London, Royal College of Nursing.

Stilwell B. (1989) Patient attitudes to a highly developed role – the nurse practitioner, *Recent Advances in Nursing,* **12**, pp. 82–100.

Touche Ross (1994) *Evaluation of Nurse Practitioner Projects,* London, NHS Executive South Thames and Touche Ross Management Consultants.

United Kingdom Central Council (1992) *The Scope of Professional Practice,* London, United Kingdom Central Council.

United Kingdom Central Council (1994) *Standards for Post Registration Education and Practice,* London, United Kingdom Central Council.

CHAPTER 22

Changing practice: the negotiated order perspective and the development of the nurse practitioner role

Shirley Reveley

Introduction

The expansion of the nursing role has been an important feature of health care in recent years, stimulating much debate, in which the role of the nurse practitioner has been central. The pressures on health-care provision have provided both threats and opportunities for health-care professionals to change their ways of working and adopt innovative approaches to patient care. The nurse practitioner role, in terms of its innovative nature and its potential for pushing back the boundaries of nursing practice, has become a test bed for the carving out of new roles and redefining territories. It is a role that impacts significantly on the work of both nurses and doctors, and has developed in a range of health-care settings, such as mental health care, learning disabilities, hospitals, both inpatient and outpatient, alternative community settings and general practice (Watson et al. 1994).

The integration of the role of the nurse practitioner is of general concern within the nursing and medical professions, and is of particular importance to nurse practitioners themselves, who wish to see the role being officially sanctioned by the United Kingdom Central Council (UKCC) for Nursing, Midwifery and Health Visiting. However, changing nursing practice does not happen overnight; it takes time – often years – for a new nursing role to become established as part of the social order of nursing. The number of nurse practitioners in the UK has increased rapidly over the past 15 years, and

particularly during the last 5 years, though it is impossible to record exact numbers as there is no register or record of nurse practitioners and the diversity of the nurse practitioner role makes it difficult even to define what a nurse practitioner is. It is clear though that nurse practitioners, in both hospital and community settings, appear to be rapidly becoming an integral part of the British health-care system. Nurse practitioners have come a long way from the early pioneering days of Stilwell et al. (1987) and Burke-Masters (1986), to become a major force for change within nursing.

In order to explain how the nurse practitioner role is becoming such an important part of the social order of nursing, this chapter will utilize the theoretical perspective of negotiated order developed by Anselm Strauss and his colleagues (Strauss et al. 1963) and applied to nursing by Svensson (1996) and Allen (1997). The chapter will begin by outlining the negotiated order perspective and noting its application to nursing. The developing role of the nurse practitioner will then be analysed within the negotiated order perspective and finally the usefulness of this approach will be discussed. Allen (1997) points out that sociologists tend not to spell out what they mean by negotiations and concludes that the term is actually being used as shorthand for social interaction. In this chapter I shall refer to negotiations as those interactions that take place between the nurse practitioner and the doctors at a face-to-face level and that are overt. Negotiations will also be included that involve nurses and other people and which take place outside the immediate clinical area, but which further the nurse practitioner movement. In this way a new social order becomes created and continually reconstituted (Strauss *et al.* 1963; Allen 1997).

The negotiated order perspective

Central to sociological discourse is the issue of social order and, more specifically, how order and stability are maintained in the face of change. The negotiated order perspective is an approach that owes much to the early work of sociologists operating within the social interactionist paradigm, particularly the symbolic interaction framework developed by George Herbert Mead and his followers. The negotiated order perspective came to the fore in the 1960s, largely as a result of the work of Anselm Strauss in his study of two psychiatric hospitals in the USA (Strauss *et al.* 1963). Strauss summarizes the negotiated order perspective as follows. All social order is negotiated; these negotiations take place in a patterned and systematic fashion; their outcomes are temporarily limited; the negotiated order constantly has to be reconstituted as a basis for concerted action; the negotiated order on any day consists of the sum total of the organization's rules, policies and local working understandings or agreements; and finally, any change arising within or imposed on the order will require renegotiation to occur (Dingwall and Strong 1985). This approach thus eliminated the need for a distinction between the formal and informal organization – 'the informal ultimately shapes the formal and vice versa' (Day and Day 1977, p. 126).

Strauss *et al.* (1963) enunciated three concepts in negotiation:

- *Negotiation*, which refers to different types of interaction and strategies used by people.
- *Negotiation context*, which refers to the balance of power between participants, for example, issues such as the legal position of nurse practitioners, their cost-effectiveness, patient satisfaction, treatment outcomes, roles and responsibilities of other professionals and supervision arrangements
- *Structural context*, which includes factors such as age and sex of participants, national policies, economics

Negotiation context and structural context provide a way of specifying the conditions which directly influence the negotiations that take place. There are apparently stable features of an organization such as the rules, policies, work groups, hierarchies, ideologies of participants, career lines and the division of labour that provide the *organizational*

background though these are not permanently binding (Strauss *et al.* 1963). Negotiation processes provide the *foreground*. People give and take, stake claims, make bargains (either implicitly or explicitly). Negotiations occur when rules and policies are not inclusive, when there is uncertainty and disagreements, and when there is change:

> When new understandings are reached, they invariably offset previous tangential agreements (Maines and Charlton 1985, p. 278).

The negotiated activity therefore reacts in turn upon previously created rules and procedures, illustrating the temporal dimension of structure and the reflexivity or connectedness between structure and process.

Day and Day (1977) describe the negotiated order approach as an interactional model which allows for a processual and emergent analysis of the way in which the division of labour and work is accomplished in large organizations. It addresses the problem of how order is maintained in a particular organization in the face of the many changes, both internal and external, that have to be dealt with. As an illustration from health care, the group general practice is a complex organization that has to maintain order in the face of numerous changes and challenges and brings together professionals and support workers from various educational and professional socialization backgrounds and with various degrees of experience, all working to a common goal of caring for sick people, or those who think they are sick (Chisolm 1997).

The Weberian model of a bureaucratic organization such as the NHS would emphasize the structures that are in place to achieve the organization's goal, such as the lines of command, communication channels and so on (Coates 1991). However, a look beneath the surface of general practice or any hospital reveals that there may not be one single common goal; indeed, there may be several different goals held by different professionals or the same professional may have goals that compete. The GP, for example, may be concerned with restoring the patient to full health as far as is possible; the health promotion practice nurse may be concerned with the prevention of illness; the midwife may see her role as dealing with women undergoing the normal physiological and social function of having a baby; and a health visitor may be concerned with the health of the practice population as a whole. Thus:

> There are cleavages along the lines of the division of labour and in terms of the actual goal of better care for patients (Maines and Charlton, 1985, p. 276).

Who decides which of these goals should have priority? How are decisions arrived at? Weber's rational bureaucratic theory would point to the rules of the organization for an answer but not everyone knows all the rules; the rules may be ambiguous; people may not know when or how to apply the rules. Protocols, or clinical guidelines, are a case in point; nurse practitioners (and others) are urged to work to protocols in the interests of patient safety, but not every condition is amenable to management by protocols, for example a sore throat. Moreover, what happens when a patient does not fit the protocol or guidelines? A nurse practitioner working with several doctors, each of whom has different ways of working and their own tried and tested remedies, must try to work with enough flexibility to maintain professional relationships – no easy task. Thus negotiation must take place; rules are fudged or bent in the interests of getting the job done, or even to suit someone's vested interests (Stelling and Bucher 1972).

The negotiated order perspective then rejects the traditional rational bureaucratic conception of organizational authority. Whilst Stelling and Bucher's (1972) study of several hospital wards in the USA showed that some sectors of the organization were clearly bureaucratic, this model could not explain the everyday processes of social control. Thus the authors argue that social control rests in and takes place through political processes. This accords with the findings of Strauss et al. (1963) who state that:

> Except for a few legal rules, which stem from state and professional prescription, and for some rulings pertaining to all of [a hospital], almost all of these house rules are much less like commands, and much more like general understandings: not even their punishments are spelled out; and mostly they can be stretched, negotiated, argued, as well as ignored or applied at convenient moments (p. 165).

Within the negotiated order perspective the concepts of temporality and situational context are emphasized, and the notion of power and power relationships is seen in terms of the situational context pertaining at any one time. This implies that the nurse – or the doctor – may be in control depending on specific circumstances. Svensson (1996) and Allen (1997) make the case for employing the negotiated order perspective as an appropriate framework for understanding doctor–nurse interactions. Svensson studied nurse–doctor interaction on contemporary hospital wards and argued that three major changes in the negotiation context have altered the relationship between doctors and nurses dramatically:

- The increased prevalence of chronic illness, which has shifted the emphasis from preventing death to handling life; this introduces a social element into health care
- The shift from a system of task allocation to team nursing, in which the nurse in charge of a small

group of patients discusses their care directly with the doctor rather than through the ward sister
- The introduction of the 'sitting round', wherein nurses and doctors discuss patients before going on to the walking round

Svensson argues that these changes have given nurses space to influence patient care decisions directly and interpret organizational rules.

The shortcomings of this study are that first, Svensson was studying doctor–nurse relationships but undertook interviews with nurses only, and that he relied solely on interview data which cannot be read as literal descriptions of reality (Silverman 1993). Allen (1997) built on Svensson's work but looked at factors in the hospital ward that inhibited, rather than promoted, negotiations 'but which nevertheless resulted in modification of the medical–nursing division of labour' (p. 501). Allen used observation in addition to interviewing both doctors and nurses and argued that as a result of recent policy initiatives there would be an increased need for inter-occupational negotiations and associated tensions at the boundary between nursing and medical work (p. 516). However, though supported in interviews, observation demonstrated little evidence of negotiation or interoccupational strains on the wards. Allen suggests that this is because staff developed strategies to manage the tensions associated with the social organization of hospital work such that non-negotiated informal boundary-blurring was a taken-for-granted feature of normal nursing work. Thus, Allen argues that formal organizational structures can be modified in the absence of face-to-face negotiations (p. 514).

Negotiated order and the nurse practitioner role

Doctor–nurse relationships are important to the success of the nurse practitioner role, regardless of setting, not least because of the relative power between doctors and nurses, i.e. the capacity of a person (the doctor) to define the nature of a problem and the means by which that problem is handled (Stelling and Bucher 1972). Doctors have to be prepared to loosen their hold on the issues of diagnosis and prescription if nurse practitioners are to undertake total responsibility for patient care. The negotiated order perspective implies that power is involved in all negotiations and it could be argued that a successful outcome of negotiation results from agreeing, either overtly or otherwise, on a shift in the balance of power between one or more individuals.

Research by the author which evaluated the impact of a nurse practitioner on primary health care illustrates the point (Chapter 21). A student nurse practitioner in a group general practice and her medical mentor entered into a learning contract about the development of her role. Face-to-face negotiations took place about the limits and content of the nurse practitioner role in discussions between the nurse practitioner, her mentor, and the other doctors and nurses in the practice setting. These negotiations set the ground rules but also tested the boundaries between nursing and medicine as supervision of the nurse practitioner's practice involved dialogue with doctors about diagnosis and treatment decisions, usually in the form of the nurse practitioner justifying her decisions. The balance of power thus rested with the doctors. However, as the role developed and trust and confidence in the nurse practitioner's skills and abilities increased, she gained increasing independence and autonomy and more say in relation to decisions about patient care, until she reached a stage of being monitored rather than supervised. Thus negotiations impacted on practice and practice impacted on negotiations in a dialectical process, which is an important feature of the negotiated order perspective.

Stelling and Bucher (1972) studied several hospital wards and developed three concepts for analysing social control in organizations. The first they termed *elastic autonomy* – autonomy that is neither fixed nor inherent in any given position; it is contingent on assessment of the person's professional competence. Autonomy in this sense refers to the capacity of a person to define the nature of a problem and the means by which that problem is handled. Elastic autonomy can expand or contract, for example in the case of a student nurse practitioner, his or her autonomy is ideally expanding as s/he develops confidence and competence, but should there be a negative event with a patient, or a new doctor coming on the scene who is wary of the nurse practitioner role, then that autonomy may well contract. What usually happens according to Stelling and Bucher (1972) is that autonomy in such a situation is held steady, not being allowed to expand further. This may happen to nurse practitioners – they are allowed so much autonomy and no more.

The second concept is that of *accountability*, which is closely linked to responsibility. Individuals can be called upon to justify their actions and explain and account for their decisions. It is linked to autonomy in so far as a nurse cannot be held accountable for something over which s/he has no control. Nurse practitioners, in common with all other registered nurses, are accountable for their actions under their professional code of conduct (United Kingdom Central Council 1992). Thus no one can cover the nurse practitioner and it is no defence to say s/he is working on the doctor's instructions (United Kingdom Central Council 1996).

The third concept is *monitoring* – checking whether or not a person is competently performing his or her work. A monitor need not be a superior and monitoring is not the same as supervision because the person being monitored is still accountable. Nurse practitioners need to be closely supervised in the early days of learning the role, but later move to being monitored. This monitoring can be done by peers, or as in one study of the introduction of the nurse practitioner role into a large group practice, it may be undertaken on a daily basis by doctors who discuss with the nurse practitioner a sample of patients she sees each day (Reveley 1997).

Patients of course also negotiate. This can be overt, as when a patient asks for information and discusses the outcome and alternatives, or more covert, as when a patient refuses to see the nurse practitioner. Strauss (1978) says patients stretch limits by persuasion, covert manipulation and requesting.

Doctors also negotiate on behalf of the nurse practitioner; for example, in the early days of the pilot study referred to above, at least two hospital consultants were upset at receiving referrals from a nurse practitioner. Letters were exchanged and eventually an agreement was reached whereby the referral letters were signed by the GPs 'on behalf of the nurse practitioner'. The nurse practitioner still made all the decisions about referral and wrote the letters, but they were countersigned by the GP (Reveley 1997).

It could be argued that negotiations that take place locally within a specific setting have no impact beyond that setting (Maurin 1980). To a certain extent this is true; the nurse practitioner role is negotiated at practice level to take account of particular patient needs. In this situation negotiating the work of the nurse practitioner involves negotiating *around* the rules (Maurin 1980), resulting in an informal achievement of objectives. The fact that 'there is a need to negotiate around the rules in health care suggests there are certain structural limits' (p. 330). However, taking account of the total contextual framework of the nurse practitioner movement, it shows that negotiations about structural factors are also taking place.

Negotiated order at the macro level

Maurin (1980) points out that the levels at which negotiations have taken place need to be differentiated as the resulting social change will differ with the level. Negotiation *about* the rules (Maurin 1980) of nurse practitioner practice takes place at different levels and in different arenas. For example, debates in the professional literature about the nature and extent of the nurse practitioner role, discussions regarding the division of labour between doctors and nurses, papers presented at professional conferences and so on are all examples of how negotiation occurs and there is currently an abundance of this type of activity in relation to the role of the nurse practitioner in modern health care. At government level negotiations take place about skill mix in health care, the role of the nurse and pharmacist in prescribing, whether GPs should be salaried or self-employed and many other issues which are all forms of the negotiating process. These negotiations *about* the rules (Maurin 1980) occur at policy-making level and may result in policy changes and institutionalization, or, in Busch's (1982) terms, *sedimentation*.

Busch (1982), following Strauss *et al.* (1963), analysed the agricultural sciences in terms of the structure, negotiation contexts and negotiations in his work, including the balance of power, language and communication. He looked at how the negotiated structure was created and used the term sedimentation to describe the process whereby negotiations become part of the structural context. When the outcome of a previous negotiation becomes taken for granted and its origins are no longer questioned, sedimentation has occurred. He uses an example from science, suggesting that scientists 'know' how to conduct an experiment. Today, the issue is 'settled' but in earlier times this had to be negotiated. An example from nursing would be observation of patients. Nurses 'know' how to take temperatures and measure blood pressure. This settled into nursing practice many years ago but before then this was in the medical domain and the change had to be negotiated by nurse reformers.

The concept of sedimentation then can be used to describe the process whereby roles become sedimented into a health-care system. There are many examples of this, such as the role of doctors in British society, which has gone virtually unchallenged for many years. Looking at this from a historical perspective shows that this role had to be negotiated vigorously and became sedimented over time, helped by structural changes such as the Medical Registration Act of 1858. Negotiations also took place at the inception of the NHS when doctors negotiated their independent practitioner status. Low morale among GPs in the post-war years led to a recruitment crisis in general practice which resulted in negotiations that culminated in the Family Doctor's Charter of 1966. This introduced the 70% reimbursement for employed practice staff which provided the negotiation context for the development of practice nurse roles.

The practice nurse role was hard-fought during the 1980s; resentment and confusion were apparent in many ways. Over the last decade, and particularly since the introduction of the GP contract (Department of Health 1990 and the Welsh office 1989), the role of the practice nurse has become sedimented into primary health care nursing. This was helped by the Council's Standards for Education and Practice following Registration (United Kingdom Central Council 1994) which was the outcome of years of negotiation. Similarly, the attachment of district nurses and health visitors to general practices in the 1974 NHS restructuring took many years of negotiation before it became a taken-for-granted aspect of health care. It can be argued that the role of the nurse practitioner is undergoing a process of sedimentation within the structural and negotiation context of health care that will eventually result in a new social order.

Busch (1982) further suggests that sedimentation of negotiations into structure may continue to be taken for granted or may be 'stirred up'. An example of this would be the challenges to medicine (Gabe *et al.* 1994) since the 1960s that have 'stirred up' the whole debate about medical dominance (Freidson 1970). He also states that negotiations occur not just internally but between other institutions as well.

Negotiations on the role of the nurse practitioner can be seen to be taking place in the institutions of medicine, nursing, pharmacology, radiography and education, amongst others. Thus, its effects are far-reaching and it is perhaps not surprising that the UKCC is reluctant to sanction the new social order by sedimenting it within UKCC regulations until all negotiations are complete. However, the negotiation context of health care will continue to change and result in further changes and this includes further negotiations about roles and role boundaries.

Busch (1982) argues that, whilst the agricultural sciences are homogeneous in some respects, they are heterogeneous in other important ways. Thus he concludes that:

> Even within 'the same' organizational context, different subgroups may be involved in different negotiations and have differing extra-organizational concerns (p. 43).

This argument can be applied to general practice, which is both homogeneous and heterogeneous. The homogeneity can be found in the following: the concept of general practice is well-established in British health care; practices all work within the administrative structure of the NHS; they emphasize a service orientation and they share an image of a unified service. However, there are important differences: some are group practices, some single-handed, some have been fundholding, others not; some are located in rural areas, others in urban areas and inner cities; some have a primary health care team, others do not; some have a practice manager, in others the GP principal acts as manager. This does not take into account the fact that professionals attached to GP practice usually have managers from a different sector of the service (with a community orientation rather than practice population orientation), thus even within an apparent universally similar organization the negotiation context for the integration of new roles is fraught with difficulty.

Hall and Spencer-Hall (1982) studied two American school districts to discover the extent to which the negotiated order perspective could explain how these two school systems were organized. One of the arguments that they put forward was that history and tradition constrain negotiations. They say that:

> Community members and schools' participants develop 'patterns and perceptions' about the systems that condition them not to question or offer alternatives (p. 57).

There are parallels here with work on doctor–nurse interactions and the professional socialization of nurses that teach them to obey doctors and encourage passivity so that negotiating may seem to be useless. Nurse practitioners negotiating around the rules in the practice situation (be it hospital ward or general practice) do not challenge the overall structure of medical–nursing boundaries. Their negotiations permit exceptions to the rules but do not substantially challenge medical authority (Maurin 1980). Moreover, some things are not up for negotiation; Svensson (1996) suggests that meta-rules will evolve regarding what is legitimate to negotiate and the forms these negotiations take, while Hunter (1994) argues that the overall balance of power still lies with the doctor.

Doctors are able to shape the health-care agenda through the mechanism of 'the third dimension of power' (Lukes 1977). This means that the exercise of power need not be openly displayed or in situations of actual conflict; rather, the effective use of power is to prevent conflict arising in the first place. Whilst one person may exercise power over another by getting that person to do what he or she does not want to do, power can be exercised over an individual in such an insidious way that his or her very wants are shaped by the one with the most power.

Hall and Spencer-Hall (1982) could have been discussing a hospital or busy health centre when they reported that the daily life of a large school building is characterized by ritual, practicality, segmentation and superficial, intermittent interaction. The following account from Maines and Charlton (1985) is immediately recognizable as applicable to the health service as well as the educational environment they were writing about:

> The day is divided up into periods, and teachers rarely see their colleagues. Off periods and lunches are short and hectic, and at the end of the day most teachers prefer to leave as soon as possible. Administrators, meanwhile, are in other buildings or in their offices so they have little interaction with either students or teachers. In other words most work is done in isolation, and contact between participants is limited. Administrators assume things are functioning smoothly unless they hear otherwise, and the consequent lack of attention and interest, combined with insistence on following the chain of command, limit the potential for negotiation (p. 287).

Hall and Spencer-Hall (1982) said that those who are without power, or who perceive themselves as powerless clearly restrained *themselves* (p. 58). The parallels with health care are clear; personnel work in isolation in their own consulting rooms and wards, the day is divided into surgery periods and visiting times, and breaks are hurried. Face-to-face contact only takes place if there is an issue to be clarified or a problem solved; otherwise each professional assumes the others are doing all right; the focus is on getting through the work. With the introduction of nurse practitioner this way of working is disturbed; space for the new worker, both physical and psychological space, has to be negotiated. An important factor is finding time to teach, supervise and monitor a new nurse practitioner. Another problem is how to negotiate the role in terms of other nursing roles within the practice or hospital.

In the face of such a major change to the social order of the general practice, or indeed the hospital ward, how is the nurse practitioner role negotiated and how can the negotiated order perspective help us to understand this? In its broad sense the concept of negotiation includes three variables. One is the degree of consensus. When there is complete agreement or complete disagreement in a situation, no negotiation can take place. Thus there has to be some degree of consensus. There must also be some degree of exchange but there can be variations in frequency, intensity and duration of exchanges. Negotiations must also include the use of strategies. According to Maines and Charlton (1985):

> These three elements – degree of consensus, degree of exchange, and use of strategies – can then systematically incorporate a wide range of behaviour, which has the virtue of allowing the analyst to make a greater number of linkages between negotiations and the larger social contexts in which those negotiations take place (p. 296).

There needs to be a good degree of consensus in the practice setting regarding testing out the nurse practitioner role. Also, there should be some degree of exchange; for example, doctors have to be prepared to exchange some of the time that they would spend with patients for time spent with the nurse practitioner for purposes of teaching and supervision. There also has to be some exchange – or at least relinquishing – of tasks such as assessing, diagnosing and prescribing for patients.

Hall and Spencer-Hall (1982) suggest a set of circumstances that, at least in their study, affect the occurrence and extent of negotiations.

- Activities that are variable, individualized, publicly performed and involve team work and co-ordination are more open to negotiation than those that are routinized and performed individually in isolation. Doctoring and nursing are carried out publicly, involve teamwork and co-ordination, thus the work of doctors and nurses should be open to negotiation and Hall and Spencer-Hall go on to say that if people are publicly accountable and must act under unclear conditions, it seems logical they will negotiate
- The bigger and more complex the organization, the greater the degree of negotiation, because larger organizations are more likely to have critical masses of individuals who can act as effective units. People feel freer to act in their own subunits because they are not so easily monitored. Smaller, simpler organizations, they argue, should have fewer separate interests, less autonomy and be easier to manage and monitor. It would appear from this second set of conditions that the nurse practitioner role is more likely to be open to negotiation in hospitals rather than general practices because hospitals are larger and more complex and so are likely to have critical masses of individuals who can act as effective units. However, nurse practitioners in the UK began in small units, for example Barbara Stilwell worked in a two-GP practice (Stilwell *et al.* 1987) and Barbara Burke-Masters in a solitary role in the community (Burke-Masters 1986). Many nurse practitioners successfully negotiate the role in small practices and units
- Equality, dispersion of power and efficaciousness are conducive to negotiations, while strong asymmetry, concentrated power and fatalism are not. Power constrains the occurrence as well as the results of negotiation. However, ineffective power is conducive to power by subordinates. Thus people who view themselves as effective and their organization as successful are more likely to engage in negotiations whilst failure and a sense of weakness lead to retreat and accommodation
- Leadership that allows delegation of authority and tolerates individuality and the development of autonomy will encourage negotiations more than leadership that centralizes authority and is bureaucratically rigid and authoritarian. Dominance suppresses involvement and therefore negotiation. Nurse practitioners then must develop professional confidence and assertiveness if they are to be successful in their negotiations with doctors who have more status, power and self-confidence
- An organization that is planning or undergoing change will show negotiation more than one that tends towards stability or emphasizes tradition. It also creates conditions where staff feel there are possibilities for other changes. More effort is needed to control the change but it should show evidence of negotiation. Programmes never go as they were intended as new contingencies appear and there is a need to fit practice to the theory. Organizations undergoing change may be more conducive to more change, but some individuals within them may retreat into traditional practices if innovation is not handled properly. This may explain why some nurse practitioners experience resentment from other nurses in the team (Stilwell 1982; Kaufman 1996)
- Professionals are more likely to enter into negotiations than semiprofessionals because they have more status, power and self-confidence, which leads them to assert themselves, make suggestions, create situations and seek dominance. Semiprofessionals (and the authors include nurses in this category) are more insecure in their status and training and are aware of the bureaucratic constraints on their actions, thus are more likely to defer to 'full professionals'. It seems, therefore, that power-sharing and good leadership will promote autonomy and allow for effective negotiations so that nurse practitioners are enabled to flourish
- The greater the focus of organizational attention and commitment of resources, the less the degree of negotiation; having a moderate number of issues with moderate intensity is more likely to generate a greater degree of freedom. Negotiation strategies may be used, wittingly or unwittingly, to ensure the smooth integration of the nurse practitioner into the existing nursing team. For example, in the study referred to previously (Reveley 1997), there appeared to be several processes that helped to sediment the nurse practitioner into that particular primary health care team, such as:

- Risk limitation
- Locating the nurse practitioner role closer to that of the GP rather than the nurses. This seemed to reduce the threat to existing nursing roles as the nurses did not believe their established roles were being eroded
- Using the nurse practitioner as a 'back door' to the GP
- Valuing the different skills amongst the various nurses meant nurses could maintain their specialist focus and thus their sense of professional identity

Oberschall (1974) suggested that:

> Conditions which favour challenge to an insti-
> tutionalised order are those which signal relaxation of
> social control so that the risk/reward ratio changes for
> some group (quoted in Maurin 1980, p. 326).

The risk/reward ratio related to nurse practitioners
has changed. For example, extensive research in the
USA and UK (Touche Ross 1994; Coopers and
Lybrand 1996) has demonstrated that nurse practitioners are safe, effective and appreciated by patients.
The problems of recruitment into general practice
and the reduction in junior doctors' hours has meant
that the medical profession, if not all nurses, is finding
the nurse practitioner role valuable and acceptable.
The *Scope of Professional Practice* (United Kingdom
Central Council 1992) has also provided a framework
for expanding nursing roles. These structural factors
provide the space (Svensson 1996) for nurse
practitioners to negotiate around the rules.

Criticisms of the negotiated order perspective

One frequent criticism of the negotiated order
approach is an implicit assumption that everything
is negotiable and therefore little account is taken of
structural constraints on social action (Benson 1977a,
1977b, 1978; Day and Day 1977; Dingwall and Strong
1985). However, Strauss does mention the constraints
of organizational policies and rules and
organizational hierarchies shaping patterns of
negotiation (Allen 1997). In a later work he addresses
the criticisms overtly:

> Negotiation does not explain everything; it is always
> found in conjunction with other processes, other
> alternatives for getting things done – notably coercion,
> persuasion or manipulation (Strauss 1978, p. 234).

Subsequently, several studies explored the dialectic
relationship between structural constraints and
negotiative processes (Busch 1982; Hall and Spencer-
Hall 1982; Svensson 1996). Another criticism is the
terminology relating to negotiations. The term
negotiation is itself ambiguous. Allen (1997) found
that negotiation can refer to brokering, mediation,
collusion, bargaining, compromising, reaching
formal or informal agreements, trading off and
making a deal. Strauss (1978) says there are sub-
processes to negotiation, which he identifies as
making trade-offs, obtaining kickbacks, compromising towards the middle, reaching negotiated
agreements and paying off debts. Moreover, he
suggests that negotiations can be one-shot, repeated,
sequential, serial, multiple or linked and can vary
in time from immediate to long-term. This apparent
lack of clarity may detract from the utility of the
negotiated order approach.

Conclusion

This chapter has examined the emerging role of the
nurse practitioner in the British health-care system
from the negotiated order perspective. It is suggested
that this perspective provides a useful framework
for analysis of the development of nurse practitioners
because it allows for greater insights into how
organizations have to change in order to make room
for new roles.

Dingwall and Strong (1985, p. 206) argue that the
Weberian model of a bureaucracy emphasizes the
character of formal organizations as rational, rule-
governed and goal-oriented. Disillusionment
experienced by researchers studying formal
organizations from within a bureaucratic framework
led to attempts to divide the organization into formal
and informal aspects in order to accommodate the
problem of anomalous findings when trying to study
an organization in terms of its structures and
achievement of goals, without considering how those
structures became constituted in the first place. In
other words, they argue, the social organization also
needs to be taken into account. The negotiated order
approach explores the social organization of nursing
and medicine from a micro perspective. Because
there is no official standard of education and practice
of nurse practitioners, the role must be negotiated
in each and every health-care setting where nurse
practitioners are trying to carve out a niche for
themselves. At the macro level the social organization
of nursing is being disturbed because of the
introduction of the nurse practitioner role. Negotiations at different levels and in different arenas
are taking place that will eventually lead to the
sedimentation of the role into mainstream nursing.

References

Allen D. (1997) The nursing–medical boundary: a negotiated
order?, *Sociology of Health and Illness*, **19**(4), pp. 498–520.

Benson J.K. (1977a) Organisations: a dialectic view,
Administrative Science Quarterly, **22**, pp. 1–21.

Benson J.K. (1977b) Innovation and crisis in organisational
analysis, *Administrative Science Quarterly*, **18**, pp. 5–18.

Benson J.K. (1978) Reply to Maines, *Sociological Quarterly*,
19, pp. 497–501.

British Medical Association (1995) A charter for the family
doctor service, *British Medical Journal* (Suppl **1**), pp.
89–91.

Burke-Masters (1986) The autonomous nurse practitioner:
an answer to a chronic problem of primary care, *Lancet*,
1 (8492), p. 1266.

Busch L. (1982) History, negotiation and structure in
agricultural research, *Urban Life*, **11**, pp. 368–384.

Chisolm, J. (1997) *The Future of General Practice*, Paper
presented at the University of Lancaster, 25 November,
Unpublished.

Coates D. (1991) *Running the Country*, London, Hodder &
Stoughton, Open University.

Coopers and Lybrand (1996) *Nurse Practitioner Evaluation Project Final Report*, NHS Executive.

Day R., Day J.V. (1977) A review of the current state of negotiated order theory: an appreciation and a critique, *Sociological Quarterly*, **18**, pp. 126–142.

Dingwall R., Strong P.M. (1985) The interactional study of organisations: a critique and reformulation, *Urban Life*, **14**(2), pp. 205–231.

Freidson E. (1970) *Profession of Medicine*, New York, Dodd Mead.

Gabe J., Kelleher D., Williams G. (eds.) (1994) *Challenging Medicine*, London, Routledge.

Hall P.M., Spencer-Hall D.A. (1982) The social conditions of the negotiated order, *Urban Life*, **11**(3), pp. 328–349.

Hunter D. (1994) From tribalism to corporatism: the managerial challenge to medical dominance. In: Gabe J., Kelleher D., Williams G. (eds.) *Challenging Medicine*, London, Routledge.

Kaufman G. (1996) Nurse practitioners in general practice: an expanding role, *Nursing Standard*, **11**(8), pp. 44–47.

Lukes S. (1977) *Power: A Radical View*, London, MacMillan.

Maines D.R., Charlton J.C. (1985) *The Negotiated Order Approach to the Analysis of Social Organization*, Foundations of Interpretive Sociology: Original Essays in Symbolic Interaction. Studies in Symbolic Interaction, Connecticut: JAI Press.

Maurin J. (1980) Negotiating an innovative health care service. In: Roth J. (ed.) *The Sociology of Health Care: Professional Control of Health Services and Challenges to Such Control*, vol. 1, Connecticut, JAI Press.

Oberschall A. (1974) *Social Conflict and Social Movements*, New Jersey, Prentice Hall. Cited in: Maurin J. (1980) Negotiating an innovative health care service. In: Roth J. (ed.) *The Sociology of Health Care: Professional Control of Health Services and Challenges to Such Control*, vol. 1, Connecticut, JAI Press.

Reveley S. (1997) *Introducing the Nurse Practitioner into General Medical Practice: The Maryport Experience.* Carlisle, University College of St Martin North Cumbria Health Authority.

Silverman D. (1993) *Interpreting Qualitative Data: Methods for Analysing Talk, Text and Interaction*, London, Sage Publications.

Stelling J., Bucher R. (1972) Autonomy and monitoring on hospital wards, *Sociological Quarterly*, **13**, pp. 431–446.

Stilwell B. (1982) The nurse practitioner at work, *Nursing Times*, **78**(43), pp. 1799–1803.

Stilwell B., Greenfield S., Drury V.W.M., Hull F.M. (1987) A nurse practitioner in general practice: working style and pattern of consultations, *Journal of the Royal College of General Practitioners*, **37**, pp. 154–157.

Strauss A. (1978) *Negotiations: Varieties, Contexts, Processes and Social Order*, San Francisco, Jossey-Bass.

Strauss A., Schatzman L., Ehrlichh D., Bucher R., Sabshin M. (1963) The hospital and its negotiated order. In: Freidson E. (ed.) *The Hospital in Modern Society*, New York, Free Press.

Svensson R. (1996) The interplay between doctors and nurses – a negotiated order perspective, *Sociology of Health and Illness*, **18**(3), pp. 379–398.

Touche Ross (1994) *Evaluation of Nurse Practitioner Projects*, London, Touche Ross Management Consultants Ltd.

United Kingdom Central Council (1992) *The Scope of Professional Practice*, London, United Kingdom Central Council.

United Kingdom Central Council (1994) *The Future of Professional Practice: The Council's Standards for Education and Practice Following Registration*, London, United Kingdom Central Council.

United Kingdom Central Council (1996) *Guidelines for Professional Practice*, London, United Kingdom Central Council.

Watson P., Hendey N., Dingwall R. (1994) *Role Extension/Expansion with Particular Reference to the Nurse Practitioner*, Nottingham, School of Social Studies, University of Nottingham.

Index

Page numbers printed in **bold** type refer to figures; those in *italic* to tables